2025

ADVANCES IN COSMETIC SURGERY

Gregory H. Branham, MD

Jeffrey S. Dover, MD, FRCPC

Shilpi Khetarpal, MD, FAAD

Smita R. Ramanadham, MD, FACS

Allan E. Wulc, MD, FACS

ELSEVIER

Publishing Director, Medical Reference: Dolores Meloni
Editor: Taylor Hayes
Developmental Editor: Sukirti Singh

Editorial Office:
Elsevier, Inc.
1600 John F. Kennedy Blvd,
Suite 1800
Philadelphia, PA 19103-2899

International Standard Serial Number: 2542-4327
International Standard Book Number: 13: 978-0-443-34699-6

EDITORS

GREGORY H. BRANHAM, MD
Chief Medical Officer, Barnes-Jewish West County Hospital, Creve Coeur, Missouri; Professor and Chief,Facial Plastic and Reconstructive Surgery, Department of Otolaryngology-HNS, Washington University School of Medicine, St Louis, Missouri

JEFFREY S. DOVER, MD, FRCPC
Director, SkinCare Physicians, Chestnut Hill, Massachusetts; Associate Clinical Professor of Dermatology, Yale University School of Medicine, New Haven, Connecticut; Adjunct Associate Professor of Dermatology, Brown Medical School, Providence, Rhode Island

SHILPI KHETARPAL, MD, FAAD
Associate Professor of Dermatology, Cleveland Clinic Cleveland, OH, USA

SMITA R. RAMANADHAM, MD, FACS
SR Plastic Surgery, East Brunswick, New Jersey

ALLAN E. WULC, MD, FACS
Associate Clinical Professor, Department of Ophthalmology, University of Pennsylvania, Philadelphia, Pennsylvania; Adjunct Associate Professor, Department of Otolaryngology, Temple University, Philadelphia, Pennsylvania

CONTRIBUTORS

ANUREET K. BAJAJ, MD, MBA
Private Practice, Plastic Surgeon, Bajaj Plastic Surgery, Oklahoma City, Oklahoma, USA

ERIC J. BELTRAMI, MD
Resident Physician, Department of Dermatology, Boston Medical Center, Boston, Massachusetts, USA

GREGORY H. BRANHAM, MD
Professor and Chief,Facial Plastic and Reconstructive Surgery, Department of Otolaryngology-HNS, Washington University School of Medicine, St Louis, Missouri; Chief Medical Officer, Barnes-Jewish West County Hospital, Creve Coeur, Missouri

NAOMI F. BRIONES, MD, FACMS, FAAD
Dermatologist, Private Practice, Wenatchee, Washington, USA; Department of Dermatology, University of California-San Diego, San Diego, California, USA

CAT N. BURKAT, MD, FACS
Professor, Oculoplastics, Orbital, and Cosmetic Facial Surgery, Department of Ophthalmology and Visual Sciences, University of Wisconsin-Madison, Madison, Wisconsin, USA

ANDREA CACCIARELLI, MD
Plastic Surgeon, JFK University Medical Center, Hackensack Meridian Health, Edison, New Jersey, USA; Clara Maass Medical Center, Montclair, New Jersey, USA

BEATRICE CHING-CHEN GO, MD
Resident, Department of Otorhinolaryngology–Head and Neck Surgery, University of Pennsylvania, Philadelphia, Pennsylvania, USA

KATHLEEN COERDT, MD
Resident Physician, Department of Dermatology, Cleveland Clinic Foundation, Cleveland, Ohio, USA

ALEXA J. COHEN, MD
Resident Physician, Department of Dermatology, Boston Medical Center, Boston, Massachusetts, USA

KEVIN B. COPPELSON, MD, DDS
Oral and Maxillofacial Surgeon, Private Practice, The Breathe Institute and Greater Ventura Oral and Facial Surgery, Los Angeles, California, USA

JEFFREY S. DOVER, MD, FRCPC
Director, Department of Dermatology, SkinCare Physicians, Chestnut Hill, Massachusetts, USA; Associate Clinical Professor, Department of Dermatology, Yale University School of Medicine, New Haven, Connecticut, USA; Adjunct Associate Professor, Department of Dermatology, Brown Medical School, Providence, Rhode Island, USA

TRINA G. EBERSOLE, MD
Assistant Professor, Division of Plastic and Reconstructive Surgery, Department of Surgery, Washington University, Saint Louis, Missouri, USA

JOHN P. FEZZA, MD
Director, Department of Cosmetic Surgery, Center for Sight, Sarasota, Florida, USA

REED M. FEZZA, MS
Department of Cosmetic Surgery, Center for Sight, Sarasota, Florida, USA

KATERINA GALLUS, MD
Private Practice, Voluntary Faculty, Plastic Surgery Division, University of San Diego, San Diego, California, USA

DAVID A. GOODMAN, MD, MS
Retired - Director of Anesthesia Services, Department of Anesthesiology, Abington Surgical Center, Willow Grove, Pennsylvania, USA

JENNIFER GREER, MD, MA
Private Practice, Plastic Surgeon, Greer Plastic Surgery, Mentor, Ohio, USA

MILAN MINESH HIRPARA, BA
Research Fellow, Department of Dermatology, University of California, Irvine, Irvine, California, USA

SWATI KANNAN, MD, FACMS, FAAD
Associate Professor, Department of Dermatology, University of California-San Diego, San Diego, California, USA

ALEXANDRA M. KEANE, MD
Resident, Division of Plastic and Reconstructive Surgery, Department of Surgery, Washington University, St Louis, Missouri, USA

GRACE C. KEANE TAHMASEB, MD
Resident, Division of Plastic and Reconstructive Surgery, Department of Surgery, Washington University, St Louis, Missouri, USA

SHILPI KHETARPAL, MD, FAAD
Associate Professor of Dermatology, Cleveland Clinic, Cleveland, OH, USA

JAMES J. LAW, MD, MSP
Fellow, Department of Ophthalmology, Lions Eye Institute, Albany Medical College, Albany, New York, USA; Oculoplastics, Orbital, and Cosmetic Facial Surgery, Department of Ophthalmology and Visual Sciences, University of Wisconsin-Madison, Madison, Wisconsin, USA

WENDY LEWIS, BA
Founder and President, Wendy Lewis & Co Ltd, New York, New York, USA

SAMUEL J. LIN, MD, MBA
Associate Professor, Director of Aesthetic Surgery, Program Director, Fellowship Co-Director, Division of Plastic Surgery, Beth Israel Deaconess Medical Center, Harvard Medical School, Boston, Massachusetts, USA

ANNE SUN LOWERY, MD
Resident, Department of Otorhinolaryngology–Head and Neck Surgery, University of Pennsylvania, Philadelphia, Pennsylvania, USA

KIRKLAND N. LOZADA, MD
Clinical Associate Professor, Division of Facial Plastic and Reconstructive Surgery, Department of Otorhinolaryngology–Head and Neck Surgery, University of Pennsylvania, Bryn Mawr, Pennsylvania, USA

DIMITRIOS MAVREAS, DDS, MS, PhD
Private Practice, Chalandri, Greece

NATASHA MESINKOVSKA, MD, PhD
Vice Chair of Clinical Research, Department of Dermatology, University of California, Irvine, Irvine, California, USA

MORGAN MURPHREY, MD, MS
Part Time Instructor, Department of Dermatology, Massachusetts General Hospital, Harvard Medical School, Physician Scientist, Wellman Center for Photomedicine, Massachusetts General Hospital, Boston, Massachusetts, USA

KEVIN H. NGUYEN, DO, MS
Resident Physician, Department of Dermatology, Larkin Community Hospital-S Miami, South Miami, Florida, USA

MEGAN NGUYEN, BA
Student Researcher, Department of Dermatology, University of California, Irvine, Irvine, California, USA

LILY PARK, DO, FAAD
Voluntary Assistant Professor, Touro University California, College of Osteopathic Medicine, Vallejo, California, USA; California Northstate University, College of Medicine, Elk Grove, California, USA; Dermatologist, Berman Skin Institute, Cameron Park, California, USA; Department of Dermatology, Larkin Community Hospital-S Miami, South Miami, Florida, USA

SUSRUTHI RAJANALA, MD
Laser and Cosmetic Dermatologic Surgery Fellow, Department of Dermatology, SkinCare Physicians, Chestnut Hill, Massachusetts, USA

SMITA R. RAMANADHAM, MD, FACS
Private Practice, SR Plastic Surgery PC, East Brunswick and Montclair, New Jersey, USA

NAZANIN SAEDI, MD
Clinical Associate Professor, Department of Dermatology, Thomas Jefferson University, Philadelphia, Pennsylvania, USA; Dermatology Associates of Plymouth Meeting, Plymouth Meeting, Pennsylvania, USA

JEFFREY SCHILLER, MD
Clinical Assistant Professor, Department of Ophthalmology, Rutgers-New Jersey Medical School, Newark, New Jersey, USA; JFK University Medical Center, Hackensack Meridian Health, Edison, New Jersey, USA

ROXANA SHIRAZI, MD
Chief Resident Physician, Department of Dermatology, Virginia Commonwealth University School of Medicine, Richmond, Virginia, USA

ALEXA B. STEUER, MD, MPH
Mohs Micrographic Surgery and Cosmetic/Laser Surgery Fellow, Department of Dermatology, SkinCare Physicians, Chestnut Hill, Massachusetts, USA

ARIANNA STROME, MD
Resident, The Ronald O. Perelman Department of Dermatology at NYU Langone Health, New York, New York, USA

NEELAM A. VASHI, MD
Associate Professor, Director of the Cosmetic and Laser Center, Founder and Director of the Center for Ethnic Skin, Department of Dermatology, Boston University School of Medicine, Boston, Massachusetts, USA

MOLLY WANNER, MD, MBA
Assistant Professor, Department of Dermatology, Massachusetts General Hospital, Harvard Medical School, Boston, Massachusetts, USA

ALLAN E. WULC, MD, FACS
Associate Clinical Professor, Department of Ophthalmology, University of Pennsylvania, Philadelphia, Pennsylvania; Adjunct Associate Professor, Department of Otolaryngology, Temple University, Philadelphia, Pennsylvania

JANE YOO, MD, MPP
Clinical Assistant Professor, Department of Dermatology, Icahn School of Medicine at Mount Sinai, Medical Director, Clinical Research Center of New York, New York, New York, USA

ARETHA ZHU, MD
Resident Physician, Institute of Ophthalmology and Visual Science, Rutgers New Jersey Medical School, Newark, New Jersey, USA

ADVANCES IN COSMETIC SURGERY

CONTENTS

VOLUME 8 • 2025

Editorial Board, *iii*

Contributors, *v*

Introduction, *xvii*
By Gregory H. Branham, Jeffrey S. Dover, Shilpi Khetarpal, Smita R. Ramanadham, and Allan E. Wulc

Preface: Welcome to 2025 and Volume VIII: Expanding Options and Improving the Care of the Cosmetic Patient, *xix*
By Gregory H. Branham

Labiaplasty: A Comprehensive Review of Indications, Techniques, and Outcomes, *1*
By Katerina Gallus

Video content accompanies this article at http://www.advancesincosmeticsurgery.com.

This article will provide a thorough review of female genital anatomy relevant to lablaplasty and clitoral hood surgery. The anatomic variation in female genital anatomy makes tailoring the procedure to the individual patient a critical component of a successful surgery and esthetic outcome. Curvilinear trim resection is the most popular labia minora reduction technique. The alternative is the wedge. Clitoral hood reduction is rarely performed as a stand-alone procedure and is an adjunct to labiaplasty surgery, no matter the technique used. Labiaplasty has a high satisfaction rate and low complication rate.

Introduction: nature of the problem, *1*
Anatomy and physiology, *2*
Indications, *3*
Consultation, *4*
Surgical technique, *5*
Trim labiaplasty, *5*
Wedge labiaplasty, *5*
Clitoral hood reduction, *6*
Postoperative care, *7*
Complications, *8*
Summary/discussion, *9*
Clinics care points, *9*
Disclosure, *9*

Update on Anesthesia and Pain Management Strategies in Cosmetic Surgery: My Approach, *11*
By David A. Goodman

Intraoperative and postoperative pain management in aesthetic plastic surgical procedures with limited use of narcotics is a major topic in both the surgery and anesthesia literature. The author describes the evolution of anesthesia and pain management in his 4 decades of practice. We've performed over 4000 cases of cosmetic surgery and mostly succeeded in limiting postoperative discomfort and narcotic usage. The article discusses the incorporation of new medications and techniques into practice and reviews the techniques of anesthetic blocks under ultrasonic guidance. Data that documents the improvements in patient care that ensued as these techniques were instituted is also provided.

Introduction, *11*
Postoperative Pain Strategies, 12
Preoperative assessment, *12*
Ambulatory enhanced recovery after surgery (ERAS) protocol, *13*
Anesthetic techniques, *13*
Our Current Perioperative Local Sedation, 14
Ultrasound-guided blocks for aesthetic surgery cases: indications and techniques, *14*

Cosmetic surgical procedures and individual anesthetic techniques by anatomic area, *18*
Data, *22*
Discussion, *22*
Summary, *22*
Clinics care points, *22*
Disclosure, *22*

Body Contouring After Massive Weight Loss, ***25***

By Jennifer Greer and Anureet K. Bajaj

Successful weight loss is achieved through bariatric surgery and medications like Tirzepatide and Semaglutide. However, this often results in significant loose skin. Developing a personalized surgical plan for body contouring to address the loose skin can have a transformative impact on a patient's quality of life.

Introduction, *25*
Preoperative Evaluation, 25
Surgical technique, *27*
Brachioplasty and Extended Brachioplasty, 27
Abdominoplasty, 27
Monsplasty, 28
Mastopexy and Augmentation/Mastopexy, 29
Thigh Lift, 30
Posterior Body Lift, 31
Reverse Abdominoplasty, 31
Bra Line Back Lift, 32
Immediate Post-Procedure Care, 32
Recovery, 34
Potential Complications, 34
Expectation Management, 34
Clinics care points, *35*
Disclosures, *35*

Nonsurgical Periorbital Rejuvenation: An Update, ***37***

By Lily Park, Kevin H. Nguyen, Naomi F. Briones, and Swati Kannan

Here we provide a concise, updated overview of non-invasive procedures for periorbital rejuvenation, including regenerative medicine modalities. We discuss managing periorbital rejuvenation with resurfacing lasers, vascular lasers, thermo-mechanical fractional injury treatment, radiofrequency, focused ultrasound, chemical peels, neurotoxin, dermal fillers, and finally, regenerative medicine, such as autologous fat transfer, platelet rich plasma, platelet rich fibrin, polynucleotide, and exosomes. By examining the benefits and limitations of each therapy, we aim to assist clinicians with the insights needed to choose the most effective treatment strategy for preriorbital rejuvenation.

Introduction, *37*
Resurfacing lasers, *38*
Overview, 38
Hybrid Resurfacing Lasers, 38
Vascular lasers, *39*
Intense pulse light, *39*
Thermo-mechanical fractional injury therapy, *39*
Radiofrequency, *40*
Focused ultrasound, *40*
Ocular safety, *41*
Chemical peels, *41*
Neurotoxins, *41*
Fillers, *42*
Hyaluronic Acid, 42
Dermal Filler Complication, 42
Poly-L-lactic Acid, 42
Calcium Hydroxyapatite, 43
Regenerative medicine, *43*
Limitation of Regenerative Medicine, 43
Autologous Fat Transfer, 43
Platelet-Rich Concentrate, 43
Polynucleotide, 44
Exosomes, 44
Summary, *45*
Clinics care points, *45*
Disclosure, *45*

The Challenging Facelift, ***49***

By John P. Fezza and Reed M. Fezza

The treatment of the obtuse, full neck is particularly challenging, and a defined jawline and cervicomental angle often requires manipulation of the deeper, subplatysmal neck structures. The causes of a full neck are multifactorial stemming from inadequate bone support, excess fat and skin and muscle laxity, and robust soft tissues. There are a wide variety of choices in rejuvenation of the jaw line, and this decision is based on anatomic knowledge, a thorough examination, sound surgical principles, as well as an understanding of the typical aging changes anticipated at various milestones.

Clinics care points, *59*
Disclosure, *59*

Chin Augmentation, *61*
By Arianna Strome, Alexa B. Steuer, Susruthi Rajanala, and Jeffrey S. Dover

As a critical part of overall facial esthetics, the chin must be considered when patients present with complaints of facial asymmetries or aging, such as jowls or an aging neck, in particular. Chin height, width, and anterior projection should be carefully evaluated, as certain augmentation modalities may be better suited to address specific anatomic deficits. Although there are rare adverse events, dermal fillers offer a minimal down-time option, often at a more affordable cost relative to invasive surgeries and have proven to be both safe and highly effective in addressing deficits in any dimension.

Introduction, *61*
Anatomic Considerations, 61
Options for Chin Augmentation, 62
Treatment selection, *63*
Procedural technique: injectable fillers, *63*
Preoperative Planning, 63
Prep and Patient Positioning, 63
Procedural Approach, 63
Immediate Postprocedural Care, 64
Clinical results in the literature, *64*
Potential complications and management, *65*
Summary, *66*
Clinics care points, *66*
Disclosure, *66*

Lasers and Lights for Acne, *69*
By Alexa B. Steuer, Susruthi Rajanala, Nazanin Saedi, and Jeffrey S. Dover

Lasers and light therapies represent important treatment options for active acne. Light-based therapies tend to involve specific porphyrins that selectively absorb various wavelengths of light, subsequently causing bacterial or sebaceous gland destruction. Through selective photothermolysis, and the absorption of specific wavelengths of optical radiation by target chromophores, lasers cause similar tissue destruction and thereby can produce a positive and targeted therapeutic effect. This article discusses the clinical results of various light and lasers therapies in acne, as well as proper patient selection, preparation, and procedural technique employed with the newly Food and Drug Administration-approved 1726 nm lasers for the treatment of active acne.

Introduction: innovative modalities for the treatment of active acne, *69*
Procedural technique, *70*
Preoperative Planning, 70
Preparation and Patient Positioning, 70
Procedural Approach, 71
Immediate Post-Procedural Care, 71
Clinical results in the literature, *71*
Lights, 71
Lasers, 72
Potential complications/risks, *74*
Summary, *74*
Clinics care points, *74*
Disclosure, *75*

Exosomes: What Is Going on?, *77*
By Milan Minesh Hirpara, Megan Nguyen, and Natasha Mesinkovska

Exosomes, nanoscale extracellular vesicles, facilitate intercellular communication by delivering bioactive molecules such as proteins, lipids, and nucleic acids to target cells. Their therapeutic potential has gained significant attention in aesthetic and regenerative medicine for applications like wound healing, skin rejuvenation, pigmentation control, and hair growth. Studies reveal their ability to promote collagen synthesis, reduce inflammation, and regulate melanogenesis leading to improved skin repair and antiaging outcomes. Although promising preclinical and early clinical results highlight their efficacy, challenges in standardization, isolation methods, and comprehensive human trials remain hurdles in translating exosome-based therapies into widespread clinical practices.

Introduction, *77*
Clinical applications, *79*
Healing and Scar Remodeling, 79
Skin Rejuvenation, 82
Pigmentation Control, 82
Hair Growth, 83
Limitations, *83*
Summary, *84*
Clinics care points, *84*
Disclosures, *84*

Combining Non-ablative Resurfacing with Radiofrequency Microneedling for Acne Scarring, *87*

By Kathleen Coerdt, Susruthi Rajanala, Alexa B. Steuer, and Jeffrey S. Dover

Acne scarring is physically and psychologically distressing to patients, and treatment of acne scarring remains a clinical challenge. Most patients have multiple types of acne scarring, so a multimodal approach to treatment is often recommended. This paper explores the role of combining non-ablative fractional lasers (NAFL) and microneedling with radiofrequency (MNRF) for the treatment of acne scarring. Combined NAFL+MNRF demonstrate promising results with significant improvements demonstrated in the literature. Further research is warranted to determine the appropriate combination regimen to integrate into clinical practice to optimize patient outcomes.

Introduction: nature of the problem, *87*
Background: monotherapy efficacy, *89*
Non-ablative Fractional Laser, 89
Radiofrequency Microneedling, 89
Non-ablative Fractional Laser Monotherapy Versus Microneedling with Radiofrequency Monotherapy, 90
Surgical technique, *90*
Pre-operative Planning, 90
Preparation and Patient Positioning, 91
Procedural Approach, 91
Immediate Post-Procedural Care, 91
Clinical results in the literature: combination therapy, *92*
Combination Non-ablative Fractional Lasers + Microneedling with Radiofrequency for Acne Scarring, 92
Adverse Effects-Combination Therapy, 94
Discussion, *94*
Summary, *94*
Clinics care points, *95*
Disclosure, *95*

Endpoints in Laser & Light-Based Devices, *97*

By Morgan Murphrey and Molly Wanner

Laser and energy-based devices interact with the skin in distinct ways. Not all interactions are created equal, and using improper settings can result in subtherapeutic, or worse, adverse outcomes. Understanding laser-tissue interactions is imperative for identifying and attaining appropriate, therapeutic endpoints. Energy-based devices that are not acting via selective photothermolysis will result in indicators that harken treatment outcomes. Warning endpoints and indicators communicate skin injury, and should promptly result in adjustment of treatment parameters.

Introduction, *97*
Laser-tissue interactions, *97*
Therapeutic endpoints, *98*
Vascular Lesions, 98
Hair Removal and Pigmented Lesions, 100
Lasers Without Specific Endpoints, 102
Warning endpoints and how to avoid them, *102*
Cooling Related Injuries, 103
Nikolsky Sign, 103
Shrinkage, Contraction, Puckering, and Charring, 103
Chrysiasis and Paradoxical Darkening, 104
Metallic Gray, Impending Epidermal Necrosis, and Pain, 104
Contact Dermatitis and Numbing Related Side Effects, 104
New frontiers and next directions, *104*
Targeting New Chromophores, 104

Endpoints Versus Indicators, 105
Endpoints and Artificial Intelligence, 105
Summary, *105*
Clinics care points, *106*
Disclosure, *106*

Adjustments to the Maxillofacial Skeleton to Improve Facial Harmony, *107*

By Kevin B. Coppelson

This article explores surgical adjustments to the maxillofacial skeleton to enhance facial harmony. It begins with an overview of the anatomy and its critical role in supporting soft tissues, influencing proportions, and maintaining balance. Principles of facial esthetics, incisor show, and lip length are discussed as guidelines for achieving optimal outcomes. Key surgical techniques are detailed. Advancements in virtual surgical planning, patient-specific hardware, and custom facial implants are highlighted. Functional considerations underscore the interplay between esthetics and functionality. Real-world case studies illustrate the transformative impact of these interventions. The article concludes with future directions.

Introduction, *107*
Anatomy of the maxillofacial skeleton, *108*
Key Structures, 108
Relationship of Soft Tissues to the Facial Skeleton, 108
Principles of facial proportions and incisor show, *108*
Ideal Facial Proportions, 108
Facial Symmetry, 109
Skeletal Proportions, 109
Control of Incisor Show, 110
Lip Length Considerations, 110
Ethnic and Gender Variations, 110
Surgical adjustments to the maxillofacial skeleton, *110*
Maxillary Adjustments, 110
Transverse Maxillary Expansion Techniques, 111
Mandibular Adjustments, 111
Additional Mandibular Procedures, 111
Zygomatic (Malar) Adjustments, 111
Virtual surgical planning and patient-specific hardware, *112*
Virtual Surgical Planning, 112
Patient-Specific Hardware, 112
Integration of Custom Facial Implants, 112
Functional considerations, *112*
Airway Obstruction and Sleep Apnea, 112
Chewing and Swallowing Difficulties, 113
Speech Disorders, 113
Temporomandibular Joint Disorders, 113
Case studies and examples, *113*
Case Study 1: Comprehensive Orthognathic Surgery for Functional and Aesthetic Improvement, 113
Case Study 2: Comprehensive Orthognathic Surgery and Custom for Post-Trauma Jaw Asymmetry and Sleep Apnea, 114
Case study 3: Orthognathic Reconstruction for Severe Mandibular Hypoplasia and Upper Airway Resistance Syndrome, 116
Summary and future directions, *118*
Clinics care points, *118*
Disclosure, *118*

Facial Rejuvenation and Orthodontics; Is There a Connection?, *121*

By Dimitrios Mavreas

Facial aging involves changes in the craniofacial skeleton, soft tissues, smile, and teeth. Orthodontic treatment can address these changes by improving directly dental and smile esthetics, and skeletal alignment and indirectly the surrounding soft issues. The guidelines for orthodontic management of the aged face aim at increasing lower face height, and volumizing the dentoalveolar part of the face. Combining orthodontics with other medical disciplines can yield synergistic effects, rejuvenating faces and improving overall well-being. Case studies demonstrate the positive impact of orthodontic treatment on facial esthetics.

Introduction, *121*
Bone changes of the midface and the mandible, *122*
Soft tissue changes, *122*

Smile/teeth changes, *122*
Rejuvenation and orthodontics—guidelines, *123*
Case 1, *124*
Case 2, *124*
Discussion, *125*
Summary, *129*
Clinics care points, *129*
Disclosure, *129*

Whitnall's Ligament Suspension Repair of Involutional Ptosis—The Old Is New, ***133***

By Jeffrey Schiller and Andrea Cacciarelli

This procedure has supplanted Muller's muscle conjunctival resection (MMCR) and levator aponeurotic advancement in my practice, which is a mixed cosmetic and functional blepharoplasty practice. It is more reliable and stable over time than aponeurotic surgery and does not require the second internal incision as with MMCR with its attendant concerns regarding direct contact with the ocular surface. It is a valuable adjunct to the cosmetic blepharoplasty surgeon's armamentarium with a low complication rate and a high rate of patient and surgeon satisfaction.

Causes of involutional ptosis, *134*
Anatomy of Whitnall's ligament, *134*
Whitnalls Ligament and Ptosis Repair, 136
Techniques for correction of involutional ptosis, *136*
Surgical technique, *137*
Summary, *139*
Clinics care points, *139*
Disclosure, *139*

Filler Rhinoplasty, ***141***

By Beatrice Ching-Chen Go, Anne Sun Lowery, and Kirkland N. Lozada

Nonsurgical rhinoplasty is an innovative technique that allows for temporary modification of the nose to improve esthetic appearance and function. As with any filler augmentation, a thorough understanding of complex nasal anatomy is key to obtain optimal results while reducing risk of complications. Injection strategy is dependent on overall desired goals and can vary when addressing the radix, middle vault, and tip. While the procedure has a relatively low-risk profile, rapid recognition and early intervention of vascular complications is crucial.

Introduction, *141*
Relevant anatomy, *141*
Filler selection, *142*
Patient selection, *143*
Injection technique, *144*
Radix, 145
Midvault, 146
Tip, 146
Other Applications, 148
Pros and cons, *149*
Complications, *149*
Summary, *150*
Clinics care points, *150*
Disclosure, *150*

Advances, Techniques, and Complications Associated with Adjacent Fat Transfer in Lower Blepharoplasty, ***153***

By James J. Law, Aretha Zhu, and Cat N. Burkat

By transferring volume from prominent eyelid fat pads to deficient midfacial hollows, fat transfer techniques utilized in lower blepharoplasty offer an effective method for aesthetically contouring the lid-cheek junction—an outcome not achievable with a purely subtractive approach. This article provides an anatomical foundation for the facial cosmetic surgeon performing aesthetic lower eyelid blepharoplasty in context of the aging midface. The application of adjacent fat transfer with both transconjunctival and transcutaneous approaches to lower blepharoplasty is outlined along with preoperative and postoperative considerations, complications, and guidelines for their avoidance.

Introduction, *153*
Lower eyelid surgical anatomy, *153*
Preoperative considerations for adjacent fat transfer, *155*

Surgical techniques, *157*
Transconjunctival Approach, 157
Transcutaneous Approach, 161
Adjunctive Procedures, 161
Postoperative care, *161*
Complications, *162*
Summary, *163*
Clinics care points, *164*
Proprietary interest statement, *164*
Disclosure, *164*

Aging Rhinoplasty, *169*

By Grace C. Keane Tahmaseb, Alexandra M. Keane, Samuel J. Lin, and Trina G. Ebersole

Aging rhinoplasty requires deep anatomic understanding of the effects of aging on the skin, subcutaneous tissue, cartilaginous framework, and bony structure. Elderly patients with realistic expectations should be sought after. A complete medical history should be obtained to determine fitness for surgery. The primary surgical maneuvers performed correct tip ptosis and address obstructive airway concerns. Care should be taken to avoid over-dissecting the underlying nasal framework owing to age-related attenuation of the bony and cartilaginous structure. When surgery is undertaken in a safe manner on properly selected patients, high satisfaction rates can be obtained.

Introduction: nature of the problem, *169*
Skin and Subcutaneous Tissue, 170
Cartilage Changes, 170
Nasal Dorsum, 170
Airway Concerns, 170
Skeletal Remodeling, 170
Surgical technique, *171*
Preoperative Planning, 171
Preparation and Patient Positioning, 171
Procedural Approach, 171
Immediate Postprocedural Care, 173
Rehabilitation and recovery, *174*
Clinical results, *175*
Potential complications and limitations, *175*
Summary, *176*
Clinics care points, *176*
Disclosure, *176*

Reputation Management: Best Practices to Handle Negative Reviews, *177*

By Wendy Lewis and Jane Yoo

The advent of online review websites and social media has transformed how patients choose their doctors of all specialties. Your online presence may include reviews, photos, patient outcomes, testimonials, comments on your website, social media channels, accolades as well as complaints. These outlets as well as recommendations from friends and colleagues, may be the first impression patients learn about your practice. In this robust digital climate, patients who are seeking aesthetic practices have more options than ever before. Since these procedures are generally not covered by insurance, they tend to be more careful about their choices. Aesthetic patients are often very well informed from numerous sources and do their homework about doctors and practices before making an appointment. They tend look for providers who demonstrate medical expertise in their category interest, and qualities such as empathy, good communication, accessibility, expertise, and reputation. Thus, a strong online reputation showcasing these important traits that patients are looking for can significantly influence their decisions to book an appointment. This chapter covers the most important basics of reputation management for dermatologists.

Defining reputation management, *177*
Get to know the basics, *178*
Protecting your digital footprint, *178*
Strategies for elevating your reputation, *179*
Most valuable content to elevate your practice, *179*
Monitoring your reputation online 24/7, *179*
Building long-term trust with patients, *179*
Five key strategies for reputation management, *180*
Summary, *180*
Disclosure, *180*

Social Media Dysmorphia, *183*

By Roxana Shirazi, Eric J. Beltrami, Alexa J. Cohen, and Neelam A. Vashi

Over the past decade, greater social media utilization has paralleled a heightened focus on aesthetic standards perpetuated through social media. This phenomenon has resulted in the emergence of a newly recognized entity in cosmetic dermatology, social media dysphoria. Social media dysphoria describes dissatisfaction with body image relative to and as a result of beauty ideals portrayed on social media applications and their associated photo editing technology. In this article, we will describe trends in social media utilization, review body dysmorphic disorder, define social media dysphoria, propose screening criteria for high-risk patients, and discuss best practices in managing such cases clinically.

Introduction, *183*
Epidemiology of social media, *183*
Body dysmorphic disorder, *184*
Social media dysmorphia, also known as *selfie dysmorphia*, *185*
Clinical and practical implications of social media dysmorphia, *186*
Future directions, *187*
Clinics care points, *187*
Disclosure, *188*

Advances in Cosmetic Surgery 8 (2025) xvii–xviii
ADVANCES IN COSMETIC SURGERY

Introduction

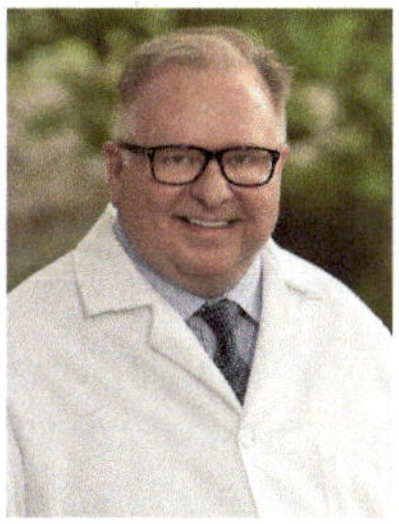

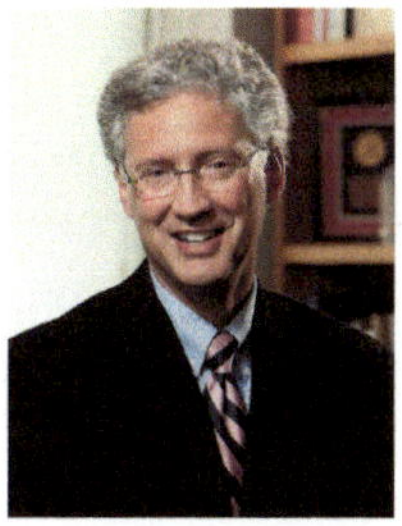

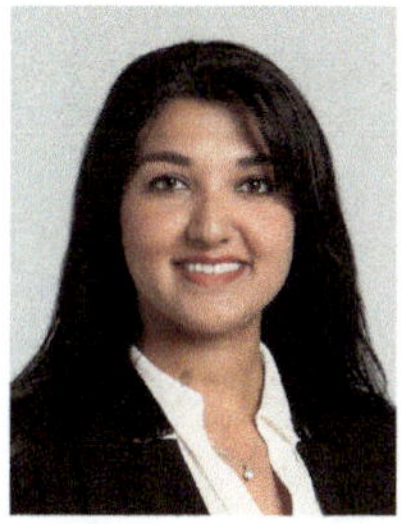

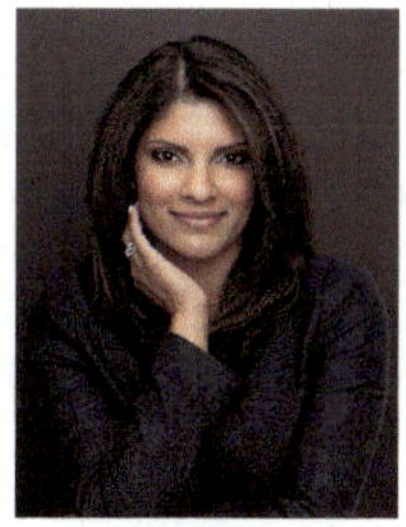

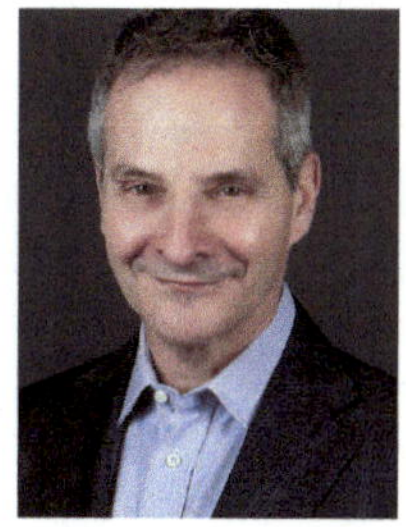

Gregory H. Branham, MD
Jeffrey S. Dover, MD, FRCPC
Shilpi Khetarpal, MD, FAAD
Smita R. Ramanadham, MD, FACS
Allan E. Wulc, MD, FACS

The desire for cosmetic surgery has infiltrated corners of society never seen before and is only expected to grow in the years ahead. As the number of cosmetic surgery procedures continues to rise throughout the world, so too do the number of specialists who perform these important procedures. When working with a patient to create their ideal image, it's critical to have the most current resources available to guide your practice and inform your decisions.

Advances in Cosmetic Surgery, now in its eighth issue, aims to highlight the year's latest advancements and breakthroughs in the field of cosmetic surgery. Experts from the four core skin specialties, including Dermatology, Plastic Surgery, Facial Plastic Surgery, and Oculoplastic Surgery, have come together to bring you, the reader, the most important advances in this rapidly evolving field.

Reviews written by leading experts in the four specialties include techniques in the field of facial contouring that include expanded injectable filler applications and modern considerations for surgical implants and surgical skeletal contouring. We explore some challenges in cosmetic surgery, including the nonideal facelift candidate and social media dysmorphia. The updates on energy devices and their use in the treatment of acne and acne scarring will expand your knowledge and enhance your options for these patients. Finally, there is an update on new postoperative pain management strategies that offer options to improve the comfort of the cosmetic procedures we perform and decrease the use of opioids in the posttreatment management of our patients.

High-quality images and videos accompany many of the articles, helping to further deepen the reader's understanding of these techniques and procedures. Whether you are planning to perform the procedures discussed here or are learning about them for the first time, we think you will find value in what this exciting series has to offer.

The editors would like to thank the authors for their insightful contributions, and all the pioneers in this field working to bring us better tools, techniques, and

https://doi.org/10.1016/j.yacs.2025.02.003
2542-4327/25/

ways of making the seemingly impossible possible for our patients.

We hope you enjoy reading this issue as much as we have enjoyed putting it together. It is our sincere hope that the articles presented here will help further break down barriers between specialties and shed new light on current cosmetic treatments.

Gregory H. Branham, MD
Facial Plastic and Reconstructive Surgery
Department of Otolaryngology–HNS
Washington University
School of Medicine
St Louis, MO, USA

Jeffrey S. Dover, MD, FRCPC
SkinCare Physicians
Chestnut Hill, MA, USA

Yale University School of Medicine
New Haven, CT, USA

Brown Medical School
Providence, RI, USA

Shilpi Khetarpal, MD, FAAD
Cleveland Clinic
Cleveland, OH, USA

Smita R. Ramanadham, MD, FACS
SR Plastic Surgery PC
East Brunswick
Montclair, NJ, USA

Allan E. Wulc, MD, FACS
Department of Ophthalmology
University of Pennsylvania
Philadelphia, PA, USA

Department of Otolaryngology
Temple University
Philadelphia, PA, USA

E-mail addresses: branhamg@wustl.edu (G.H. Branham)
jdover@skincarephysicians.net (J.S. Dover)
shilpikhetarpal@gmail.com (S. Khetarpal)
smitar2280md@gmail.com (S.R. Ramanadham)
awulcmd@gmail.com (A.E. Wulc)

Advances in Cosmetic Surgery 8 (2025) xix–xx
ADVANCES IN COSMETIC SURGERY

Preface

Welcome to 2025 and Volume VIII: Expanding Options and Improving the Care of the Cosmetic Patient

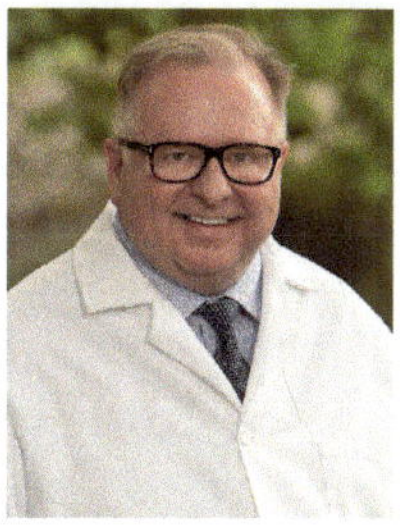

Gregory H. Branham, MD
Editor

Welcome to the eighth issue of *Advances in Cosmetic Surgery*. I, along with the diverse and very talented coeditors, Drs Jeffrey Dover, Shilpi Khetarpal, Smita R. Ramanadham, and Allan E. Wulc, have curated a group of contributors whose submissions will expand options for our patients and improve and advance their care.

Advances in Cosmetic Surgery values the expertise that is represented across the various fields who teach, practice, and do research in Cosmetic Surgery. The editorial board represents specialists from dermatology, plastic surgery, ophthalmic plastic surgery, and facial plastic surgery and offers a broad perspective in the field of cosmetic surgery. Combining expertise from diverse fields provides enhanced perspective and knowledge that will improve the care of our patients. This has been the goal of *Advances in Cosmetic Surgery* since its inception.

This issue introduces techniques in the field of facial contouring that include expanded injectable filler applications and modern considerations for surgical implants and surgical skeletal contouring. We explore challenges in cosmetic surgery, including the nonideal facelift candidate and social media dysmorphia. The updates on energy devices and their use in the treatment of acne and acne scarring will expand your knowledge and enhance your options for these patients. Finally, there is an update on new postoperative pain management

https://doi.org/10.1016/j.yacs.2025.02.001
2542-4327/25/

strategies that offer options to improve the comfort of the cosmetic procedures we perform and decrease the use of opioids in the posttreatment management of our patients.

With deep gratitude and appreciation, the editors and production staff would like to thank the expert contributors for sharing their knowledge and talent in this issue. To you, the readers, we thank you for your commitment to advancing the field of cosmetic surgery by acquiring new skills and knowledge. If you have areas that you would like us to investigate further and consider for inclusion in upcoming issues, please contact us. We hope that this issue will promote thought and consideration on how we all can improve and advance the care of our cosmetic patients.

DISCLOSURES

The author has no conflicts of interest or disclosures to disclose.

Gregory H. Branham, MD
Division of Facial Plastic and
Reconstructive Surgery
Department of Otolaryngology–
Head and Neck Surgery
Washington University
Facial Plastic Surgery Center of
Washington University
1044 North Mason Road, Suite L10
Creve Coeur, MO 63141, USA

E-mail address: branhamg@wustl.edu

Advances in Cosmetic Surgery 8 (2025) 1–9
ADVANCES IN COSMETIC SURGERY

Labiaplasty

A Comprehensive Review of Indications, Techniques, and Outcomes

Katerina Gallus, MD*
Private Practice, Restore SD Plastic Surgery, 8899 University Center Lane Suite 200, San Diego, CA 92122, USA

KEYWORDS
• Female genital anatomy • Clitoral hood reduction • Labia minora hypertrophy • Labia reduction surgery
• Clitoral hood

KEY POINTS

- Labiaplasty surgery has become a commonly performed procedure in the United States due to increased awareness and the evolution of esthetic ideals.
- Understanding the anatomy of the female genitalia and the variations is a key to planning the appropriate surgical plan for achieving an esthetic outcome in labiaplasty surgery.
- Labiaplasty is performed with a curvilinear trim or wedge reduction, both acceptable and safe procedures with a low complication rate.
- Clitoral hood reduction is a balancing procedure commonly performed with labiaplasty and limited to skin excision.
- Postoperative care and instructions are essential in ensuring the patient's timely and smooth recovery.

Video content accompanies this article at http://www.advancesincosmeticsurgery.com.

INTRODUCTION: NATURE OF THE PROBLEM

An increasing number of women seek improvement regarding female genitalia, most often with concerns about the labia minora and clitoral hood. The American Society of Plastic Surgeons annual statistics report 10,592 labiaplasties performed in 2023, which has increased since it began reporting the procedure in 2015 [1,2]. The Aesthetic Society reported 18,120 labiaplasties in 2023, a 67% increase from the number reported in 2019 [3].

The increase in awareness and demand for the procedure has been attributed to multiple factors: increasing awareness of a surgical solution, changing fashions that favor tight leggings and revealing clothes, contemporary pubic grooming, the representation of the vulva in mass media as hairless, flat, and with no protrusion beyond the labia majora, and the functional benefits of the procedure.

Historically, obstetrician-gynecologists have opposed the procedure. Genital esthetic surgery was condemned in the 2007 and 2019 American College of Obstetricians and Gynecologists (ACOG) Committee Opinion. ACOG published a formal article that vaginal rejuvenation and cosmetic vaginal procedures lacked data and efficacy to support these procedures [4]. ACOG stated that procedure risks were too high and suggested reassurance to women for the wide variability

*Corresponding author. *E-mail address:* drgallus@restoresdplasticsurgery.com

https://doi.org/10.1016/j.yacs.2025.01.003

ABBREVIATIONS	
ACOG	American College of Obstetricians and Gynecologists
HS2	Herpes Simplex 2

of female genital appearance. As such, plastic surgeons tend to lead in publications and research and offer the procedure to patients.

There is no universal esthetic standard for the ideal vulvar complex and a vast presentation of varying anatomic variations. Additionally, the ideals and esthetics of female genital surgery continue to evolve with changing fashion, lifestyles, and social trends. Surgeons need to understand anatomy, ensure that our patients have realistic expectations of results, and choose the procedure that will create balance and harmony for the individual patient.

ANATOMY AND PHYSIOLOGY

Understanding anatomy and anatomic variations can help optimize a tailored surgical approach. Normal labia minora anatomy encompasses a broad range of sizes, thicknesses, and colors.

The basic anatomy of the external female genitalia has been well described. It consists of the mons pubis, the clitoris and its overlying clitoral hood, the labia minora, and the majora.

The focus of this text is primarily on the labia minora. The labia majora are 2 folds that extend posteriorly from the mons pubis (the triangular adipose tissue just anterior to the pubic symphysis) to the perineal area. The majora can be considered empty or redundant in some patients and addressed accordingly with volume restoration or reduction.

Enveloped and medial to the labia majora are the clitoris, clitoral hood, and labia minora. The minora and majora are separated by a sulcus.

The clitoris is positioned directly under the clitoral hood. The frenula are folds of skin of varying sizes that extend from the glans clitoris to merge with the extension of the clitoral hood to form the labia minora. There can be wide variations in the clitoral hood with the presence of lateral folds, heavy folds, small hoods, and variations in continuity with the labia minora.

The clitoral hood extends laterally and superiorly to the anterior labial commissure. The inferior border extended to the junction with the labial minora. This junction is the defining point of the frenulum, which is the portion of the labia minora that extends to the clitoris. The urethral meatus can usually be found at the frenulum's apex.

The labia minora continues posteriorly from the clitoral hood toward the perineal body. The labia can join posteriorly or remain separate and attach to the perineum. Variations in size, thickness, and pigmentation occur. The presence of rugae is common in those seeking labiaplasty (Fig. 1).

The blood supply to the female genitalia consists of branches of the internal pudendal artery—the posterior labial artery and the perineal artery. This artery also gives rise to the dorsal artery of the clitoris. There are contributions from the external superficial pudendal artery via the anterior system. Georgiou and colleagues's study determined the presence of a dominant central artery, which impacts the wedge technique's healing and safety if not oriented properly [5].

The innervation of the external female genitalia is through the pudendal nerve. The superficial branch becomes the posterior labial nerve, and the deep branch becomes the dorsal nerve of the clitoris. The dorsal clitoral nerve is deep to the clitoral fascia and the tunica albuginea. If the surgeon remains superficial to dartos fascia in this region, injury to clitoral innervation is unlikely.

There is no consensus as to how to classify the appearance of female genitalia. This is partly due to commonly referred aspects of the minora as hypertrophic or enlarged. However, studies have demonstrated that variation in the labial length, width, color, rugosity of the labial skin, and clitoral size encompasses a wide spectrum of normality. Several classification systems have been proposed, addressing the ability to measure or document the size and/or location of labial protrusion.

A commonly used classification system, the Banwell Classification system, serves as a clear means of documenting the labia anatomy, educating the patient, and informing the surgeon about the best labiaplasty technique [6]. The Banwell Classification identifies the most prominent lateral point of the labia minora in either the upper, middle, or lower third of the vaginal vault. The thickness, rugosity, and pigmentation should also be noted. As with most bilateral anatomy, asymmetry is common and should be identified (Fig. 2).

The posterior attachment of the labia minor also varies. The attachment may be low (close to the perineum), medium, or high. In some cases, there is a posterior connection or posterior fourchette (Fig. 3).

The clitoral labial complex also encompasses a wide variety of anatomic variations. In most anatomic texts, the clitoral body and hood are small, but both can be enlarged. The clitoral hood can create a double fold with either horizontal or, more commonly, lateral fold

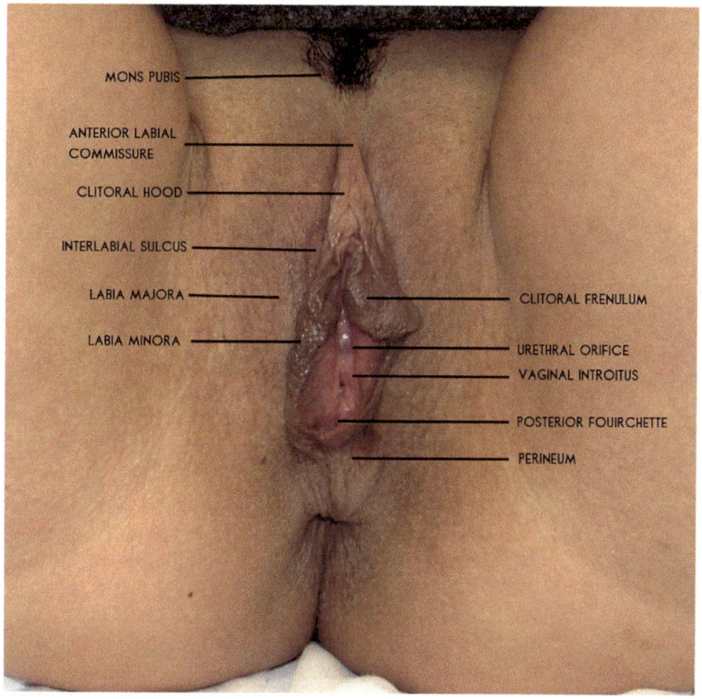

FIG. 1 Anatomy of external female genitalia.

excess. The junction between the clitoral hood and the labia minora is also varied (Fig. 4).

INDICATIONS

Most labia minora enlargement is congenital, although it can occur after childbirth, hormone therapy, weight loss, and aging. Surgical intervention is indicated when enlargement impacts self-esteem, causes discomfort, or for esthetic reasons. Contraindications include those patients with body dysmorphic disorder and those who expect the procedure to enhance their sexual lives and improve their ability to achieve orgasm. Unrealistic expectations, comorbid psychological conditions, patient confusion, active vulvovaginal diseases, coagulopathy, and smoking are other contraindications.

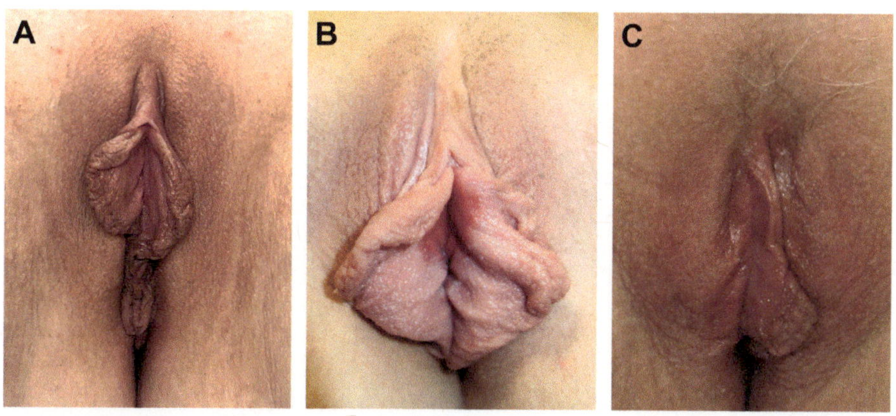

FIG. 2 Examples of Banwell Classification. (**A**) Labia upper third prominence, (**B**) labia middle third prominence, and (**C**) labia with lower third prominence.

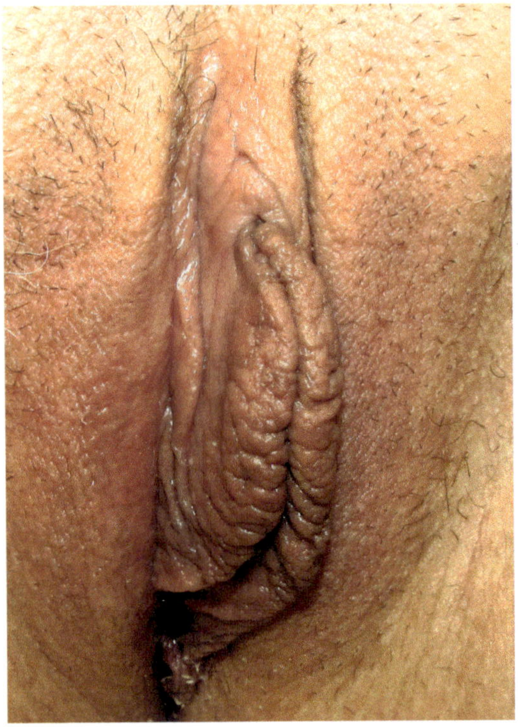

FIG. 3 Examples of variations in posterior attachment of the labia minora.

CONSULTATION

It is important to obtain a thorough, focused history and physical examination of patients. A smoking history is a contraindication to proceeding with surgery unless the patient commits to cessation for a minimum of 2 weeks before and after surgery.

It is important to screen for a history of Herpes Simplex 2 (HS2) and frequent yeast infections. Prophylactic antiviral therapy is prescribed for patients with an HS2 history, and prophylactic fluconazole is prescribed for women with frequent yeast infections.

Medical history should include parity and a history of traumatic injury. Understanding their motivations for the surgery is also important. The concept of esthetic ideals is always evolving, so the goal of the surgical outcome should be to keep in mind the patient's context of anatomic variation and seek a proportionate result that is in harmony with the patient's anatomy.

The examination occurs early in the consultation with the patient, who holds a handheld mirror so the physician and patient can be clear about the relevant anatomy. This includes the patient's goals and expectations regarding clitoral hood, anterior commissure, and labial projection. If indicated, a vaginal examination can be performed, but this is generally reserved for those seeking vaginoplasty or perineoplasty.

After the examination is completed and the patient is determined to be a suitable candidate, an explanation of the surgical technique, whether the clitoral hood should be addressed, and if there are other concerns are discussed. Before and after photos are reviewed to explain variations in anatomy and clarify goals. An explanation of the procedure, what to expect, recovery time, and postop care is reviewed. The patient is given printed and emailed information regarding the preop and postop instructions for scheduling and emailed again just before the procedure. Medications prescribed include a small amount of oxycodone and a dose of fluconazole. If the patient has a history of HSV or frequent yeast infections, the appropriate medications are ordered prophylactically. Antibiotics are unnecessary; after the first 24 hours,

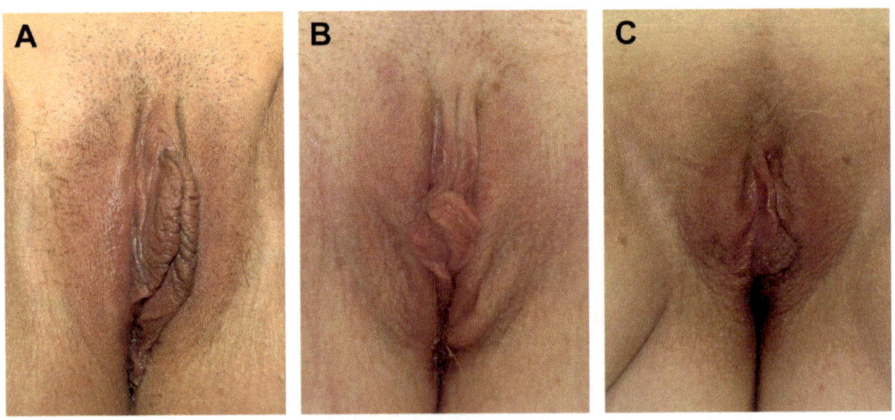

FIG. 4 Examples of variations in clitoral labial complex. (**A–C**) clitoral hood (CH) variations.

patients can take Tylenol or non-steroidal anti-inflammaotry drugs for pain. Patients are instructed to shower with an antibacterial cleanser on the morning of surgery.

SURGICAL TECHNIQUE

Getting preoperative photos in both the standing and lithotomy positions is important, taking care to pose the labia if necessary to demonstrate excess. In standing, have the patient abduct their legs to shoulder width to visualize labial protrusion (Fig. 5).

The procedure can be performed effectively under local anesthesia. General anesthesia is appropriate when combined with other surgeries.

The patient has the option to take an oral sedative if desired. However, the procedure is comfortable under local anesthesia, some patients have appropriate anxiety about the procedure, and taking an oral sedative allows them to relax. Midazolam ketamine odansetron melts (MKO melts) are an opioid-free, slow-release medication given 30 minutes before the start of the procedure. It consists of 3 mg of midazolam, 25 mg of ketamine hydrogen chloride, and 2 mg of ondansetron. Any anxiolytic is a reasonable option. Patients who choose not to take the MKO melt are often motivated by the ability to drive home themselves after the procedure.

A topical numbing cream (plasticized 23% lidocaine and 7% tetracaine) is applied to the area for 10 to 15 minutes. The patient is then placed in the lithotomy position, and the topical is removed (Fig. 6).

Markings are performed with care to evaluate for symmetry. The patient is handed a handheld mirror to review the markings, and local anesthetic is injected (Fig. 7).

Local anesthesia (1% Lidocaine and Epinephrine 1:100,000 and 0.25% Marcaine in a 1:1 ratio) with a small amount of bicarbonate solution is injected. The injection is performed with a 30-gauge needle. It begins on the mucosal side of the minora, using the least amount of local anesthesia to provide an effect without overly distorting the tissues. The injection is well tolerated due to the previously placed topical anesthesia. The local anesthetic is allowed to set for 10 minutes, during which time the patient is prepped and draped with betadine or equivalent (Fig. 8).

TRIM LABIAPLASTY

Trim labiaplasty, a curved linear resection, is performed with a simple surgical instrument set and a needle tip bovie cautery at a low setting (Fig. 9). For thicker labia, care to remove muscle is important to debulk the result. Once excision is performed and hemostasis is achieved, closure is begun. Closure is performed in layers with 5.0 Monocryl, reapproximating the mucosa. The deep layer is a horizontally oriented running suture layer to promote hemostasis and then is used as a running subcuticular suture. The edges can then be oversewn with a running 5.0 fast absorbing plain gut or 5.0 Vicryl Rapide suture very loosely to allow for edema. Before the last suture, additional local anesthesia consisting of 0.25% Marcaine is infiltrated to allow the patient to have time to travel home and take pain medications (See Video 1 Labiaplasty, Trim Technique).

WEDGE LABIAPLASTY

Wedge labiaplasty can be performed in those with radial elongation of the labia and continuous edge

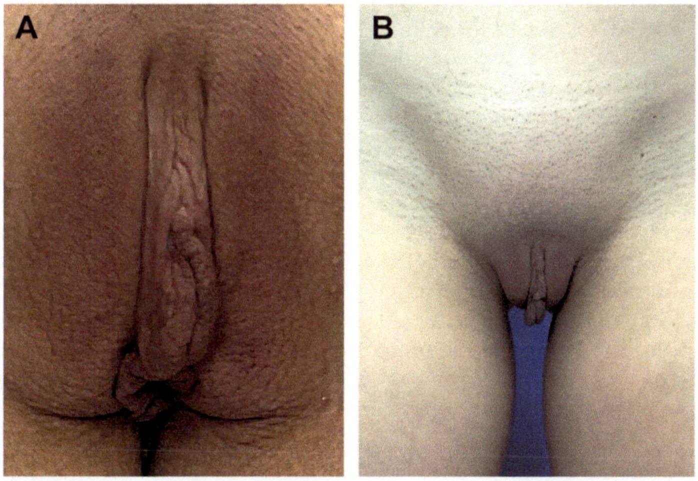

FIG. 5 Preoperative photo examples. (A) Preop lithotomy example and (B) preop standing example 1.

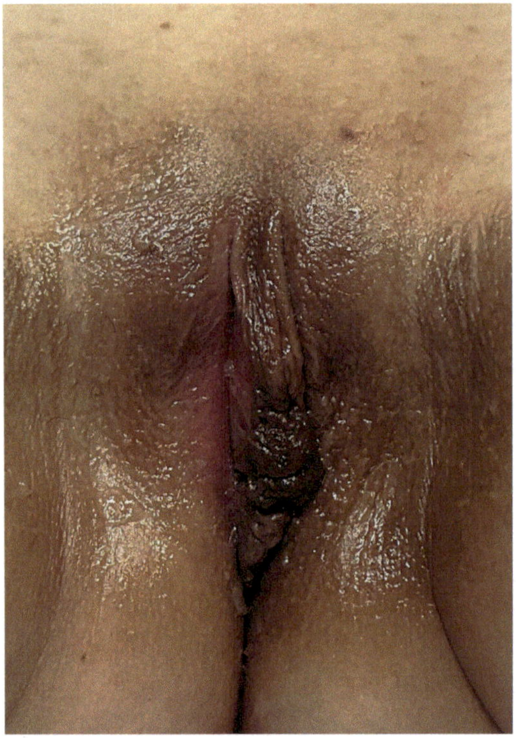

FIG. 6 Patient with numbing cream applied.

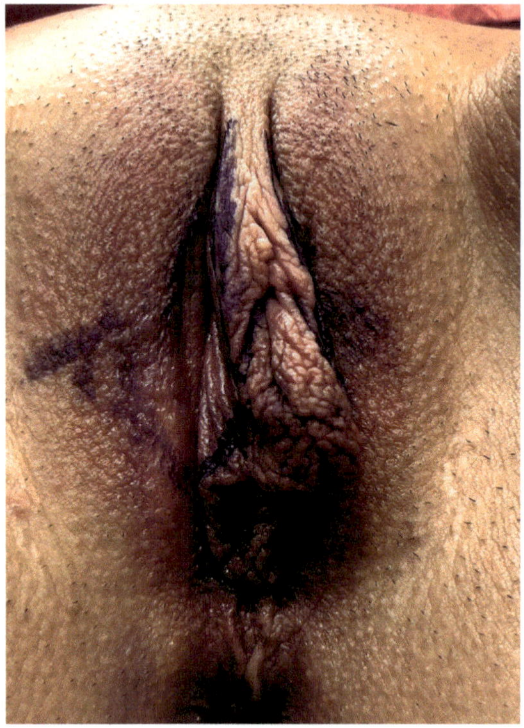

FIG. 7 Markings for curvilinear resection and clitoral hood reduction.

pigmentation that they are willing to maintain. The anterior limb is drawn first, then folded posteriorly to approximate the posterior limb of the V. The anterior limb must be greater than 0.5 cm from the urethral meatus to avoid creating distortion of the urinary stream. The 2 edges should approximate with minimal tension. Although a more anterior wedge position results in better flap perfusion, the clitoral frenulum, hood, and minora must be considered. Incisions are made with either a 15-blade or a needle-point cautery device. A full-thickness "pie wedge" of tissue is resected from the most protuberant portion of the labial minora. The wedge can be full thickness (for those with bulky or thicker labia) or a wedge that preserves the submucosa for those with thin or atrophic labia. After hemostasis, the submucosa and mucosa are reapproximated. The closure of the defect is from deep to superficial with a fine monofilament absorbable suture in an interrupted buried fashion. It is critical to approximate the leading edge precisely to prevent notching. The final layer consists of a running absorbable suture. Local anesthesia is again infiltrated. The advantages of the wedge technique include preservation of the natural edge, a shorter scar, and decreased scar sensitivity.

CLITORAL HOOD REDUCTION

An ideal configuration and relation of the glans clitoris to the hood has not been established. The innervation is generally attributed to the dorsal nerve of the clitoris, which travels deep into Buck's fascia. The procedure is performed for aesthetic reasons that fulfill the goals of the patient and is not a procedure to improve sexual stimulation. The goal is to address clitoral hood tissue that projects beyond the labia majora or bulkiness and contributes to widening the intervulvar commissure. Conservative reduction is encouraged to avoid exposure of the glans clitoris.

Markings are made to address the redundancy. This most commonly uses a paramedian vertical resection to address redundant lateral folds. The apex should not extend beyond the apex of the anterior labial commissure. The distal incision is continued medially to the labia minora when performed as a composite resection using a trim technique. When combined with a wedge technique, the medial markings do not converge.

In patients with a horizontal clitoral hood excess, the excess can be addressed with an inverted V pattern resection.

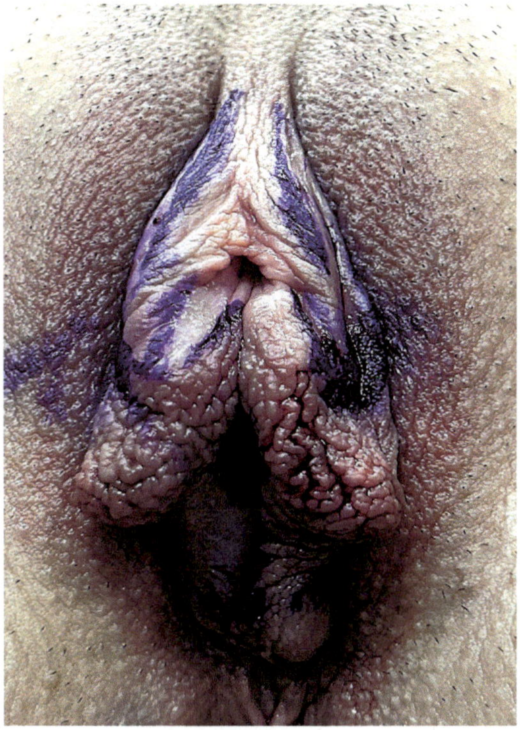

FIG. 8 Appearance after injection of local anesthesia.

With paramedical vertical excess, preserving 6 to 8 mm of tissue centrally is recommended to avoid over-resection and limit postoperative edema. The excision of the clitoral hood with any technique or modification is limited to tangential removal of skin only, taking care to avoid deeper tissues.

Sutures consist of an intracuticular running closure with 5-0 Monocryl. The final layer is a loose-running simple closure with 5.0 FA Plain Gut suture. Before the last suture, additional local anesthesia consisting of 0.25% Marcaine is infiltrated to allow the patient to have time to travel home and take pain medications.

POSTOPERATIVE CARE

The area is cleansed with saline solution. At the end of the surgery, topical bacitracin, an ABD pad, and an ice pack are applied.

The patient is discharged home with postoperative instructions (that have been previously reviewed and emailed as well as printed for them) with a home kit that includes the following:
Peri bottle
Aquaphor
Arnica supplement

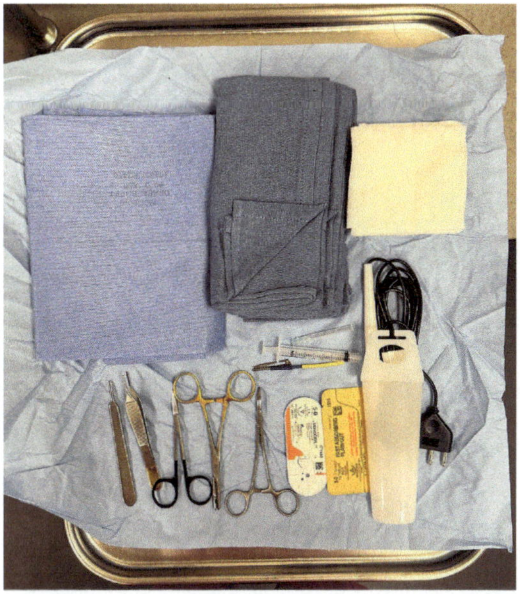

FIG. 9 Tray setup for labiaplasty.

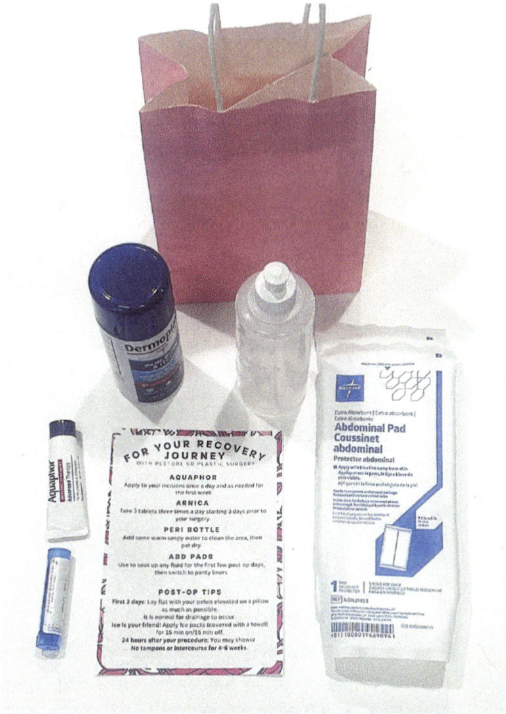

FIG. 10 Picture of postoperative kit.

Dermaplast spray
Abdominal (ABD) pads (Fig. 10)

The patient is instructed to go home immediately and remain as flat as possible with their pelvis elevated on a pillow for 72 hours as much as possible. They are advised to take their oxycodone every 4 to 6 hours for pain in the first 24 to 48 hours. The peri bottle is to be filled with warm water and sprayed over incisions after bathroom use to avoid wiping. The area is then gently pat dry with no rubbing.

The patient is advised to avoid lifting anything over 10 lbs or raise their heart rate or blood pressure for 2 weeks. The patient must not soak in a tub or Sitz bath or swim for the first 4 weeks to not weaken the sutures. After 2 weeks, they can increase their activity level, with most allowed full activity at 4 weeks. They are to refrain from intercourse, tampons, or insertion of anything else for 4 to 6 weeks. Photos are taken at 4 weeks and 3 months (Fig. 11). They are evaluated in the clinic at 1 week, 4 weeks, and, if needed, at 3 months. The sutures dissolve rapidly between 10 and 14 days and may manifest as itching and discharge. This can be alleviated with hydrocortisone cream.

COMPLICATIONS

Postoperative complications from labiaplasty include wound dehiscence, hematoma, infection, poor scarring, and over-resection or under-resection. According to the most recent review of nationally available data, the rate of complications ranges from 2% to 4% and has been quoted as 2.7% in cosmetic labiaplasty [7].

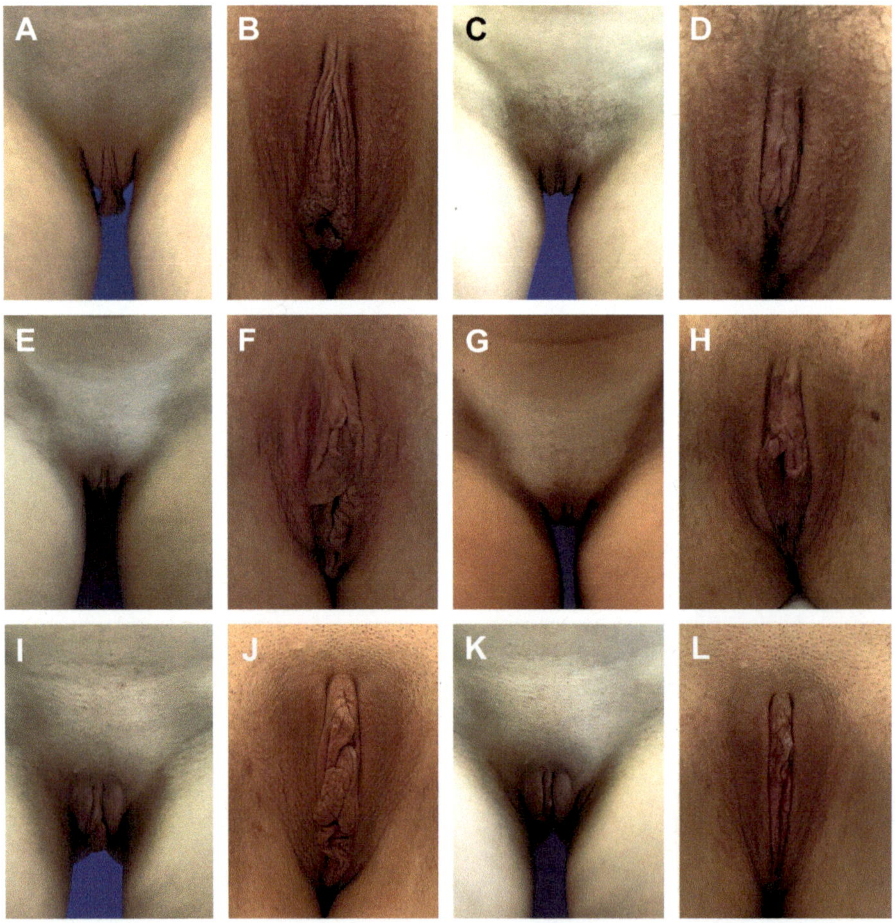

FIG. 11 Examples of before and after labiaplasty. (**A**) before standing 1x, (**B**) before lithotomy 1x, (**C**) after standing 1x, (**D**) after lithotomy 1x, (**E**) before standing 2, (**F**) before lithotomy 2, (**G**) after standing 2, (**H**) after lithotomy 2, (**I**) before standing 3, (**J**) before lithotomy 3, (**K**) after standing 3, (**L**) after lithotomy 3.

Complications are more likely to occur in smokers and those with a high body mass index (BMI).

Wound dehiscence is the most common complication noted. It is a problem for wedge labiaplasty when there is over-resection and undue tension on the closure. Scar widening, fenestrations, "coin slot," webbing, and pigment mismatch may occur with wedge labiaplasty. Curvilinear resection techniques can result in scalloping of the edge, amputation, or "penis deformity" if the clitoral hood is not addressed.

Postoperative hematomas tend to form in the first 24 to 48 hours, and the patient will complain of asymmetrical swelling and pain. Large hematomas require surgical evacuation, while smaller ones can be managed with observation. It is important to achieve meticulous hemostasis during surgery to minimize this complication.

Conservative resection will ensure that excessive skin retraction does not occur, which can lead to pain and potentially dyspareunia. Oversresection that includes clitoral hood reduction is exceedingly difficult to correct. Any revision to address minimal excess or asymmetry is deferred until the patient is at least 3 months postsurgery.

SUMMARY/DISCUSSION

The mainstreaming of labiaplasty in media and popular culture has certainly contributed to an increase in interest in pursuing the procedure. A shared decision-making approach and fully educating the patient on expected results are critical. Understanding the anatomy and applying the technique that provides a consistent and safe result for the patient while maintaining sensitivity and sexual function is paramount in achieving a high patient satisfaction rate with this procedure.

The overall satisfaction rate after labiaplasty is mostly greater than 90% [8]. The procedure is associated with a significant improvement in self-esteem and improvement in intimacy, physical discomfort, and clothing restrictions. The high patient satisfaction and low incidence of complications make cosmetic surgery of the female genitalia an accepted and often requested esthetic procedure.

CLINICS CARE POINTS

- The most common approach and easiest technique of labiaplasty to master is the trim or curvilinear resection instead of the wedge technique.
- The curvilinear resection has advantages. It allows for a larger reduction in the length and thickness of the labia minora. It also removes the hyperpigmented and rugae at the edge of the labia minora, a common patient request.
- Considering clitoral hood reduction is important in providing a balanced result that is pleasing to the patient.
- Patient-based decision-making is imperative in labiaplasty. It allows the patient to visualize the marking clearly, ask questions, and adjust the results.
- Meticulous hemostasis and precise closure accounting for postoperative edema will allow optimal results and minimize complications.

DISCLOSURE

No financial or commercial conflicts of interest or funding sources. No disclosures.

SUPPLEMENTARY DATA

Supplementary data related to this article can be found online at https://doi.org/10.1016/j.yacs.2025.01.003.

REFERENCES

[1] Available at: https://www.plasticsurgery.org/news/plastic-surgery-statistics?sub=2016+Plastic+Surgery+Statistics. Accessed November 16, 2024.
[2] Available at: https://www.plasticsurgery.org/news/plastic-surgery-statistics. Accessed November 16, 2024.
[3] Available at: https://www.theaestheticsociety.org/media/procedural-statistics. Accessed November 16, 2024.
[4] Committee on Gynecologic Practice. Elective female genital cosmetic surgery: ACOG Committee Opinion, Number 795. Obstet Gynecol 2020;135(1):e36–42.
[5] Georgiou CA, Benatar M, Dumas P, et al. A cadaveric study of the arterial blood supply of the labia minora. Plast Reconstr Surg 2015;136(1):167–78.
[6] Furnas HJ, Canales FL, Pedreira RA. The safe practice of female genital plastic surgery. Plast Reconstr Surg Glob Open 2021;9(7):e3660.
[7] Wells MW, Chang IA, Wu RT, et al. Labiaplasty: analysis of the national surgical quality improvement program database. Aesthet Surg J 2022;42(7):771–80.
[8] Géczi AM, Varga T, Vajna R, et al. Comprehensive assessment of labiaplasty techniques and tools, satisfaction rates, and risk factors: a systematic review and meta-analysis. Aesthet Surg J 2024;44(11):NP798–808.

Advances in Cosmetic Surgery 8 (2025) 11–23
ADVANCES IN COSMETIC SURGERY

Update on Anesthesia and Pain Management Strategies in Cosmetic Surgery

My Approach

David A. Goodman, MD, MS
Department of Anesthesiology, Abington Surgical Center, 2701 Blair Mill Road, Suite 35, Willow Grove, PA 19090, USA

KEYWORDS
• Pain management • Plastic surgery • Ultrasound guided blocks • ERAS • TIVA • LMA

KEY POINTS

- How to use enhance recovery after surgery (ERAS) protocols to provide a limited to narcotic free anesthetic for plastic surgical cases. Describe what medications are used and why.
- Describe each of the different ultrasound-guided blocks to provide pain relief during the procedure as well as into the postoperative period to limit narcotic usage.
- Describe the different types of anesthesia that can be used for outpatient plastic surgery and expand on what medications and techniques can be used.
- Describe the advantages of using a laryngeal mask anesthesia versus endotracheal intubation for plastic surgery procedures, specifically for head and neck surgeries.
- A discussion on the use of long-acting amide anesthetics such as Exparel (Pacira, Tampa, Fl) based on current literature and personal experience.

INTRODUCTION

This article describes my approach to the practical management of perioperative and postoperative anesthetic and pain management in patients undergoing common cosmetic surgical procedures.

I will discuss how my approach has evolved, both in conjunction with the evolution of my specialty and also because of my interaction with the aesthetic plastic surgeons with whom I have worked for the past 35 years. We have instituted ERAS protocols originally described for the hospital setting to avoid the potential for postoperative nausea and vomiting and narcotic abuse. When possible, we avoid endotracheal intubation, laryngeal mask anesthesia (LMA), and instead use total intravenous sedation for the majority of our aesthetic cases. Our approaches are described for some of the most common cosmetic procedures done at our center.

The author provides a summary of the types and techniques of ultrasound-guided blocks that he has personally performed, which have been transformative to our practice and to the cosmetic plastic surgeons with whom the author has worked at our center. These blocks are performed after the induction of anesthesia before the surgeon beginning their case. As a believer in pre-emptive anesthesia, the author believes that preventing the transmission of nerve impulses related to the surgery from the skin to the spinal cord to the brain and blocking the release of hormone-like substances that are released in

E-mail address: snoozydoc@comcast.net

https://doi.org/10.1016/j.yacs.2024.12.004 www.advancesincosmeticsurgery.com
2542-4327/25/

ABBREVIATIONS

Dex	dexmedetomidine
ESP	erector spinae plane
LA	local anesthetic
LMA	laryngeal mask anesthesia
PACU	postoperative anesthetic care unit
PIFP	pectointercostal fascia plane
PMM	pectoralis major muscle
TP	transverse process

response to surgery (such as prostaglandins), gives rise to less pain at the conclusion of the surgical procedure. Regional blocks enormously reduce postoperative discomfort. We suggest the possibility that these blocks could enjoy wider use in cosmetic surgical practice to reduce narcotic usage and to enhance patient satisfaction. They virtually eliminate the need for intraoperative and postoperative narcotics with their known incidence of postoperative nausea and vomiting as well as addiction. There is a learning curve to these techniques that can easily be mastered by most anesthetic providers.

Techniques of anesthetic blocks under ultrasonic guidance are reviewed and our protocols for many of the most commonly performed cosmetic procedures done at our surgical center is discussed. The author provides data that documents the improvements in patient care that ensued as these techniques were instituted.

Every anesthesiologist and every cosmetic surgeon will have preferences based on their training, their experience, new techniques and technologies as they emerge, and on the evolving medical literature. Herein described is our individual approach that has been instituted successfully. Where appropriate, we provide evidence-based literature that agrees with our approach. We also discuss approaches that are conflict with our approach and provide clinical experience to justify it.

Aesthetic surgical procedures include all facial and eye plastic surgical procedures, (including rhinoplasty, blepharoplasty and face and neck lift) and breast and body procedures (including breast augmentation, breast reduction, and mammoplasty, abdominoplasty brachioplasty, thigh lift, and various subcutaneous energy-based treatments).

We will describe our.

1. Preop assessment for patients accepted at surgical center including a discussion of American Society of Anesthesiologist (ASA) risk assessment, marijuana use, glucagon-like peptide (GLP)-1 medications and obesity.
2. ERAS protocols
3. Our intraoperative measures for airway and anesthetic management that will discuss whether to use an oral airway, LMA, flex LMA, or endotracheal intubation. LMA inflation pressures/volumes will also be discussed.
4. Our techniques of ultrasound guided blocks. Types of ultrasound machines available (standalone vs handheld).
5. Our IV sedation protocols

Before instituting the changes to anesthesia practice in 2014, almost 100% of patients getting aesthetic surgery procedures received narcotic, whether in the operating room (OR), the postoperative anesthetic care unit (PACU), or at home. Since 2018 when we began tabulating our data, in over 4000 cosmetic surgical cases the use of narcotics has gone from 97% to 3% of patients, with widespread patient and surgeon acceptance.

Postoperative Pain Strategies

New nerve blocks, such as ultrasound-guided PECS blocks by Bianco [1] in 2011 followed by other fascia plane blocks are used to limit narcotic use and aid in postoperative pain relief.

PREOPERATIVE ASSESSMENT

All patients before coming to the surgical center do an online comprehensive assessment of their medical conditions, medications, allergies, and anesthetic history of problems. Specific questions about cannabis use and whether it is medical or recreational and frequency are also asked. These are usually done at least 5 days before surgery so that if any significant problems are noted they can be addressed. A preoperative nurse initially goes through the data and if any specific abnormalities are noted they have an anesthesiologist sign off on the case. If further information is required, it can then be done in a timely manner before the surgical date. Sometimes if the information is not received the surgeon is notified and the case may then be rescheduled for when the information becomes available. This has led to a very rare history of cancellation on the day of surgery.

As cannabis use has become more widespread, we noticed that these patients had more anesthetic complications than nonusers. These included difficulty in inducing an anesthetic state whether sedation or general anesthesia (GA), more propofol needed, some arrythmias, and respiratory difficulties due to hyperreactivity [2–4]. Cannabis users may have difficulty with postoperative pain and a potential for higher pain scores and increased opioid requirements. We instituted a policy that required all cannabis users, some medical users excluded after discussion with the patient, to stop their usage 3 days before their surgery [5,6].

As GLP-1 medication usage has increased, especially for its use for weight loss, we saw instances of aspiration that required emergency intubation and transfer to the hospital. As these medications can cause a delay in gastric emptying [7–9], we instituted a policy of a 2-day clear liquid diet to give an extra day for elimination of solids. On the day of surgery, an ultrasound of the stomach was performed if the anesthesiologist had that skill. If it was determined that the stomach was *empty*, the case was performed as though the patient was not on a GLP-1 medication. If the anesthesiologist was not skilled in performing ultrasound of the stomach, then many of these patients were performed under endotracheal intubation that would have otherwise been performed under sedation. This was left to the discretion of the anesthesiologist involved.

Obesity is an obvious problem in the United States. At the surgical center, we actually perform preop and postop bariatric surgical endoscopies. We have performed those in patients with body mass index (BMI) as high as 65. Most of our stretchers and OR tables can handle up to at least 750 pounds. All of the following procedures have been performed in obese patients at the center after a careful medical and anesthesia physical evaluation by the anesthesiologist taking care of the patient. In some of these patients who would typically be done with deep sedation an LMA is used instead. We do not use a specific cut off of BMI. All necessary difficult intubation equipment is available the same as at the main hospital.

AMBULATORY ENHANCED RECOVERY AFTER SURGERY (ERAS) PROTOCOL

ERAS protocols (Guidelines—ERAS Society [erassociety.org]) for [10] mainly inpatient procedures have been developed by the ERAS Society in order to reduce narcotic usage, decrease recovery time for patients, and allow for a better outcome. At the author's outpatient surgical center, we modified these to virtually all the procedures done there.

The patients are encouraged to take 1000 mg acetaminophen at home before coming to the center. At the center, most are given 100 mg celecoxib po. For breast and abdominal plastic cases, 100 mg gabapentin po is also given. For the facial cosmetic cases, many of our surgeons prescribe gabapentin (Neurontin) in doses of 100 to 300 mg as well as Aprepitant 40 mg to be taken at home before coming to the center. Further specifics of the different cases will be discussed in the section under each procedure.

ANESTHETIC TECHNIQUES

Over the 35+ years this author has been in practice, inhalation agents have evolved from Halothane[R], Ethrane[R], and Forane[R] to Sevofluorane[R], which is now used primarily at our center. In 1989 propofol was introduced and replaced Sodium Thiopental as the primary agent used for sedation and for GA. The unique rapid on and off mechanism of propofol allowed its use from deep sedation to a form of *general anesthesia without a breathing tube*. With its introduction, cases needing anesthesia changed from a Versed-fentanyl or Versed-ketamine based anesthetic with the surgeon injecting local anesthesia to a propofol-fentanyl or propofol-ketamine combination.

We currently use ketamine preferentially over fentanyl because of its unique properties as a pain reliever and because, unlike fentanyl, it does not depress respirations. Initial IV dosing of 5 to 20 mg accompanied by propofol (dosing) prevents the dysphoric issues and hallucinations associated with the drug. This allows for the surgeon to inject the surgical field with local anesthetic without patient movement. For areas where local anesthetic may not be sufficient, ketamine supplemented with propofol or a small dose of dexmedetomidine (Dex) 5 mcg IV (see below) can be given to allow the surgery to proceed without patient movement.

LMA has been a staple in our ambulatory surgery practice and is the preference for some of our cosmetic surgeons. While some anesthesiologists feel that LMA should only be used for cases under a certain number of hours, 2 to 3 [11], there is no literature or studies to confirm this, we have not found that its use to be a deterrent even in cases that last as long as 8 hours. The advantages of LMA are numerous. It avoids risks to the vocal cords, has a lower incidence of laryngospasm during emergence, and doesn't require visualization of the vocal cords on insertion. While LMA does have a greater incidence of coughing, and sore throat, these issues resolve quickly following surgery [12]. Rarely, a patient may develop a more severe problem, but this is equally the case with endotracheal intubated patient. Care must be taken to properly inflate the LMA (30 mL air for a 3, 40 for a 4, and 50 for a 5) the same as an endotracheal tube (ETT). Problems tend to occur due to too high of a pressure in the cuffs against the tissue over the duration of the procedure. In appropriate patients, and with discussion with the surgeon, in some patients we will use the flexible LMA so that the surgeon can suture it to a tooth and drape it into the field so they can move it around during the case.

The risk of aspiration is theoretically described as a greater possibility with LMA and potentially worse in patients with gastroesophageal reflux disease (GERD). It is worthwhile to note that we have not seen aspiration in over 1600 cases since LMA was introduced into our practice. Our technique for placement of patients with a history of GERD is to elevate the back of the OR table 15–20° for the case. This will help prevent passive regurgitation in those that are prone to it such as the obese and morbidly obese.

Our Current Perioperative Local Sedation

The introduction of Dex in 1999 allowed us to avoid LMA and do many cases under deep sedation. This is accomplished with a bolus of propofol, 50 to 100 mg at a time, combined with ketamine 5-10 mg IV for the surgeon to inject the local. A continuous infusion of low dose propofol, dose varies with patient and placement of local. Also, an infusion of ketamine (0.25 to 1 mg/kg/hr.) is also started. If the patient does seem to respond despite the infusions, a 10 to 20 μg bolus of Dex is given, and the surgeon injects more local anesthesia into the field.

Many of these spontaneously breathing patients need an oral airway to avoid obstruction.

Typically, depending on the extent of the head and neck surgery, nasal canula delivery of oxygen at 3 to 5 L/min allows oxygenation in breast and body cases. Lower flows (2 L or less) in facial plastic surgery cases can be used. The anesthesia provider must communicate directly with the surgeon in these latter cases and potentially shut off O_2 flow when safe to allow for cautery or laser treatments such as for laser blepharoplasty or for laser resurfacing. In these latter cases, O_2 is turned off and a small 5 to 10 mg bolus of ketamine is given.

Another combination we have used successfully in practice involves continuous infusions of ketamine and Dex. Neither causes respiratory depression, and each has side effects opposite of the other, so they tend to cancel each other out. Ketamine can cause tachycardia, hypertension, and an increase in tracheal secretions, while Dex causes bradycardia, hypotension, and a decrease in secretions. We use this technique in patients where the surgeon wishes to avoid any breathing devices, including oral airway such as rhinoplasty or lip lifts. In these cases, the provider must watch the patient's O_2 saturation to keep it above 90% when the oxygen dissociation curve starts its decline, so the surgeon can use the Bovie around the airway as well as laser to the face without a fire risk.

ULTRASOUND-GUIDED BLOCKS FOR AESTHETIC SURGERY CASES: INDICATIONS AND TECHNIQUES

Since 2014, we have used ultrasound guided blocks to dimininsh postoperative discomfort successfully as an accompaniment to cases performed under local with sedation with the above-described techniques.

At our institution, we have come to prefer ropivacaine over bupivacaine for the local anesthetic for blocks due to its lesser cardiac toxicity. The concentration varies with the maximum based on the patient's weight and other local the surgeon may inject and may vary from 0.2% to 0.5%. All blocks this author performs have dexmethasone added to them to prolong their duration [13]. In addition, the erector spinae plane blocks used for the breast implant removal cases have Dex 10 mcg per 20 mL of local added to prolong the block of the larger spinal nerve segments.

Not all of my colleagues add adjuvants to their blocks. This author finds that steroids significantly add to the duration of block and patient satisfaction on postoperative phone calls done on days 1 to 3; before their use this author found less satisfaction and greater opioid use (unpublished data).

- Erector spinae plane (ESP)
  - Indications
    - T2 (neck, shoulder, arm, clavicle)
    - T4 (chest)
    - T5 (breast implant removal) combined with PECS1
    - T9 (abdomen)
    - L2 (laminectomy, thigh lift, hip)
    - L4 (hip, knee)
  - Additives in solution
    - Dexamethasone 4 mg per 20 mL local anesthetic (LA)
    - Dex 10 mcg per 20 mL LA
  - Volume/dose
    - 10 to 15 mL LA per side
    - 20 mL LA per side
    - If doing a combined breast and abdomen procedure then 15 mL LA per needle
  - Effectiveness
    - Depending on what spinal area you are targeting, it spreads 5 to 6 segments around the injection site. As an example, if injection is done at T5 in a cephalad to caudad direction I would expect T3 to T7 or T8 distribution
  - Complications
    - Hematoma, local anesthetic toxicity, pneumothorax (Figs. 1 and 2)

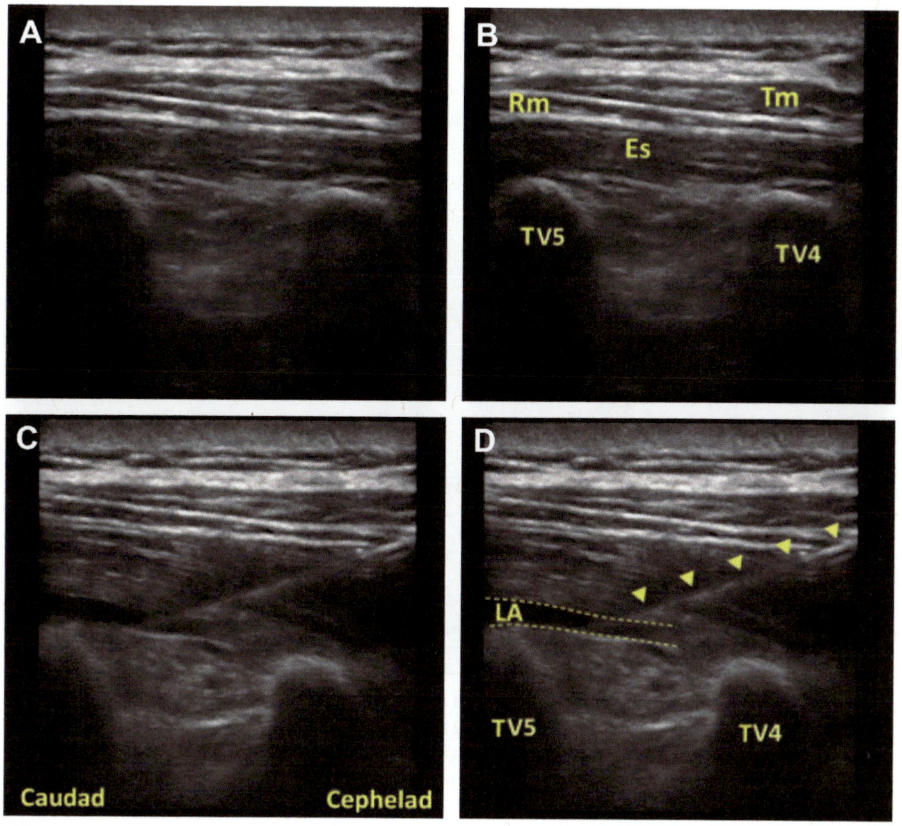

FIG. 1 (**A**) Sonographic anatomy for ESP block. (**B**) Tm, trapezius muscle; Rm, rhomboid major muscle; Es, erector spinae muscle; TV4 & TV5, TP of the fourth & fifth thoracic vertebrae respectively. (**C, D**) Ultrasound guided ESP block showing location of needle (*arrows*) and LA deposited deep to the Es. (*Data from* Hamilton DL*, Manickam B. Erector spinae plane block for pain relief in rib fractures. https://doi.org/10.1093/bja/aex009.)

An ESP is done with the patient in either a sitting, lateral, or prone position. The block can be done under local anesthesia, sedation, or under GA. This is based on the institutions set up. At our institution, all were done in the OR under either sedation or GA before the surgeon starting. This author prefers the block to be performed under GA as it does not require the patient's cooperation when using ultrasound. This procedure can be performed at any level of the spine from T2 to Sacrum. An ultrasound needle is placed to the appropriate transverse process (TP) and the appropriate amount of local anesthesia is placed. Dosing and amount will be determined by procedure, patient's weight, and any other local that the surgeon may place during the case.

- PECS1 & 2 (PECS2 incorporates PECS1 in the block without moving the needle).
  - Indications
    - PECS1: Port placement, pacemaker, supplement for ESP for breast implant removal cases to get the brachial plexus nerves
    - PECS2: Breast cases on breast without previous surgery, axillary dissections
  - Additive in solution
    - Dexamethasone 4 mg per 20 mL LA
  - Volume/dose
    - PECS1: 10 mL LA
    - PECS2: 20 mL LA for the deep part and 10 mL LA for PECS1 part
  - Effectiveness
    - The PECS1 block typically will block the medial and lateral pectoral nerves
    - PECS2 also blocks multiple levels of the anterior thoracic spinal nerves in the chest

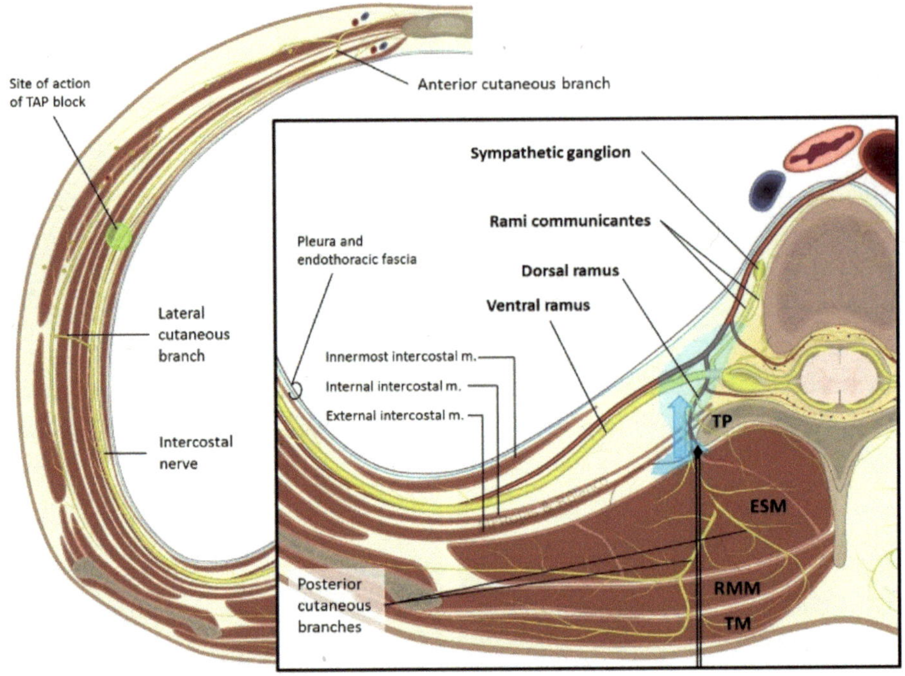

FIG. 2 Anatomy of the ESP block. LA (in *blue*) injected anterior (deep) to the ESM spreads in a craniocaudal direction along this tissue plane. It also spreads anteriorly through the connective tissue spanning the TP and enters the thoracic paravertebral space to anesthetize not only the ventral ramus and dorsal ramus of the spinal nerve, but also the white and gray rami communicantes that carry the preganglionic and postganglionic sympathetic fibers to and from the sympathetic ganglia. The ESP block thus has the potential to provide both somatic and visceral analgesia of the trunk. The proximal site of action blocks afferents from posterior, lateral, and anterior branches of the ventral ramus, resulting in extensive somatic analgesia. The TAP block, by contrast, acts more peripherally and provides only somatic analgesia to the anterior abdomen. (*Blue arrow*) local anesthetic spread. RMM, rhomboid major muscle; TM, trapezius muscle. (*Adapted and reproduced with permission from Maria* Fernanda Rojas Gomez; (Bonvicini, D., Boscolo-Berto, R., De Cassai, A. et al. Anatomical basis of erector spinae plane block: a dissection and histotopographic pilot study. J Anesth 35, 102–111 (2021). https://doi.org/10.1007/s00540-020-02881-w).)

- Complications
  - Hematoma, local anesthetic toxicity, pneumothorax (Fig. 3)

PECS blocks were first described by Bianco in 2011 [1]. PECS1 block is done with an ultrasound needle placed between the pectoralis major muscle (PMM) and minor muscles. In the context of this article, it is done as part of a sequence of blocks for breast surgeries. A PECS2 block is a PECS1 with the addition of the needle being placed between the pectoralis minor and serratus plane muscles. This author recommends PECS2 block only be performed in a breast that has not been previously operated on nor had radiation. This author's experience early after PECS2 was described on a patient with previous radiation was poor distribution of the local anesthetic to the thoracic nerves but a block of the brachial plexus. He believes this is due to the tissue planes being disrupted or nonexistent due to the radiation. No tissue planes in the fascia lead to the local going the path of least resistance. In this case out to the axilla and the brachial plexus nerves.

- Serratus Plane (also known as PECS3)
  - Indications
    - Tissue expander removal and implant, transverse rectus abdominus muscle (TRAM) flap, implant removal, previously operated breast, axillary dissection
  - Additives in solution
    - Dexamethasone 4 mg per 20 mL LA
  - Volume/dose
    - 15 to 20 mL LA
  - Effectiveness
    - Will block multiple anterior intercostal nerve segments

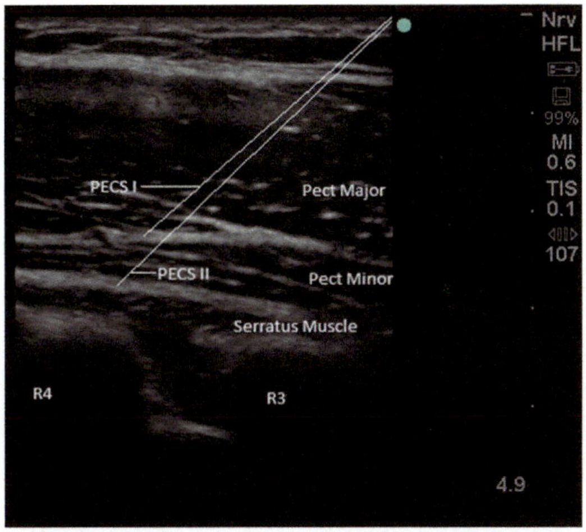

FIG. 3 PECS1 & 2 with needles labeled. r3, rib 3; r4, rib 4. (*Data from* PECS1&2: Ortiz, James, MD., ASRA Pain Medicine Update. Aug 7, 2019.)

- Complications
  - Hematoma, local anesthetic toxicity, pneumothorax (Fig. 4)

A Serratus Plane block is performed with the patient either supine or lateral at the either rib 4 with the injection going cephalad to caudad, or at rib 7 with the injection going caudad to cephalad. This would be operator preference and sometimes dictated by the patients' anatomy or previous procedure. Typical volume of local anesthetic is 15 to 20 mL.

- Pectointercostal fascia plane (PIFP)
  - Indications
    - Cardiac surgery, as an additional block to PECS2 for breast procedures
  - Additives in solution
    - Dexamethasone 4 mg per 20 mL LA
  - Volume/dose
    - 10 mL LA
  - Effectiveness
    - Block multiple levels of deep intercostal nerves to medial part of breast and nipple
  - Complications
    - Hematoma, local anesthetic toxicity, pneumothorax (Fig. 5)

PIFP is a block done in conjunction with other blocks for breast surgery, especially if the nipple is involved. This block is combined with either a PECS2 or serratus plane block to make sure the medical breast and nipples are anesthetized. The block is typically done using an ultrasound needle placed either at or between rib 4 and 5. The target is between the pectoralis major and intercostal muscles to get the deep intercostal nerve that the other blocks do not get. Typical local anesthetic volume will be 10 mL. Concentration is based on what the other blocks are being performed.

- Subcostal transverse abdominus plane (TAP)
  - Indications
    - Abdominal surgeries above the umbilicus, combined with TAP or Quadratus Lumborum (QL) for abdominoplasty
  - Additives in solution
    - Dexamethasone 4 mg per 20 mL LA
  - Volume/dose
    - 20 mL LA per side if only block, 15 mL per side if combined with another block
  - Effectiveness
    - Blocks T6/7 to T10 intercostal nerves to skin
  - Complications

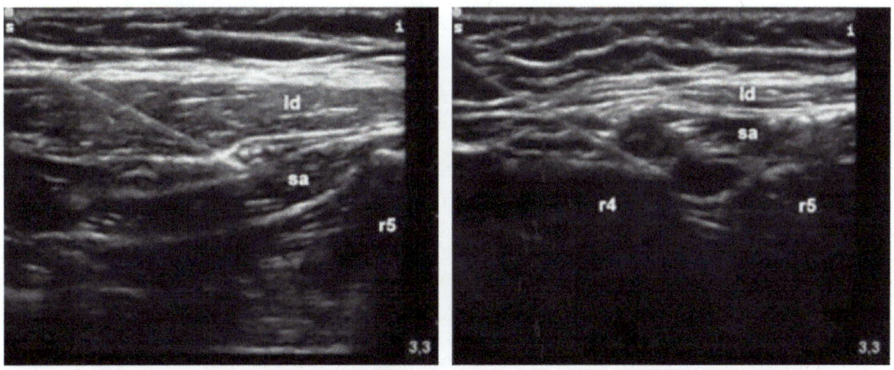

FIG. 4 Sonographic images when the planes above (*left*) or below (*right*) the serratus muscle are dissected using LA. The latissimus dorsi muscle (ld) lies superficial to serratus anterior (sa). In both options, the needle is directed passing the fourth rib (r4) toward the fifth rib (r5). (*Data from* Serratus Plane: Blanco R, Parras T, McDonnell JG, et al. Serratus plane block: a novel ultrasound-guided thoracic wall nerve block. Anaesthesia 2013;68:1107–1113. https://doi.org/10.1093/bja/aex013.)

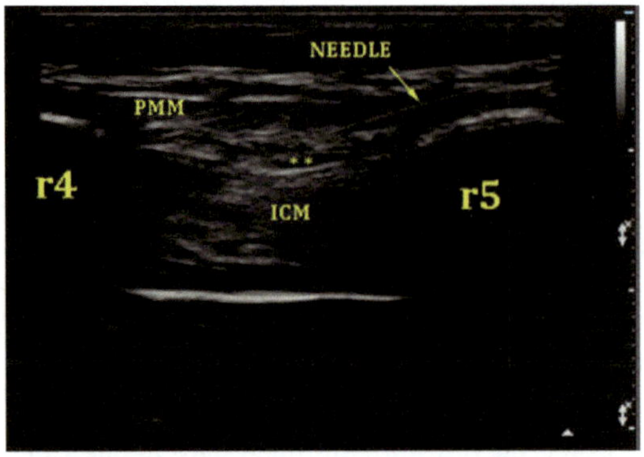

FIG. 5 Ultrasound image of the anterior thoracic wall showing LA infiltration (*yellow asterisks*) of the ribs (r4 and r5) and PMM. ICM, intercostal muscle. (*Data from* Pectointercostal fascia plane: de la Torre PA. A novel ultrasound-guided block: a promising alternative for breast analgesia. Aesthet Surg J 2014l;34(1):198–200. https://doi.org/10.1177/1090820X13515902.)

    - Hematoma, local anesthetic toxicity, bowel perforation (Figs. 6 and 7)

This author uses this block for upper abdominal surgery and as part of a combination block with QL for abdominoplasties. The ultrasound needle is placed at the junction of the rectus abdominus muscle and the internal oblique muscle. A typical volume of LA is 15 to 20 mL. Concentration is based on what the other blocks in the sequence are getting.

- QL 1 (Lateral QL)
  - Indications
    - Abdominal surgery (hernia, cesarean section, abdominoplasty, bowel repair), hip surgery
  - Additives in solution
    - Dexamethasone 4 mg per 20 mL LA
  - Volume/dose
    - 20 mL LA per side if only block, 15 mL per side if combined with another block
  - Effectiveness
    - Can block T6 to L1 nerves to skin as well as ilioinguinal, iliohypogastric, and genitofemoral nerves
  - Complications
    - Hematoma, LA toxicity, bowel perforation (Fig. 8)

The QL block that this author uses for abdominal cases is the lateral QL, or QL1. It is performed with an ultrasound needle at the junctions of the transverse abdominus muscle/fascia and the QL muscle. 15 to 20 mL of the local anesthetic is injected. Concentration is based on what the other blocks in the sequence are getting or maximum concentration based on the patient's weight if the only injection for lower abdominal surgeries.

COSMETIC SURGICAL PROCEDURES AND INDIVIDUAL ANESTHETIC TECHNIQUES BY ANATOMIC AREA

- Eye and facial plastic surgical procedures

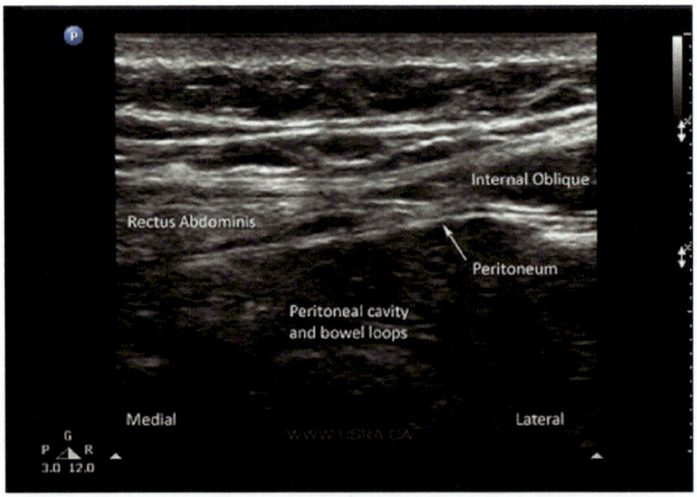

FIG. 6 Subcostal TAP between rectus abdominis and internal oblique muscles. (*Data from* Subcostal TAP: Niraj G, Kelkar A, Powell R. Ultrasound-guided Subcostal Transversus Abdominal Plane Block. International Journal of Ultrasound and Applied Technologies in Perioperative Care. 2010;1(1):9–12.)

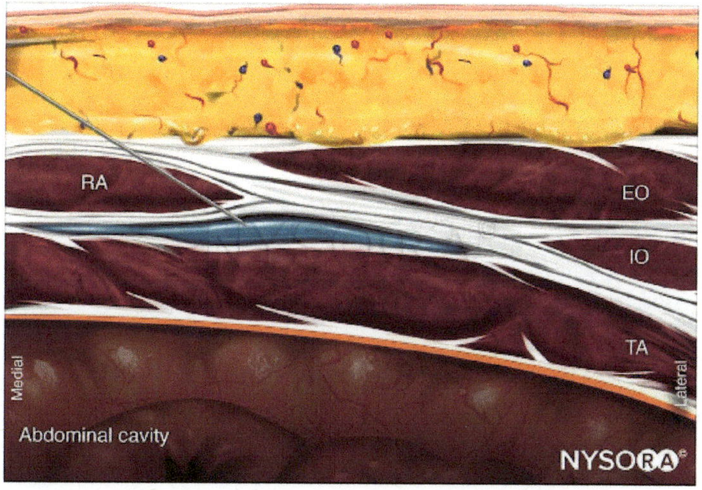

FIG. 7 NYSORA illustration of subcostal TAP. EO, external oblique muscle; IA, internal oblique muscle; RA, Recuts abdominus muscle; TA, transverse abdominus muscle. (*Data from* Subcostal TAP: Truncal and Cutaneous Nerve Blocks - NYSORA.)

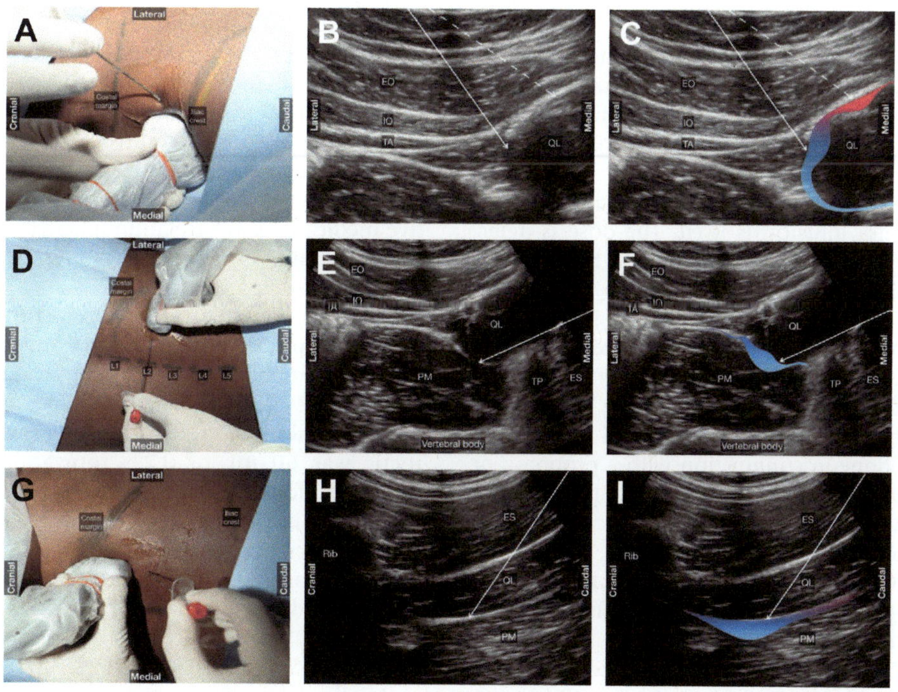

FIG. 8 ABC-lateral, DEF-anterior, GHI-posterior. Lumbar spine 1,2,3,4,5. *Arrows* in (**B, E, H**) are the target area for the block. *Arrows* in (**C, F, I**) is the local anesthetic flow. (**A-C**) lateral quadratus lumborum block; (**D-F**) anterior quadratus lumborum block; (**G-I**) posterior quadratus lumborum block. (*Data from* Quadratus Lumborum: Elsharkawy H, El-Boghdadly K, Barrington M. Quadratus Lumborum Block Anatomical Concepts, Mechanisms, and Techniques. Anesthesiology 2019;13(2):322-335.)

Eye and facial plastic surgical procedures at our surgical center, facelifts, neck lifts, midface lifts, blepharoplasties, rhinoplasty, lip lift, laser resurfacing, and endoscopic facial surgical procedures are performed. They may last anywhere from 1 to 8 hours. The anesthesia used varies based on the procedure, patient preference, surgeon's preference, and anesthesia evaluation of the patient's risks. Typical morbidly obese patients are done with either a light sedation, spontaneously breathing propofol-ketamine or sometimes ketamine-dexmedetomidine infusions, and possibly the placement of an LMA.

Preop: The patients are pretreated before blepharoplasty with acetaminophen 1000 mg (500 for renal patients), celecoxib 100 mg, and gabapentin 100 mg. Gabapentin 300 mg is used for all other head and neck procedures. Many with a previous history of postoperative nausea and vomiting also get Emend preop. None of the patients typically get narcotic medication.

The cases that are expected to last greater than 3 hours or the patient is on some type of sedative or antidepressant at home may also receive Versed 1 to 2 mg IV in the OR at the beginning of the case. For all these cases, the surgeon injects local anesthesia. All nonintubated or LMA cases typically get oxygen supplementation via nasal or oral canula at low flows (1–3 L/min). If a patient has a history of postoperative nausea and vomiting, propofol infusion of 25 to 50 mcg/kg/hr. is used.

For those patients not getting an inhalational anesthetic a propofol infusion is used. The dose is determined by patient response, typically 100 to 150 mcg/kg/min. Ketamine is used initially as a small 5 to 10 mg bolus for the surgeon to inject local anesthesia and then either by periodic as needed boluses or by infusion of 0.25 to 1 mg/kg/hr. If we elect to use Dexmedetomidine we give it as a small 5 mcg bolus or occasionally (obese patients) as an infusion of 0.5 mcg/kg/hr. This is done in conjunction with a propofol, or ketamine infusion in dosing as described above, based on the anesthesiologists and CRNA preference.

- Brachioplasty (9 cases)

Preop: Modified ERAS protocol consisting of acetaminophen 1000 mg (500 for renal patients), celecoxib 100 mg, and gabapentin 100 mg.

Intraop: The author's approach combines a GA with LMA and US-guided T2 ESP block. In the OR, the patient is induced with propofol 200 to 300 mg and ketamine 10 mg IV while on their side and the LMA placed.

The block is then performed with 15 mL per side of 0.375% ropivacaine mixed with 4 mg dexamethasone. The injection is done in the caudad to cephalad direction. No narcotics are given.

Postop: If a patient has discomfort in the PACU, an additional 100 mg Gabapentin po and 15 to 30 mg ketorolac (Toradol IV) is given. In our experience, these have not required PACU narcotics or narcotics at home the next day.

- Breast reduction (129 cases)

Preop: Modified ERAS protocol consist of acetaminophen 1000 mg (500 for renal patients), celecoxib 100 mg, and gabapentin 100 mg.

Intraop: The patient is induced with propofol 200 to 300 mg and ketamine 10 mg IV and an LMA placed. The US-guided block for these patients is either a PECS2 block in combination with a PIFP block or a serratus anterior block and PIFP in combination. The size of the breast is a determining factor as the serratus block sometimes has less tissue to traverse than the PECS2 and this author finds it safer to perform for that reason.

A total volume of 20 mL + 10 mL 0.2% ropivacaine per side with a total of 8 mg dexamethasone added to the local anesthetic. Each of the 30 mL will have 4 mg dexamethasone in it. Of these patients, 8 received OR narcotics (25–50 mcg fentanyl), and 10 received them in the PACU (0.2 mg Dilaudid as needed).

Postop: For a complaint of a burning sensation in the PACU, gabapentin 100 mg po was given. Toradol 15 to 30 mg IV is given at the discretion of the PACU nurse. Only 17 (13%) required narcotics at home.

- Breast Augmentation (319 cases)

Preoperative modified ERAS protocol. The preoperative medications are acetaminophen 1000 mg (500 for renal patients), celecoxib 100 mg, and gabapentin 100 mg.

Intraop: The patient is induced with propofol 200 to 300 mg and ketamine 10 mg IV and an LMA placed. For these patients, US-guided block was a combination of a PECS2 block (20 mL local per side) and PIFP (10 mL local per side). The total volume of block anesthetic was 60 mL of 0.2% ropivacaine with 8 mg dexamethasone.

Postop: Before 2023, 13 (~4%) patients received OR narcotics and 14 (~4%) in the PACU. Since the beginning of 2023 no narcotics have been given. An additional dose of gabapentin 100 mg po was given in the PACU for any complaints usually which were of a burning nature. Toradol 15 to 30 mg IV was given at the discretion of the PACU nurse.

- Breast implant removal (1355 cases) [5].

Is a complex and challenging procedure because all patients have had prior surgery, and the tissues have been disrupted either by implant leakage or by capsular scar tissue. Almost all of the data for these cases was performed by a single surgeon, Dr Brian Buinewicz. Initially, all procedures were performed under general anesthesia but as our protocols have developed we have moved from LMA to IV sedation with an oral airway. Also, the type of blocks used has evolved over time as we have discovered that some blocks in some patients are more useful.

Preop: Modified ERAS protocol. These patients all received acetaminophen 1000 mg and celecoxib 100 mg in preop. gabapentin 100 mg was added to the routine in 2019.

Intraop: In 2021, we began to use total intravenous anesthesia (TIVA) (for all these procedures and stopped using anesthetic gases in almost all patients). Our infusion now consists of a background of 1 mg/kg/hour of ketamine and a propofol infusion titrated to patients' need (80–200 mg/kg/min), aiming for the smallest doses possible. A reduction in narcotic usage was seen from 18% [14] (prior to 2021) to 2.6% (since beginning of 2021) of patients. Patients surveyed went from 38% having moderate (35%) to severe (3%) pain on the next days' postoperative phone call to 16% (15/1%). LMA was placed only in those patients that had obstructive airways unrelieved by placing an oral airway.

Initially all patients received an ultrasound-guided block that consisted of a serratus plane (20 mL), PECS1 (10 mL) and PIFP (10 mL) block per side. This consisted of a mixture of 0.2% ropivacaine and a total of 8 mg dexamethasone. As our experience developed, we've gone to performing ESP blocks at the T4 level (injecting cephalad to caudad) in conjunction with the PECS1 block. 20 mL of a mixture of 30 mL 0.375% ropivacaine with 4 mg dexamethasone is injected for the ESP block and 10 mL for the PECS1. There was a reduction of narcotic need from 27% to 12% of patients. With the introduction of Dex to our center, we've begun employing it initially with only IV boluses of 10 μg IV prn, to also adding 10 mcg per 20 mL to the LA block mixture.

Our experience with postoperative pain surveys in PACU and on day one postoperatively led us to understand that most postoperative pain was related to discomfort under the breast. We've therefore attempted to get better spread and switched to a T5 ESP block instead of the T4 block.

Currently the technique is to start the patient in the right lateral decubitus position, begin TIVA with propofol and ketamine infusions, perform the T5 ESP block, turn the patient supine, continue infusions, place the PECS1 blocks, and then start the surgery. If the patient seems to respond at the beginning, a small bolus of 10 to 20 mcg Dex IV is given. Any patient airway obstruction is initially handled with an oral airway. Supplemental oxygen is given by nasal canula.

Postop: Supplementation with Dex in the OR has led to a decrease in narcotics in the PACU from ~3% to ~2%. The switch from T4 to T5 ESP saw a reduction in PACU narcotics from 5.9% to 2.8%. With the institution of the T5 ESP block, no patient has had severe pain the next day. Only 30 of 191 (16%) patients took narcotics at home, down from 61 or 184 (33%) since the change in block level.

In the PACU, if needed for any burning sensation, an additional 100 mg gabapentin po is given. For a pain level above 5, 15 to 30 mg of ketorolac (Toradol IV) is given. At the PACU nurses' discretion, 0.2 mg hydromorphone (Dilaudid) IV prn is also available.

- Abdominoplasty ± Liposuction (169 cases)

Preop: Modified ERAS protocol. These patients all received acetaminophen 1000 mg and celecoxib 100 mg in preop. gabapentin 100 mg was added to the routine in 2019.

Intraop: The technique for abdominoplasty depends on whether it is performed as a stand-alone procedure or as an addition to some type of breast surgery. All patients are given the acetaminophen, celecoxib, and gabapentin combination as previously described. All patients were placed under general anesthesia with either an LMA or Endotracheal tube at the anesthesiologist's preference. Most of the author's cases were performed with an LMA. All patients received an ultrasound-guided block. This was either a T8 or 9 ESP with 20 mL 0.375% ropivacaine with 4 mg dexamethasone per side, or a combination of a Subcostal TAP block and lateral QL block with 15 mL per site per side of a mixture of 30 mL 0.2% ropivacaine + 4 mg dexamethasone per syringe. Narcotics were given at the discretion of the CRNA.

Postop: In the PACU, an additional 100 mg gabapentin po was given for a burning sensation, and 15 to 30 mg ketorolac (Toradol) IV given for pain level above 5. Narcotics 0.2 mg IV hydromorphone (Dilaudid) prn was given at the PACU nurses discretion.

- Thigh lift (4 cases)

This author wrote a case report [15] on performing L2 ESP for thigh lift surgery.

Preop: All patients were given the acetaminophen 1000 mg, celecoxib 100, and gabapentin 100 mg combination as previously described.

Intraop: All patients were placed under general anesthesia with an LMA. All procedures were done by Dr Brian Buinewicz. The patient was brought into the OR and placed on their side, general anesthesia with

10 mg ketamine and appropriate dose of propofol was given to allow LMA placement. An L2 ESP block then was performed with 10 mg 0.2% ropivacaine + 2 mg dexamethasone per side via an ultrasound needle. The patient was then turned supine for the surgery. Postop: None of the patients were given narcotics at the surgical center and none took any at home. 2 took nothing but acetaminophen at home for postoperative pain.

DATA

The author has kept unpublished data on all ultrasound-guided block patients performed at the Abington Surgical Center since 2014. He personally has performed blocks on 9382 patients encompassing 19,866 blocks. Results reflect the addition of the PIFP block to breast cases in 2018, ES in April 2018, and gabapentin routinely in 2020. There were about 33% of patients that were lost to follow-up despite phone calls and having a self-addressed envelope with appropriate questions to be filled out and returned. The author can only assume that the patients did well as there was no negative feedback from the surgeons about any particular patient where postoperative follow-up was unsuccessful.

DISCUSSION

There is a learning curve for the surgeon, anesthesiologist, CRNA, and PACU staff to get comfortable with some of the techniques I have described. This author always gave the discretion of using narcotics in the OR to the CRNA in the room. Because of this, as new CRNAs came to the surgical center to work, they had not had any experience with our techniques. Many routinely gave some narcotic at the beginning of the case as was their *routine*. My overall statistics are somewhat skewed because of this as less narcotics could have been and over time, all CRNA's adopted our protocol of no to minimum narcotics, and only if necessary due to an ineffective ultrasound-guided block or due to the fact that some of the patients came to the surgical center already on daily dosing of narcotics for chronic pain and required it due to narcotic tolerance.

At our institution we do not use the BIS^{R} monitor for anesthetic depth [16].

I would be remiss if I did not discuss Exparel^{R}, liposomal bupivacaine. There is controversy in the literature [11,17,18] over the benefits of various long-acting anesthetics and their benefit and their duration for postoperative pain relief. It has not been introduced at our center. Also, other LA, if used, can dissolve the liposomes and cause release of a toxic dose of bupivacaine.

We specifically use ropivacaine over bupivacaine for its safety profile.

SUMMARY

In this article, I describe how anesthesia and postoperative pain management have evolved and are currently performed for cosmetic surgery patients in a free-standing outpatient surgical center. Modified ERAS protocols that were customized by the author are detailed. The goal of these protocols is to reduce narcotic usage intraoperatively and postoperatively. The combination of the preoperative medications acetaminophen, celecoxib, and gabapentin along with ultrasound guided fascia plane blocks for many of the cases done before the start of surgery, allows for this success. Narcotic usage in our center has decreased from 97% to 3% at the center.

With regard to airway management, oral airways or LMA were used in the majority of cases in combination with a propofol based anesthetic. A Dex and ketamine combination has worked well for patients undergoing facial cosmetic surgery. It has been rare that a patient required an endotracheal tube.

We describe in detail our approaches to the blocks.

CLINICS CARE POINTS

- Using multimodal preoperative treatments and ERAS protocols decreases postoperative pain.
- Preemptive analgesia at the beginning of a procedure helps to decrease postoperative pain and anesthetic needs.
- Use of laryngeal mask anesthesia instead of an endotracheal tube is a consideration based on preoperative anesthetic evaluation.
- Fascia plane blocks at the beginning of a procedure will decrease postoperative pain requirements and may lessen narcotic needs intraoperative and postoperative.

DISCLOSURE

Nothing to disclose.

REFERENCES

[1] Blanco R. The 'pecs block': a novel technique for providing analgesia after breast surgery. Anaesthesia 2011;66:847–8.

[2] Lynn RSR, Galinkin JL. Cannabis, e-cigarettes and anesthesia. Curr Opin Anaesthesiol 2020;33(3):318–26, PMID:32371642.

[3] Lee BH, Sideris A, Ladha KS, et al. Cannabis and cannabinoids in the perioperative period. Anesth Analg 2024; 138(1):16–30.

[4] Shah S, Schwenk ES, Sondekoppam RV, et al. ASRA Pain Medicine consensus guidelines on the management of the perioperative patient on cannabis and cannabinoids. Reg Anesth Pain Med 2023;48(3):97–117, Epub 2023 Jan 3. PMID: 36596580.

[5] Echeverria-Villalobos M, Todeschini AB, Stoicea N, et al. Perioperative care of cannabis users: a comprehensive review of pharmacological and anesthetic considerations. J Clin Anesth 2019;57:41–9.

[6] Huson HB, Granados TM, Rasko Y. Surgical considerations of marijuana use in elective procedures. Heliyon 2018;4:e00779.

[7] Silveira SQ, da Silva LM, de Campos Vieira Abib A, et al. Relationship between perioperative semaglutide use and residual gastric content: a retrospective analysis of patients undergoing elective upper endoscopy. J Clin Anesth 2023;87:111091.

[8] Fujino E, Cobb KW, Schoenherr J, et al. Anesthesia considerations for a patient on semaglutide and delayed gastric emptying. Cureus 2023;15(7):e42153.

[9] Mizubuti GB, Ho AM, Silva LMD, et al. Perioperative management of patients on glucagon-like peptide-1 receptor agonists. Curr Opin Anaesthesiol 2024;37(3): 323–33.

[10] Yu SH, Beirne OR. Laryngeal mask airways have a lower risk of airway complications compared with endotracheal intubation: a systematic review. J Oral Maxillofac Surg 2010;68(10):2359–76.

[11] Bertram-Ralph E, Maguire O, Columb M, et al. Liposomal bupivacaine defining efficacy, how effective is effective? Editorial. Eur J Anaesthesiol 2023;40:622–3.

[12] Simon LV, Torp KD. Laryngeal mask airway. In: StatPearls [Internet]. Treasure Island (FL): StatPearls Publishing; 2024. Available at: https://www.ncbi.nlm.nih.gov/books/NBK482184.

[13] Pehora C, Pearson AME, Kaushal A, et al. Dexamethasone as an adjuvant to peripheral nerve block. Cochrane Database Syst Rev 2017;(11):CD011770.

[14] Katsnelson JY, Goodman DA, Patterson CK, et al. Regional pain blocks and perioperative pain control in patients undergoing breast implant removal with capsulectomy. Aesthet Surg J Open Forum 2022;4:ojac079.

[15] Goodman DA. Erector spinae block at L2 for thigh lift surgery, a new application. J Clin Anesth 2019;52:82.

[16] Lewis SR, Pritchard MW, Fawcett LJ, et al. Bispectral index for improving intraoperative awareness and early postoperative recovery in adults. Cocharane Database of Systematic Reviews 2019;9. https://doi.org/10.1002/14651858.CD003843.pub4:Art No: CD003843.

[17] Ilfeld BM, Eisenach JC, Gabriel RA, et al. Clinical effectiveness of liposomal bupivacaine administered by infiltration or peripheral nerve block to treat postoperative pain A narrative review. Anesthesiology 2021;134: 283–344.

[18] Kim D, Liu J, Beathe JC, et al. Interscalene brachial plexus block with liposomal bupivacaine versus standard bupivacaine with perineural dexamethasone A noninferiority trial. Anesthesiology 2022;136:434–47.

Advances in Cosmetic Surgery 8 (2025) 25–35
ADVANCES IN COSMETIC SURGERY

Body Contouring After Massive Weight Loss

Jennifer Greer, MD, MA[a,*], Anureet K. Bajaj, MD, MBA[b]
[a]Private Practice, Greer Plastic Surgery, 6101 Heisley Road, Mentor, OH 44060, USA; [b]Private Practice, Bajaj Plastic Surgery, 8106 N May Avenue, Suite B, Oklahoma City, OK 73120, USA

KEYWORDS
• Bariatric surgery • Medical weight loss • Skin removal • Body contouring

KEY POINTS
- *Personalized Surgical Planning*: Creating a custom plan to address loose skin after significant weight loss can greatly improve a patient's quality of life.
- *Preoperative Evaluation*: Assess the patient's health, expectations, goals, and optimal surgery timing, while planning procedures based on patient needs and recovery capacity.
- *Treatment Areas*: Body contouring targets areas like the arms, abdomen, breasts, and thighs, which can be treated together or staged based on surgery time.
- *Recovery Preparation*: Patients should allow adequate recovery time, including time off work, to ensure optimal results and reduce the risk of complications.

INTRODUCTION

More patients are achieving successful weight loss thanks to bariatric surgery and medications like Tirzepatide and Semaglutide. However, this often results in significant loose skin. Developing a plan to address this can seem daunting, but by discussing the patient's goals, evaluating medical conditions that may impact healing, and educating them on available procedures, you can create a personalized surgical plan to meet their needs.

Preoperative Evaluation

Medical and pre-operative considerations

Before undergoing body contouring procedures, patients should be in overall good health. Significant contraindications include known cardiac disease such as uncontrolled hypertension, arrhythmias, or the presence of pacemakers/defibrillators, as well as uncontrolled diabetes, typically indicated by an HbA1C greater than 7%. Nicotine use, whether from smoking or vaping, is another contraindication due to its negative impact on wound healing and increased risk of infection. Patients who smoke or vape should be advised to stop for at least 4 weeks prior to surgery, as well as for 4 to 6 weeks after surgery. Compliance can be verified with a urine cotinine test.

Additionally, patients should be at a stable weight for at least 3 months. This ensures that they are not continuing to lose weight, which could impact the results of body contouring procedures. Rather than relying on strict body mass index thresholds, the decision to proceed with surgery should be based on a realistic assessment of the patient's ability to maintain long-term weight loss. During the physical examination,

*Corresponding author. 6101 Heisley Road, Mentor, OH 44060. *E-mail address:* jgreer@greerplastics.com

https://doi.org/10.1016/j.yacs.2025.01.004 www.advancesincosmeticsurgery.com
2542-4327/25/

ABBREVIATIONS	
ASC	ambulatory surgery center
FDL	Fleur-de-lis

specific areas of fat distribution should be evaluated, as each patient's body stores fat differently. Even if a patient is not at their ultimate goal weight, certain areas may show minimal fat, such as the upper arms, which might not benefit much from additional weight loss.

Patients who have gone through bariatric surgery are at risk for protein deficiency—*Protein deficiency (serum albumin <3.5 mg/dL) remains the most severe macronutrient complication associated with malabsorptive surgical procedures* [1]. Post-bariatric surgery patients are advised to take in 60g to 80g per day of protein, or 1g/kg to 1.5 g/kg of ideal body weight to support wound healing. This same recommendation applies to patients on medications like Semaglutide and Tirzepatide, which suppress appetite and can make it harder for patients to meet their nutritional needs. Protein supplements, such as whey protein, may also be helpful.

A discussion of the pre-operative evaluation would not be complete without a discussion of deep vein thrombosis (DVT) risk and prevention. Patients are typically assessed for their risk of DVT using the Caprini score during the preoperative visit. All patients with a Caprini score of 7 or higher are given subcutaneous enoxaparin starting on the first postoperative day [2].

Surgical planning and procedure selection

When considering body contouring procedures, it is important to assess the patient's specific concerns and priorities. In our experience, the most common areas for skin removal include the upper arms (brachioplasty), breasts (mastopexy, augmentation, or reduction), abdomen (abdominoplasty), and thighs (thigh lift). While many patients do not specifically request a posterior body lift, it is essential to evaluate the back and assess it as part of a comprehensive, circumferential approach. For optimal results, the back and trunk should often be addressed together, and it may be beneficial to stabilize the trunk with these procedures (abdominoplasty and posterior body lift) prior to proceeding with additional procedures since the abdomen and back will impact the breast and thighs. The patient's goals should guide the procedure selection, but these and other anatomic considerations also play a role. For example, brachioplasty and mastopexy are often performed together due to their proximity.

In evaluating the patient's body, both subcutaneous and visceral fat must be considered. Subcutaneous fat is assessed by skin pinch, while visceral fat can affect the results of abdominoplasty and is evaluated by having the patient relax and contract their abdominal muscles to assess the degree of abdominal prominence. Diastasis (separation of abdominal muscles) may also contribute to a prominent abdomen, and in cases where visceral fat is limiting results, patients with significant skin overhang may still benefit from improved body contouring assuming that appropriate expectations are set preoperatively. It is important to review preoperative photos with the patient to discuss what is realistically achievable and then set expectations accordingly.

Combining and staging procedures

When planning the sequence of procedures, it is crucial to balance the patient's priorities with total operative time. The American Society of Plastic Surgeons recommends a maximum of 6 hours for surgeries performed in an ambulatory setting. While combinations of procedures that target anatomically close areas (such as brachioplasty with mastopexy) often make sense, the patient's preferences and anatomic considerations should dictate the final plan. In some cases, it is beneficial to stabilize the trunk first before performing procedures on other body areas, such as the breast or thighs. A circumferential body lift or trunk stabilization may improve the overall outcome and serve as a foundation for addressing other areas later.

When discussing the timing of the staged procedures, patients should be advised to wait at least 3 to 6 months between stages to allow for proper recovery. This also provides an opportunity for revisions or touch-ups if needed. In some cases, staging can be based on anatomic proximity and patient preferences, with related surgeries being grouped together, while more distant procedures (eg, brachioplasty and thigh lift) can still be safely performed in a single operative session.

Surgical location—ambulatory surgery center versus inpatient hospitalization

In recent years, the majority of body contouring procedures are being performed in *ambulatory surgery centers* (ASCs) or office-based operating rooms, as opposed to inpatient settings. The safety of performing these procedures in an outpatient setting has been well-established, with studies showing similar outcomes to inpatient procedures. In fact, ASCs have several advantages: they provide a more intimate, patient-focused environment, reduce costs, and allow for quicker recovery due to the ability for early mobilization. While these procedures were once commonly performed in the hospital setting, ASCs have proven to be a safe and effective alternative that offers patients greater convenience and more personalized care. Procedures performed in an ASC are reserved for patients ASA III or less; therefore, patients with multiple medical comorbidities may benefit from a procedure performed in a hospital.

SURGICAL TECHNIQUE

Brachioplasty and Extended Brachioplasty

Brachioplasty removes the excess skin of the upper arm, sometimes extending the incision across the elbow to address the lower arm. Patients see an improvement in how clothing fits over the upper arm, especially with more form-fitting clothing such as blazers and may feel more comfortable in sleeveless clothing. The greatest downside to brachioplasty is the scarring, since the scars fade less than those from other skin-removal operations.

Traditional brachioplasty extends from the axilla to the elbow. The extended brachioplasty continues the incision inferiorly along the lateral chest, curving into the inframammary crease (Deborah White M.D., Deborah White M.D. Plastic Surgery, email, October 20, 2020). This extension removes excess skin over the lateral chest, which may spill over the bra or form a roll along the inframammary crease (Fig. 1A, B).

Mini-brachioplasty uses an incision along the axillary crease to remove skin, but it is less effective for post-bariatric patients as it only targets the upper third of the arm. It is also prone to wound healing issues but can be a useful revision option for patients who have had a full brachioplasty and developed additional skin laxity over time.

Markings

Brachioplasty markings are made with the patient standing and arms outstretched at shoulder height. Initial markings are done with the elbow extended to relax the triceps, creating more laxity over the posterior arm. The incision is centered midway between the bicipital groove and the posterior arm to ensure the scar is hidden when the arm is relaxed. Areas of excess fat, often above the elbow, are marked for potential liposuction to improve contour. For extended brachioplasty, the markings extend down the lateral chest and curve into the inframammary fold. The axilla should not have significant skin removed to avoid webbing, and a Z-plasty is rarely needed if minimal skin is excised.

Positioning

The patient is positioned supine with the elbows extended and shoulders abducted at 90°, using regular arm boards. Intravenous access should be placed in the dorsum of the hand with a heplock attached. If an extended brachioplasty is being done, taping the breasts in a medial position will improve exposure. The arms are prepped circumferentially, and the hands can either be covered with stockinette or simply toweled off.

Skin excision is performed using the avulsion method described by Hunstad and colleagues [3] A superwet rather than tumescent technique is used to limit the amount of wetting solution left after aspiration. Aspiration is performed aggressively under the planned area of skin excision with the purpose of debulking subcutaneous adipose tissue and dissecting out the deep plane. Once aspiration is complete, the skin is incised down to the level of aspiration and avulsed using a kocher clamp. Hemostasis is obtained with cautery. Closure is performed in layers with absorbable sutures.

Once skin closure is complete the incisions are dressed with a self-adhesive mesh combined with 2-octyl cyanoacrylate (Prineo). The patient is then placed in compression sleeves or a dressing with an ACE wrap.

Abdominoplasty

Abdominoplasty allows for repair of rectus diastasis and effectively removes excess skin over the lower abdomen. Many patients have excess skin superior to the umbilicus in both the horizontal and vertical dimensions. Fleur-de-lis (FDL) abdominoplasty removes this skin by adding a vertical incision as well, and should be a consideration in patients who have lost 50 pounds or more. Although the vertical scar is visible in a 2-piece bathing suit, scars in this location fade with time. The FDL abdominoplasty has the additional benefit of creating a neo-umbilicus [4], which looks natural because the scar goes through, rather than around it.

Markings

Patients are marked for the abdominoplasty while standing. Skin is first retracted superiority to expose the mons pubis. The mons may become ptotic after pregnancy and weight loss, so upward traction on the area while marking is critical to correct the ptosis. The horizontal incision will fall within the hair-bearing skin, approximately 5 to 7 cm superior to the vulvar cleft. The incision curves gradually upwards on each side, crossing the anterior-superior iliac spine. The midline is marked from the xiphoid to the mons. For

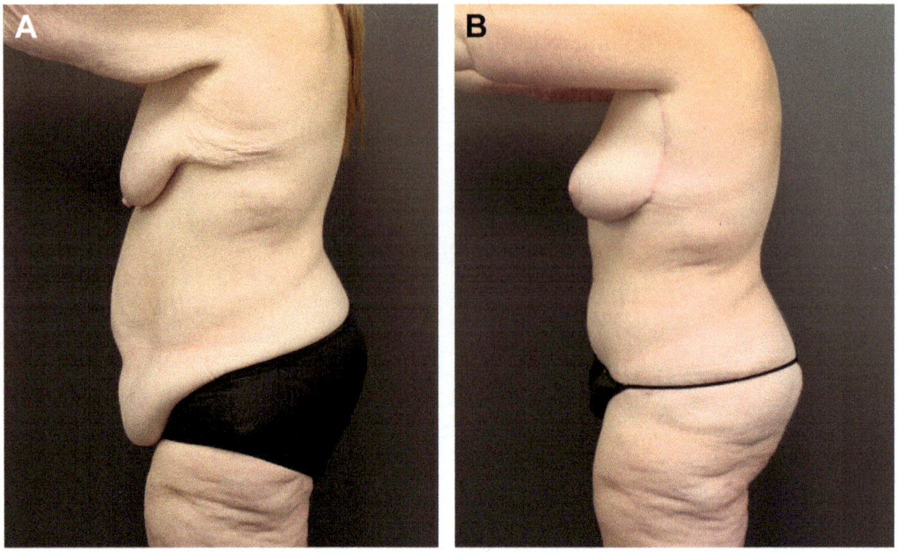

FIG. 1 **(A)** Before view of a 43 year old patient with excess skin over the lateral chest. **(B)** The same patient 6 weeks after extended brachioplasty with excision of skin over the lateral chest.

an FDL abdominoplasty, the vertical skin excision is initially marked with the patient standing, and then adjusted once on the operating room (OR) table.

Positioning

Abdominoplasty is performed with the patient supine—the bed should be checked to ensure that it flexes at the appropriate point. If the patient is placed in the lithotomy position for a concurrent thigh lift, one must be cognizant of the fact that the lithotomy position has risks related to prolonged positioning including neuropraxia, DVT, and strain on the hip joint. For this reason, it may be advisable to reposition and drape the patient after the abdominal surgery is completed, depending on planned total surgical time.

Because the lower abdominal incision is marked with upward tension on the skin to maintain a low position of the incision after closure, the lower aspect of the skin flap often overlays the inguinal lymph nodes. Placing vertical tension on the skin flap using Kochers will help maintain the correct plane of dissection and avoid damaging the lymphatics. After removal of the excess skin the rectus diastasis is repaired. Progressive tension sutures using 2-0 polydioxanone (PDS) in a barbed suture are placed between the Scarpa's fascia and anterior rectus sheath to advance the skin flap and close dead space (Fig. 2). Patients are then flexed at the waist to allow proper placement of the umbilicus. For the FDL abdominoplasty, the umbilical tabs are tacked to the anterior rectus sheath with three 3-0 nylon sutures (Fig. 3). The Scarpa's fascia is then closed with 2-0 PDS barbed sutures, and the skin with 4-0 monoderm barbed suture.

Monsplasty

The mons is ideally addressed during abdominoplasty, though it can be treated separately if the patient has already had an abdominoplasty procedure. After weight loss, patients often have a prominent mons due to skin laxity and fat distribution. The goal of monsplasty is to create a flatter contour below the abdomen (Fig. 4A–F), but this may be limited if the pubic bone itself is prominent, as it often remodels during obesity but remains prominent after weight loss. This should be assessed during the consultation so patients are informed about the expected outcome.

Markings for monsplasty are drawn with the patient standing. Ptosis of the mons is actually in a forward-facing vector rather strictly vertical, causing the vulvar cleft to be oriented in parallel to the floor rather than the native vertical orientation. Therefore, it is important to rotate the excess skin back into its normal position rather than providing only upward traction. Marking the horizontal skin incision approximately 5 to 7 cm superior to the vulvar cleft will place the incision in the appropriate position to rotate the mons back into its upward position. Adding a short incision inferiorly along the inguinal crease on each side allows the

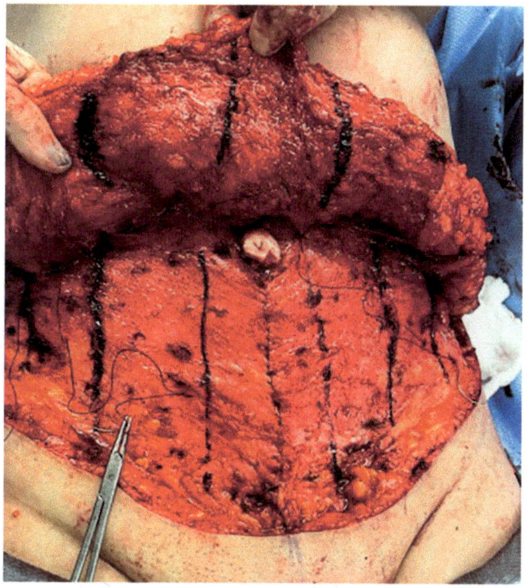

FIG. 2 Progressive tension sutures are placed in rows down the abdomen to close off potential dead space and take tension off the skin closure.

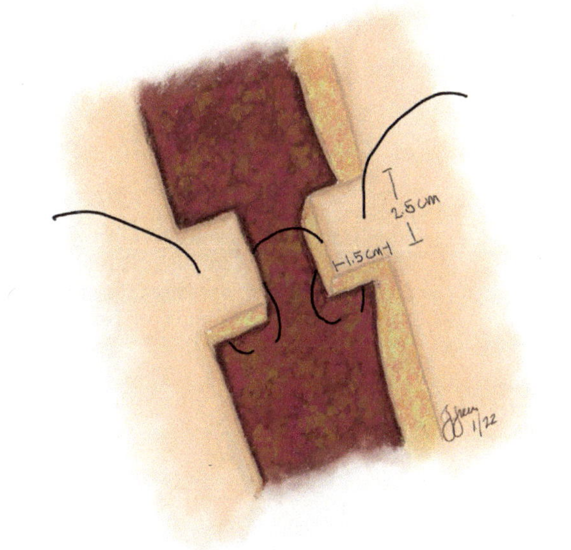

FIG. 3 Inset of the neo-umbilicus. 3-0 nylon sutures are placed through the skin, into the anterior rectus sheath, then back through the skin exiting in the dermal level of the skin tab before crossing to the contralateral skin tab.

horizontal skin excess to be removed as well. Liposuction extending down into the superior aspect of the labia majora will remove the excess adipose tissue.

Closure of the monsplasty is performed as part of the lower abdominal incision when combined with an abdominoplasty. If performed separately, the skin above the mons should be removed up to the level of the abdominoplasty scar.

Mastopexy and Augmentation/Mastopexy

After significant weight loss, patients often experience reduced breast volume, particularly in the upper breast, with remaining tissue concentrated in the lower pole. Surgical options depend on the desired size and appearance. For those with disproportionately large breasts after weight loss, a reduction or mastopexy that removes lower pole tissue is recommended. For patients wishing to maintain their size, a mastopexy with autoaugmentation is appropriate [5]. This technique, developed by Ribeiro, involves relocating tissue from the lower pole to the upper pole using an inferior pedicle, elevating the nipple on a superior-medial pedicle, and securing the inferiorly-based tissue to the pectoralis fascia beneath the nipple. Patients should be aware that this approach does not provide the same upper pole fullness as breast augmentation. P4HB can be used for additional soft tissue support in these cases.

Women who desire a larger breast size or desire more upper pole fullness are candidates for an augmentation-mastopexy. The authors' preferred method is the total submuscular augmentation and mastopexy previously described by Dr Holly Casey Wall [6]. This technique leaves the costal insertion of the pectoralis major muscle intact to support the inferior position of the implant, rather than relying on an inframammary crease, which is often attenuated and inferiorly displaced secondary to weight-loss.

A comprehensive explanation of the technique can be found in the referenced article, but we will summarize a few key points. The patient is marked sitting up. The midline is marked, as well as the breast meridian (extending from the mid-clavicle inferiority to the nipple) and the inferior border of the pectoralis major muscle. The new nipple position is marked along the breast meridian where it intersects with the inferior border of the pectoralis muscle.

The implant is placed through a periareolar or vertical incision, using a horizontal myotomy in the pectoralis muscle to gain access to the subpectoral plane. The myotomy is repaired in a vertical fashion. Once the implants are placed, the patient is sat up on the OR table to mark the planned tissue removal for the mastopexy. This is done by medially and laterally displacing the

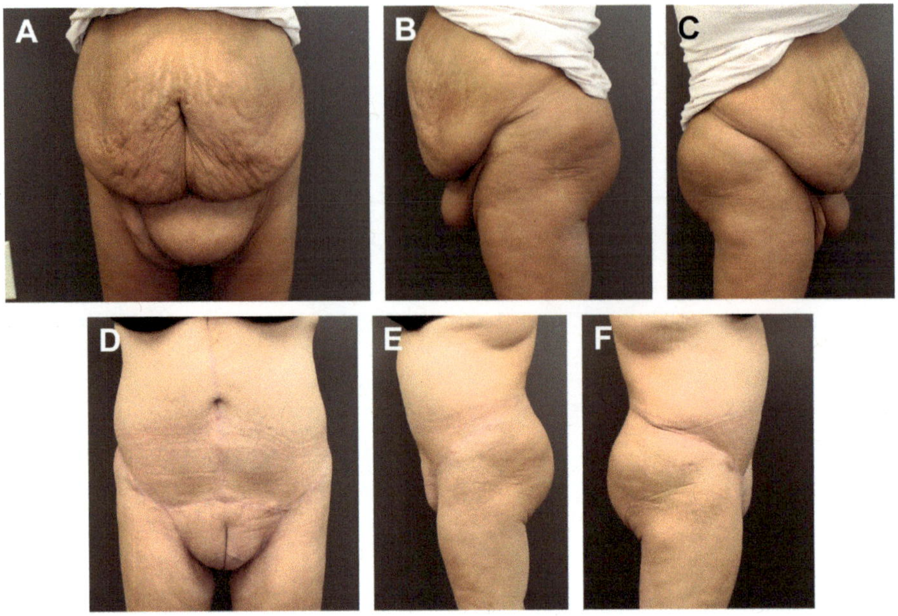

FIG. 4 Front (**A**) and lateral (**B, C**) preoperative photos of a 45 year old patient who had fleur-de-lis abdominoplasty with monsplasty and medial thigh lift. Note the extensive ptosis of the mons. Front (**D**) and lateral (**E, F**) 3 month postoperative views of the same patient, showing correction of the ptotic mons.

lower pole of the breast to mark the extent of tissue removal between the nipple and inframammary fold. Once supine, the nipple is elevated on a superior-medial pedicle. The excess tissue between the nipple and inframmary fold is removed, and the medial and lateral breast pillars are approximated with 2-0 PDS. Next the excess tissue and skin along the IMF is removed, setting the new position of the IMF at the bottom of the implant, rather than in its slightly lower native position. It is critical to remove as much ptotic tissue as possible so that the remaining breast tissue follows the contour of the implant, rather than dropping off the implant. Similar to other skin-removal procedures, incisions are closed in layers with absorbable sutures (Fig. 5A–D).

Thigh Lift

A thigh lift improves excess skin over the proximal thigh, with several variations depending on skin distribution. Patients often pull upward on their thigh skin to envision a smooth result, but it is important to manage expectations, as this does not account for loss of skin elasticity.

The medial thigh lift removes skin from the upper inner thigh using a crescent incision in the groin crease. This incision is prone to complications like wound dehiscence and widening of the mons. To prevent scar migration, it is helpful to tack the distal skin flap to the pubic bone.

If excess skin extends lower on the thigh, a vertical extension will address the medial thigh excess, and a hockey stick extension carrying the incision across the anterior knee, superior to the patella, may be added to address the excess skin over the knee (Fig. 6A–D).

The spiral thigh lift extends the incision laterally along the outer thigh to address excess skin over the outer thigh (Fig. 7A, B) addressing skin laxity there.

An APEX thigh lift [7] extends the incision along the posterior buttock crease and addresses the posterior thigh.

However, all thigh lift variations primarily target the proximal thigh and may not fully address laxity in other areas.

Thigh lifts can be performed alone or in combination with other procedures. Incisions along the inguinal crease can also flatten the mons, and a spiral thigh lift incision can merge with the lateral abdominoplasty incision. Marking for the procedure is done with the patient standing, but the planned skin excision should be rechecked once the patient is in lithotomy position, as hip adduction reduces the amount of skin that can be removed.

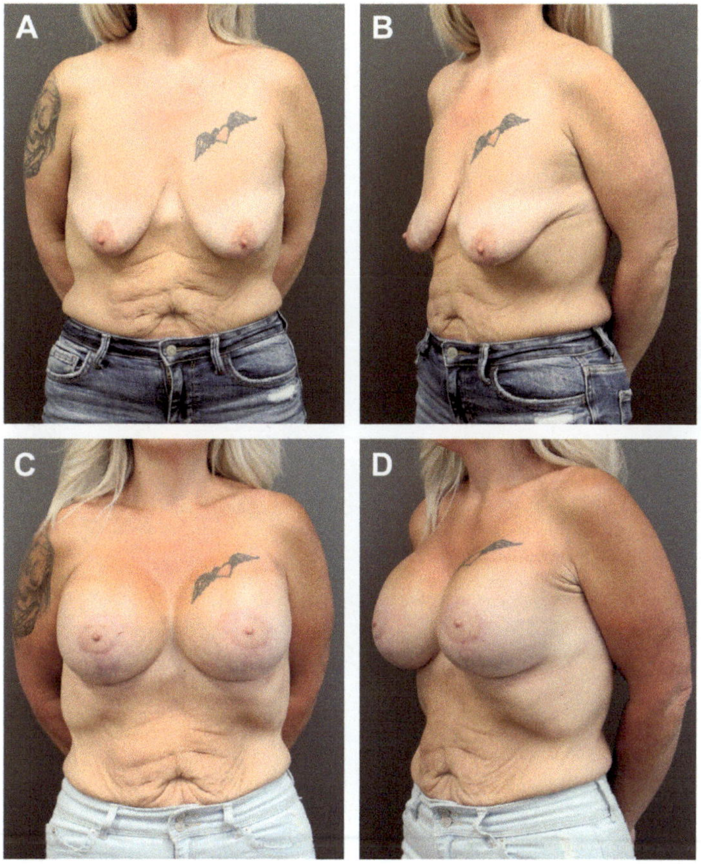

FIG. 5 (**A** and **B**) preoperative photos of a woman in her 40s who wanted fuller breasts after losing 100lbs as a result of gastric bypass surgery. (**C** and **D**) 3 month postoperative photos after placement of 580 mL silicone implants under the muscle and mastopexy.

The surgical technique is similar to brachioplasty, often involving liposuction to create a deep plane for skin removal. Liposuction is also recommended on the lateral thigh and around the knee to enhance contour. For patients with significant lipodystrophy, it may be beneficial to stage the procedure by performing liposuction to reduce thigh volume before proceeding with skin excision.

Posterior Body Lift

Posterior body lift is often performed at the same time as abdominoplasty, but may also be staged separately without difficulty. The goal of posterior body lift is to remove loose skin over the lower back, thereby lifting the buttocks. Patients are marked in the standing position, similar to other body contouring procedures and then placed prone for surgery. The incision is contoured along the upper border of the buttock. Minimal skin is removed in the midline since their area generally has less laxity and over resection can result in wound dehiscence (Fig. 8A–D). The skin is undermined with aggressive liposuction in the same fashion as brachioplasty and thigh lift. When done in conjunction with abdominoplasty the skin excision is carried as far anteriorly as possible, and the open area is covered with large occlusive dressings prior to flipping the patient supine. Closure is performed in layers in a similar fashion to other procedures.

Reverse Abdominoplasty

Reverse abdominoplasty is a surgical technique designed to remove excess skin from the upper abdomen. It can be performed as a standalone procedure or combined with traditional abdominoplasty, or

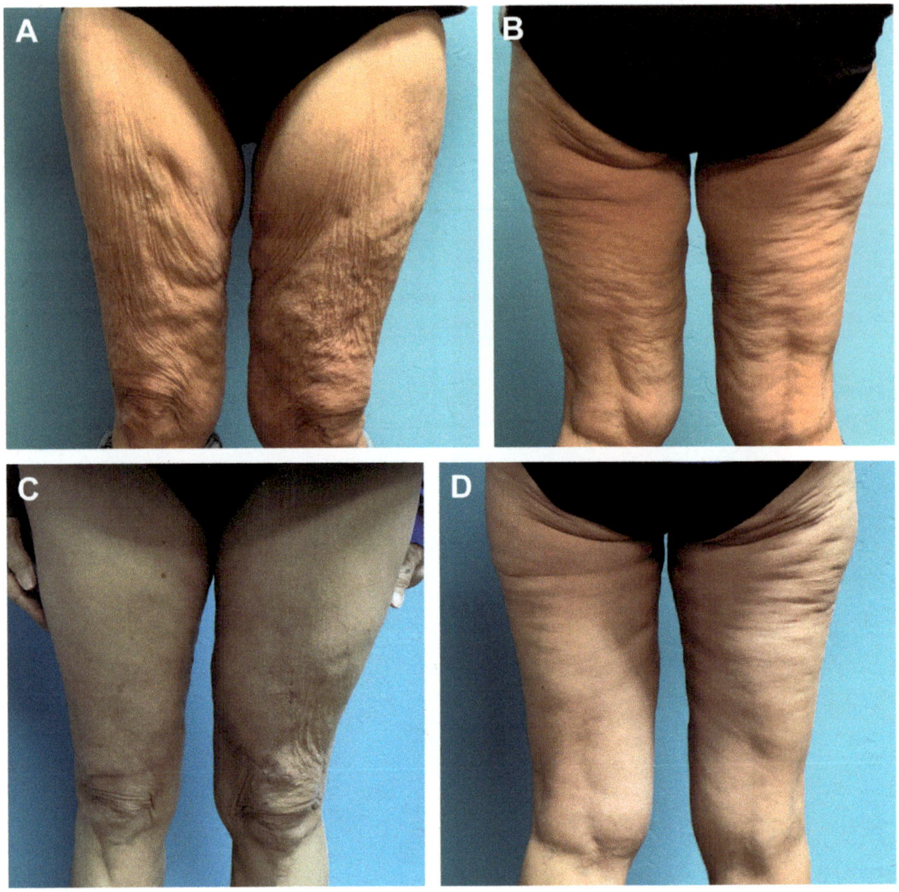

FIG. 6 (**A** and **B**) Front and posterior preoperative view of medial thigh lift. (**C** and **D**) Front and posterior postoperative view of medial thigh lift with hockey stick extension.

even as a follow-up to an FDL abdominoplasty to address any remaining loose skin. The incision is made along the inframammary crease, and extends across the midline with the midline portion drawn as a W. A critical component of the reverse abdominoplasty is securing the deep layers of the incision to the rib periosteum to maintain the position of the inframammary crease. This is typically done using a 2-0 Vicryl or PDS suture to ensure proper tissue support, preserve the aesthetic contour, and decrease the risk of inferior scar migration.

Bra Line Back Lift

The bra line back lift, as described in the literature [8], is a procedure designed to address excess skin across the upper back. It is particularly useful when skin extends too far posteriorly to be removed through the lateral chest incision of an extended brachioplasty, or when the excess skin is not fully addressed with a posterior body lift. The incision is strategically placed along the bra line, ensuring it remains well-concealed under most bras or swimsuits, providing both aesthetic and functional benefits.

Immediate Post-Procedure Care

Drains and dressings

Drains are rarely used for most procedures including thigh lifts, brachioplasties, and mastopexy. Occasionally, they may be used for an abdominoplasty; however, with the use of progressive tension sutures, they may be reserved for patients with a body mass index above 30 kg/m^2.

Post-operative instructions

After surgery, patients are typically fitted with either compression garments or dressings, depending on the

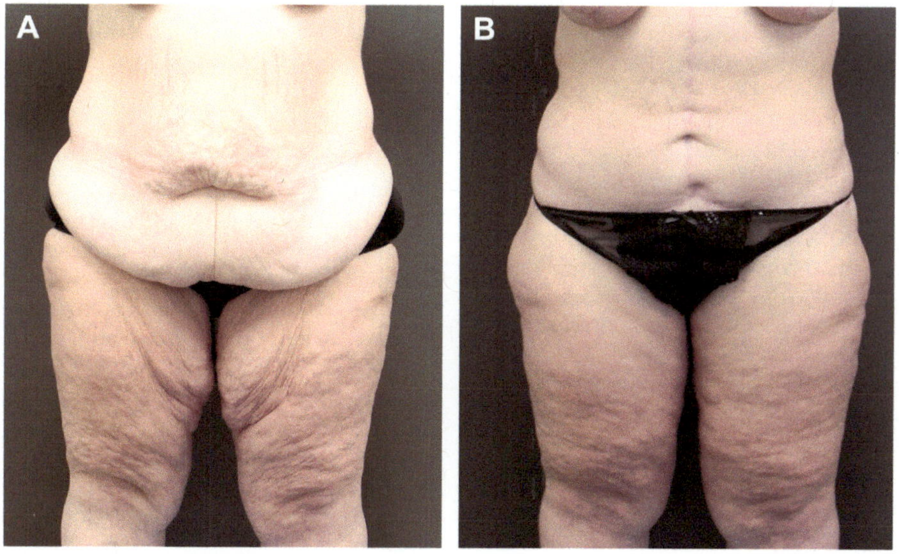

FIG. 7 (**A**) Preoperative photo of a patient in her 40s who lost 120lbs. (**B**) 10 months postoperative from fleur-di-lis abdominoplasty and spiral thigh lift.

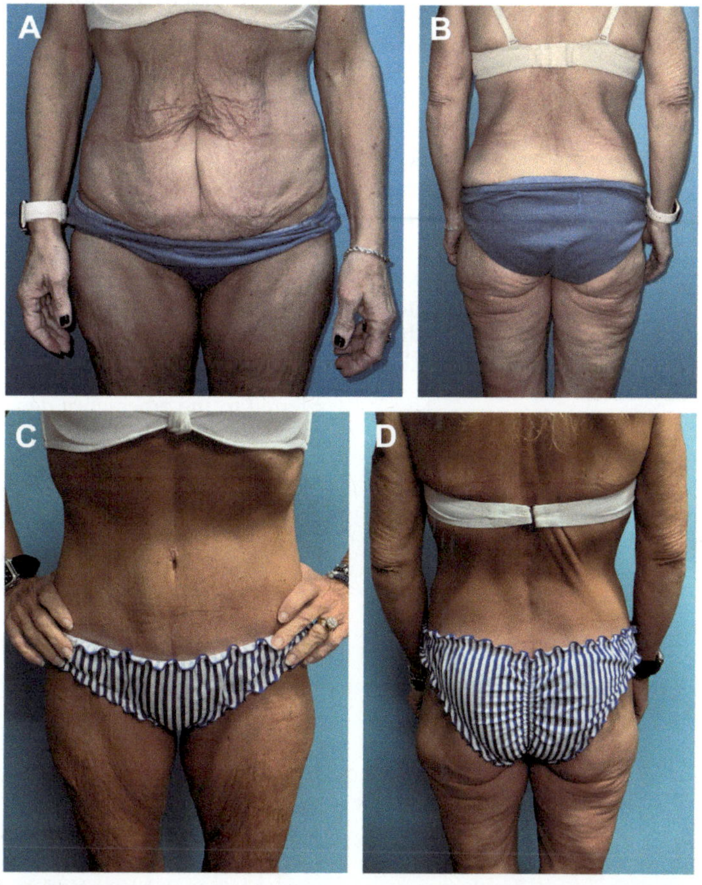

FIG. 8 (**A** and **B**) preoperative view circumferential body lift. (**C** and **D**) postoperative view circumferential body lift.

procedure. For abdominoplasty and posterior body lifts, a compression garment is used. Patients undergoing breast surgery are generally provided with a post-surgical bra. For brachioplasty and thigh-lift procedures, the initial dressings include fluffs, Kerlix rolls, cling rolls, and ACE wraps. These dressings are removed and reapplied during the first post-operative visit. After the first week, patients who had thigh lifts or brachioplasty can transition to compression sleeves and/or leggings. Post-operative compression garments can be beneficial to the patient—while there are no conclusive data regarding seroma prevention, they do provide extra support for patients, and many patients like the feeling of extra security that they provide.

Patients are discharged home postoperatively and are seen in the clinic within the first 24 to 48 hours following surgery. Patients are instructed to ambulate for 5 to 10 minutes every 2 hours while awake to help minimize the risk of DVT.

Pain management

Thanks to the implementation of Enhanced Recovery After Surgery protocols, opioids are no longer the primary medication for pain management. Instead, pain control is achieved through a combination of scheduled non-opioid medications, such as celecoxib, gabapentin, and acetaminophen, along with as-needed oxycodone and a muscle relaxant. For abdominoplasty surgeries, a TAP block may be performed intraoperatively, while PEC blocks can be used for breast surgeries. For other procedures, postoperative pain is managed with local infiltration of liposomal bupivacaine. Patients remain in their compression garments or dressings until their first postoperative visit, which typically occurs within 24 to 48 hours of surgery. After this visit, they are cleared to shower.

Recovery

Recovery will vary depending on the surgical procedure or combination of surgical procedures. Most procedures will necessitate 5 to 7 days off of work, and longer for combined procedures. If used, drains are removed when drain output decreases to 30 mL/day for 2 continuous days.

Patients should avoid any sustained cardiovascular exercise for the first 3 to 4 weeks postoperatively, as the increased edema caused by this activity can cause wound dehiscence and delayed healing. For similar reasons, patients are given a lifting restriction of no more than 10 pounds for 2 weeks and then this restriction is increased to 15 pounds. After 4 weeks, patients can gradually begin to increase their activity level.

After 3 to 4 weeks, patients may begin using a silicone-based scar gel to the incisions daily, preferably twice a day. They should also be instructed to massage their scars regularly.

Potential Complications

Delayed healing is the most common concern requiring additional attention postoperatively. First steps include discussing nutrition intake, and if the patient quit smoking prior to surgery, whether there has been a relapse. Activity restrictions should also be revisited if edema is more than expected. Conservative wound care includes dressing changes that maintain a moist healing environment without causing maceration. Topical hypochlorous acid spray (sold under the brand name Microcyn or Briotech) applied to open areas can help decrease bacterial colonization to optimize wound healing.

Seroma is also a well-known complication of skin removal surgery. Diagnosis can be made based on clinical examination, but point-of-care ultrasound is useful to confirm diagnosis and guide aspiration. Aspiration should be performed 2 to 3 times a week until the seroma resolves. An alternative option for large seromas or patients who live farther away is to place a seroma catheter in the office. Instillation of a sclerosing agent such as betadine or kenalog may be useful for persistent seromas.

DVT and pulmonary embolus (*PE*) should be high in the differential diagnosis for any postoperative patient experiencing asymmetric leg swelling (symmetric edema is common postoperatively), cramping in the calves, shortness of breath, or difficulty or pain on inspiration. Any patient with these symptoms should be referred to the emergency department for evaluation.

Hypertrophic scars may occur at areas of high-tension and some patients are simply more prone to forming hypertrophic scars. Injection of triamcinolone alone or mixed 1:1 with 5-fluorouracil is an effective initial step. Fractionated laser treatments can also help remodel hypertrophic scars. If these steps do not achieve the desired improvement, scar revision can be performed under local anesthesia.

Expectation Management

Managing patient expectations is a crucial part of ensuring a successful outcome. After significant weight loss, patients often experience a loss of skin elasticity, which can lead to some skin laxity returning once the swelling from surgery subsides. In some cases, revision procedures may be needed to address this.

When discussing preoperative expectations and reviewing photographs with patients, it is helpful to show them before-and-after images of individuals with similar body types and weight loss histories. This allows patients to have a clearer understanding of what they can realistically expect from the procedure.

CLINICS CARE POINTS

- Preoperative assessment and mitigation of factors that affect healing such as elevated blood sugars, nutrition status, and smoking status is critical for a successful outcome.
- Skin removal surgery after weight loss due to bariatric surgery can be safely performed in the outpatient setting.
- Skin removal surgery should be viewed as a series of operations rather than a 1-time treatment: most patients have more problem areas than can be safely treated in a single operation, and small revisions are often necessary to achieve an optimal outcome.

DISCLOSURES

Dr J. Greer has nothing to disclose. Dr A.K. Bajaj is an investor in PatientFi and an Advisory Board Member for Allergan Aesthetics. During the preparation of this work the authors used Gen AI. After using this tool/service, the authors reviewed and edited the content as needed and take full responsibility for the content of the publication.

REFERENCES

[1] Sherf DS, Goldenshluger A, Globus I, et al. Nutritional recommendations for adult bariatric surgery patients: clinical practice. Adv Nutr 2017;8(2):382–94. Available at: https://pmc.ncbi.nlm.nih.gov/articles/PMC5347111/. Accessed November 10, 2024.

[2] Pannucci CJ, Bailey SH, Dreszer G, et al. Validation of the Caprini risk assessment model in plastic and reconstructive surgery patients. J Am Coll Surg 2011;212(1):105–12. Available at: https://pmc.ncbi.nlm.nih.gov/articles/PMC3052944/. Accessed November 10, 2024.

[3] Knotts C, Hunstad J, Kortesis B. Avulsion brachioplasty: technique overview and 5-year experience. Plast Reconstr Surg 2014;133(2):283–8. Available at: https://pubmed.ncbi.nlm.nih.gov/24469164/. Accessed November 10, 2024.

[4] Mendes FH, Donnabella A, Fagotti Moreira AR. Fleur-de-lis abdominoplasty and neo-umbilicus. Clin Plast Surg 2019;46(1):49–60. Available at: https://pubmed.ncbi.nlm.nih.gov/30447828/. Accessed November 12, 2024.

[5] Hönig J, Frey H, Hasse F, et al. Autoaugmentation mastopexy with an inferior-based pedicle. Aesthetic Plast Surg 2009;33(3):302–7. Available at: https://pubmed.ncbi.nlm.nih.gov/19225831/. Accessed November 10, 2024.

[6] Wall S, Claiborne J, Casey Wall H. Superiorly based short-scar mastopexy augmentation: a 10-year review of 1217 consecutive cases. Plast Reconstr Surg 2023;151(6):918e–30e. Available at: https://pubmed.ncbi.nlm.nih.gov/36728622/. Accessed November 10, 2024.

[7] Shermak MA. Body contouring. Plast Reconstr Surg 2012;129(6):963e–78e.

[8] Hunstad J, Chen C, Abbad T. Bra-line back lift. Clin Plast Surg 2019;46(1):77–84. Available at: https://pubmed.ncbi.nlm.nih.gov/30447831/. Accessed November 13, 2024.

Advances in Cosmetic Surgery 8 (2025) 37–48
ADVANCES IN COSMETIC SURGERY

Nonsurgical Periorbital Rejuvenation

An Update

Lily Park, DO, FAAD[a,b,c,d,*], Kevin H. Nguyen, DO, MS[d], Naomi F. Briones, MD, FAAD[e,f], Swati Kannan, MD, FAAD[f]

[a]Touro University California, College of Osteopathic Medicine, Vallejo, CA 94592, USA; [b]California Northstate University, College of Medicine, 9700 W Taron Drive, Elk Grove, CA 95757, USA; [c]Berman Skin Institute, 3581 Palmer Drive Suite 203, Cameron Park, CA 95682, USA; [d]Department of Dermatology, Larkin Community Hospital-S Miami, South Miami, FL 33143, USA; [e]Private Practice, Wenatchee, WA 98801, USA; [f]Department of Dermatology, University of California-San Diego, 8899 University Center Lane UNIT 350, San Diego, CA 92122, USA

KEYWORDS

• Periorbital rejuvenation • Cosmetic dermatology • Laser resurfacing • Radiofrequency • Neurotoxins • Fillers • Exosomes • Regenerative medicine

KEY POINTS

- Periorbital age-related issues can be managed with non-invasive procedures such as high-intensity focused ultrasound, radiofrequency microneedling, botulinum toxin, fillers, chemical peels, laser resurfacing, and regenerative medicine.
- Comprehensive treatment plans may be designed per each periorbital area of defects after addressing underlying etiologies.
- While regenerative medicine, such as fat transfer, platelet-rich concentrate, exosomes, and polynucleotides, is promising for periorbital rejuvenation, it is limited by small subject study sizes, a lack of standardized protocols, and regulatory challenges.

INTRODUCTION

The periocular region is often the first to exhibit signs of aging due to its delicate skin, thin underlying muscles, and frequent facial expressions. Factors such as genetic predisposition, sun exposure, repetitive movements, and smoking accelerate the loss of hyaluronic acid, collagen, and elastin resulting in various age-related changes, such as tear trough deformities, fat pad protrusion, rhytides, dermatochalasis, brow descent, temple hollowing, pseudoherniation of eyelid fat, involutional ptosis, elongation of the lower eyelid, photoaging, and hyperpigmentation. While surgical procedures like blepharoplasty have been the gold standard for periorbital rejuvenation, concerns about downtime, general anesthesia, and surgical anxiety often deter patients. As a result, non-surgical treatments have surged in popularity, including the growing interest in and advancements of regenerative medicine. While existing reviews on nonsurgical periorbital rejuvenation primarily focus on lasers and energy-based devices, this article expands on the topic by including an overview of regenerative medicine modalities, providing a broader presepective on emerging treatments in the field. We aim to provide a concise review of current non-invasive periorbital rejuvenation techniques, outlining their benefits and limitations to assist clinicians in selecting appropriate therapeutic approaches.

*Corresponding author. Berman Skin Institute, 3581 Palmer Drive Suite 203, Cameron Park, CA 95682, USA. *E-mail address:* DrLilyPark@gmail.com

https://doi.org/10.1016/j.yacs.2025.01.005 **www.advancesincosmeticsurgery.com**
2542-4327/25/

ABBREVIATIONS

BoTN	botulinum toxin
CaHA	calcium hydroxyapatite
CO2	carbon dioxide
Er:YAG	Erbium:Yttrium Aluminum Garnet
HA	hyaluronic acid
HIFU	high-intensity focused ultrasound
IPL	intense pulse light
KTP	potassium-titanyl-phosphate
MFU	microfocused ultrasound
PDGF	platelet-derived growth factor
PDL	pulse dye laser
PLLA	Poly-L-Lactic acid
PRF	platelet rich fibrin
PRP	platelet rich plasma
RF	radiofrequency
SOOF	sub-orbicularis oculi fat

RESURFACING LASERS

Overview

Resurfacing lasers deliver energy, instigating thermal reactions that promote dermal remodeling and collagen and elastin production.

- Based on the degree of epithelial disruption, these technologies can be broadly classified as:
  1. Ablative lasers
  2. Nonablative lasers
- Depending on the uniformity of the treatment, they can also be categorized as:
  1. Fractionated
  2. Non-fractionated

Ablative resurfacing devices vaporize the epidermis and part of the dermis to stimulate collagen production, dermal contraction, and tissue remodeling [1,2]. Full epithelial vaporization leads to significant tightening of the epidermis and dermis but is associated with prolonged downtime. Examples of ablative resurfacing lasers include the 10,600 nm carbon dioxide (CO2) laser and the 2940 nm Erbium:Yttrium Aluminum Garnet (Er:YAG) laser.

Although ablative laser resurfacing offers superior results for facial skin rejuvenation in improving texture, tone, and the appearance of wrinkles compared to other laser treatment modalities, rare but serious side effects such as lower lid ectropion along with scarring, hypopigmentation, or hyperpigmentation can occur, especially with non-fractionated CO2 lasers [3]. Increased risk of hyperpigmentation in darker skin is another limitation of fully ablative laser non-fractionated resurfacing.

Fractional laser treatments are a suitable alternative for patients with darker skin tones. Fractional ablative resurfacing utilizes fractional photothermolysis, delivering energy in a gridline-patterned of microablative columns, creating microthermal zones. This technology induces thermal injury in these zones, facilitating heat shock protein formation around the dermis and stimulating collagen formation. Meanwhile, the surrounding skin around the zones is preserved, mitigating adverse effects like scarring or prolonged downtime [2]. A study of 12 volunteers with Fitzpatrick skin types III to V and class II to IV on the Glogau wrinkle scale compared the effects of fractional Er:YAG (4 sessions, 2 weeks apart) with a single session of ablative Er:YAG laser. Both treatments showed comparable clinical improvement, though the ablative laser slightly outperformed the fractional laser. Histologic analysis revealed a significant decrease in elastin concentration and increased tropoelastin levels in both groups, with greater improvement observed after the ablative treatment. However, the fractional group experienced fewer side effects and milder erythema, with healing occurring within 2 to 4 days, whereas for the ablative group, complete re-epithelialization took 2 weeks, and erythema resolved within 1 to 3 months [3].

Nonablative resurfacing lasers induce thermal tissue coagulation without epithelial ablation and penetrate tissue deeper due to their lower water absorption coefficient than ablative lasers [4]. Thermal injury from this treatment is confined to the dermis, typically resulting in fewer side effects and a shorter recovery than ablative lasers. However, these non-ablative approaches are generally less effective than their ablative counterparts for treating rhytides [4]. Some examples of nonablative resurfacing laser devices include the 1927 nm thulium-doped laser (Fig. 1), 1565 nm, 1540 nm, and 1550 nm erbium-doped lasers, the 1540 nm Er:Glass laser, the 1440 nm Nd: YAG, and 1410 nm diode nonablative fractional laser (NAFL) [5]. Sukal and colleagues showed that 3 to 7 treatments with a 1550 nm NAFL, applied in 2 to 3 passes per area at 3 to 4 weeks intervals, resulted in eyelid tightening in all 31 patients, as assessed by 3 physicians using a 4-point evaluation scale, 3 to 4 weeks after the final treatment; additionally, 56% of the patients had increased eyelid aperture compared to their baseline [6].

Hybrid Resurfacing Lasers

Integrating ablative and nonablative fractional technologies, hybrid resurfacing lasers allow energy delivery

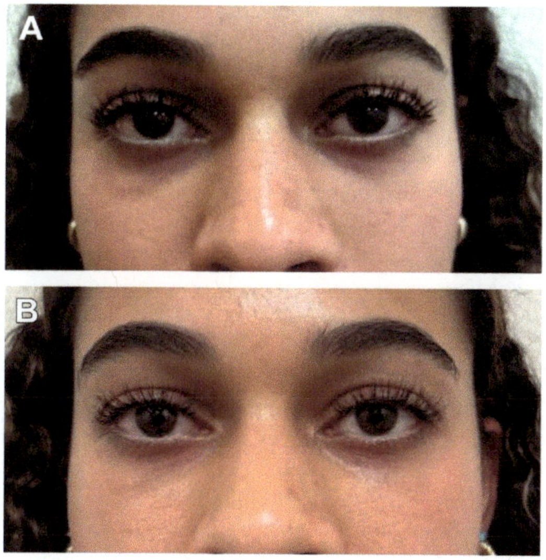

FIG. 1 18-year-old mixed female with hyperpigmentation. (A) Before treatments, (B) noticeable improvement seen at 1-month follow-up after 2 sessions of NAFL 1927 nm treatments.

at multiple depths, thus improving both superficial skin texture and deeper rhytides. Applying deeper penetrating wavelengths tightens skin laxity, while the superficial wavelengths are efficacious in addressing pigmentary and textural alteration linked to the aging process [4].

A study of 1 single-pass treatment with a CO2 and 1570-nm hybrid laser demonstrated significant periorbital rejuvenation. Mild-to-moderate erythema and crusting were seen, with an average downtime of 5.9 days [7].

VASCULAR LASERS

Various lasers can address periocular cutaneous vascular lesions by targeting the hemoglobin within the vessels, allowing for the destruction of blood vessels without epidermal changes.

Pulse dye laser (PDL), 585 nm and 595 nm, can treat the appearance of infraorbital bluish discoloration caused by vascular changes within the eyelid skin [5]. While less frequently utilized for this purpose, PDL may have unintended benefits in mild to moderate periorbital rhytides and skin rejuvenation through a heating effect in deeper skin layers that stimulates collagen remodeling and tightening through the release of growth factors [8].

Potassium-titanyl-phosphate, KTP, laser treatment can improve vascularity and pigmentation, even after a single treatment [9]. A study showed a series of long-pulsed KTP laser treatments, ranging from 3 to 6 sessions, demonstrated significant improvements in redness and pigmentation, as assessed by investigator, subject, and observer scores [8]; the treatments also showed mild to moderate improvement in skin tone and texture, with a mild improvement in rhytides, when compared to baseline photographs in a study [10].

Nd:YAG lasers also demonstrate effectiveness in periorbital rejuvenation [11].

- Q-switch Nd:YAG lasers target melanin due to their short pulse duration, reducing melanin and thus improving infraorbital hyperpigmentation [11]. Significant enhancements in skin color, erythema, melanin pigment, and lightness were seen in a photo-analysis study, following 6 sessions of fractional Q-switch Nd:YAG laser treatment administered at 2-week intervals [11].
- One to 2 treatments of long-pulsed Nd:YAG can improve the appearance of periorbital veins and is considered superior to KTP or PDL for treating periorbital veins [12]. Contact cooling and post-procedure ice packs can mitigate the risks of scabbing, minor burns, and skin darkening [12].

Q-switched ruby laser (694 nm) has also proven effective in treating infraorbital dark circles. A study observed improvement in 93% of patients treated with 8 fractional Q-switched ruby laser sessions at weekly intervals, as evidenced by before-and-after photo comparisons [13].

INTENSE PULSE LIGHT

Intense pulse light (IPL) therapy shows variable effectiveness in improving periorbital hyperpigmentation and rhytides [14–17]. Due to its inconsistent efficacy around the eyes, other modalities are generally preferred for periorbital rejuvenation.

THERMO-MECHANICAL FRACTIONAL INJURY THERAPY

Non-laser, fractional, non-ablative, thermomechanical therapy (Tixel, Novoxel, Israel) applies up to 400°C of thermal energy to targeted tissue using a titanium handpiece tip. This tip utilizes brief pulses to achieve tissue coagulation in the dermis without disrupting the epidermis, thus resulting in little to no downtime. An ocular shield is also unnecessary during treatment as no chromophore is targeted. A study involving 3 to 5 sessions of the thermo-mechanical fractional injury therapy, spaced 3 to 5 weeks apart, showed improvement in mild to moderate periorbital rhytides, comparable to the outcomes achieved with 3 to 5 sessions of 1565 nm NAFL treatment, 3 to 5 weeks apart [18].

In addition, the combination of thermomechanical therapy and topical application of 1% liquid tetracycline resulted in significant improvement in festoons, with a mean of 5.0 ± 1.9 treatments performed at intervals of 5.4 ± 1.2 weeks [19].

RADIOFREQUENCY

Radiofrequency (RF) devices emit a rapidly alternating electromagnetic current to tissue and generate heat deep in the dermis and subcutaneous fat. The lower moisture content in the epidermis increases impedance, resulting in minimal surface ablation. This makes RF devices a suitable choice for the periorbital region, especially for darker skin tones, due to the reduced risk of hyperpigmentation and scarring [20]. This energy generates thermal effects that trigger tissue remodeling, collagen contraction, and elastin production, with resultant enhancements in skin laxity, fine rhytides, skin reflectance, and hyperpigmentation.

RF devices can be subcategorized into monopolar, bipolar, or multipolar depending on electrode configuration.

The first monopolar RF device, Thermage (Solta, California, USA), was approved by the Food and Drug Administration in 2002 for periorbital rhytides and remains the only device with an indication for eyelid rejuvenation [21]. Due to considerable pain and the rare side effect of lipolysis, low-energy techniques with multiple passes were adopted [22].

For safety and tolerability in the periorbital region, transcutaneous, temperature-controlled, monopolar RF devices have been developed. These devices have automatic temperature feedback control of energy deposition at a targeted range of 40 to 45° Celsius to stimulate collagen remodeling and tightening [23].

Bipolar and multipolar transcutaneous RF methods also offer controlled, well-tolerated superficial dermal injury through selective thermal coagulation. A significant improvement in periorbital skin texture was seen in patients over 50 years old compared to those below age 50 at 6-month follow-up after 3 treatments [24].

RF with microneedling devices have been developed to deliver current through an array of needles into the skin, allowing for controlled heat penetration [5]. A fractional modification permits the electric current to be exerted only at the distal tips of the needles in the dermis or subcutaneous fat by insulating the proximal portions. The resultant sparing of the epidermis further minimizes the potential side effects of post-inflammatory pigment alteration [4].

Thus, RF devices can offer effective periorbital tightening with quick recovery and favorable side effect profiles. Full results typically appear in 4 to 6 weeks post-treatment, although multiple treatments are often needed [5].

FOCUSED ULTRASOUND

- Microfocused ultrasound (MFU) uses high-frequency acoustic waves to produce microthermal zones of injury at specific depths within the dermis, resulting in dermal tightening through neocollagenesis, while sparing the epidermis. Approved for eyebrow lifting and tightening by the Food and Drug Administration (FDA) in 2009, intense MFU with visualization (Ulthera, Mesa, Arizona) has demonstrated its efficacy and safety for eyelid rejuvenation [25].
- High-intensity focused ultrasound (HIFU) single treatment with 2.0-mm focal depth demonstrated significant improvement in periorbital rhytides, particularly in younger patients who tend to have more heat-labile collagen bonds, as opposed to the irreducible collagen multivalent cross-links found in older patients [26,27]. Upper and lower eyelid tightening using HIFU (ULTRAFORMER III, Classys, Seoul, Korea) was also observed in another study [28]. However, caution is advised to avoid delivering excessive energy to the deep subcutaneous tissue since HIFU lacks real-time imaging during treatment [27,29].
- A high-intensity, high-frequency ultrasound device (Sofwave, Tel Aviv, Israel), has been designed to deliver acoustic energy via Synchronous Ultrasound Parallel Beam technology at an approximate depth of 1.5 mm, thereby eliminating the need for depth visualization during treatment [20]. A newer handpiece applicator with 3 ultrasound transducers allows for targeted treatments in hard-to-reach areas such as around the eyes. Approved by the FDA in 2019 for reducing fine lines and wrinkles, this device can achieve periorbital rejuvenation by delivering energy through an array of parallel, geometric, 3D cylindrical-shaped thermal zones, resulting in thermal coagulation and subsequent collagen and elastin remodeling in mid-dermis [30].

OCULAR SAFETY

Improper eye shield usage can lead to complications like ectropion, visual disturbances, pain, and severe outcomes such as corneal injuries and retinal burns [31].

Longer wavelength lasers such as Er:YAG and CO2 lasers have stronger water absorption and can cause corneal injury, whereas shorter wavelength lasers (400–1200 nm) such as PDL, Alexandrite, Nd:YAG, and IPL can have retinal absorption as they predominantly target melanin [32]. Macular holes, a type of retinal damage, have been associated with 1064 nm lasers [31].

While pulling the skin away from the orbit may help reduce ocular risks, patients need to wear metal shields for resurfacing and vascular lasers when treating around the eyelid margins. However, when using RF devices around the eyelid margins, plastic protective lens shields are more appropriate, as metal eye shields can overheat and cause potential corneal damage [5].

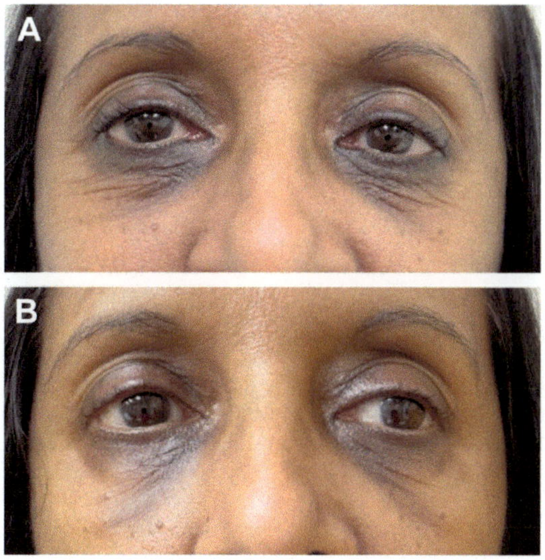

FIG. 2 62-year-old Indian female with significant lower eyelid hyperpigmentation, skin laxity, and dermatochalasis. Performed a series of 4 TCA 10% to 15% chemical peels. (**A**) Before treatment, and (**B**) 1 month after 4 sessions.

CHEMICAL PEELS

Depending on the type of peel, chemically ablating the epidermis with or without dermal injury results in varied levels of collagen production, dermal remodeling, and epithelial regeneration (Fig. 2). This process can effectively rejuvenate the eyelids and address periocular hyperpigmentation (Table 1).

Side effects include erythema, milia, scarring, corneal damage with direct contact, or uneven pigmentation [33]. Pretreatment with topical tretinoin and hydroquinone 2 to 4 weeks before chemical peels may reduce post-inflammatory hyperpigmentation and enhance peeling [34–36].

TABLE 1
Common Examples of Chemical Peels Based on the Affected Depth of Layers

Depth of Peels	Affected Layer	Common Types
Superficial	Epidermis	Glycolic acid, azelaic acid, Lactic acid 15% with trichloroacetic acid (TCA) 3.75%, TCA 10%–35%, Jessner's solution, retinoids, 5-Fluorouracil, salicylic acid, mandelic acid, pyruvic acid
Medium	Papillary dermis	35% TCA with Jessner's solution
Deep	Reticular dermis	Baker-Gordon solution, Phenol

NEUROTOXINS

There are currently 7 botulinum toxin (BoTN) preparations available in the United States, each differing in molecular weight, antigenicity, and dosing per unit. The latest BoTN, DaxibotulinumtoxinA, was FDA-approved in 2022 for treating glabellar lines, with a longer duration of up to 6 months [37].

Common treatment areas for periorbital rejuvenation include orbicularis oculi, procerus, and corrugator supercilli. The 3-point injection technique, a newly accepted technique for glabella injection, targets the bony origin of the procerus and corrugator supercilii muscles (Fig. 3). If visible muscular contraction occurs at the upper eyebrow, a subdermal injection in the medial third of the eyebrow is recommended [38].

If there is no significant lid laxity, a point just below the lateral one-third of the brows can be injected to lift the eyebrow, and the lower eyelids can be widened by injecting at the mid pupillary line, 2 to 3 mm below the lower eyelid margin, targeting the palpebral aperture to widen the eyes [1]. Injecting microdoses of dilute

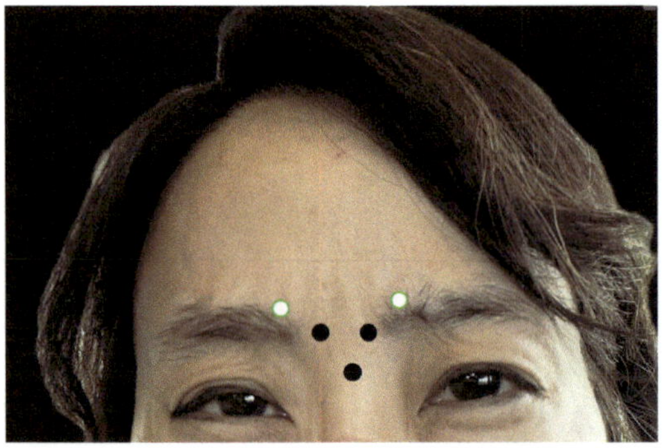

FIG. 3 The 3-point glabella and corrugator neurotoxin injection targets the bony origin (*black dots*), along with subdermal injections in the medial third of the eyebrow (*white dots*) when indicated.

BoTN into periorbital muscles has also demonstrated efficacy in periorbital rhytides [39]. Care must be taken to avoid complications like eyebrow or eyelid ptosis by understanding the facial anatomy, dosing, and injection techniques (Fig. 4).

FILLERS

Periorbital hollows can be volumized using fillers, such as in the tear trough, the nasojugal fold, and the lateral palpebromalar groove. Soft tissue fillers can improve brow contour and position and upper eyelid frame deformity as well [40].

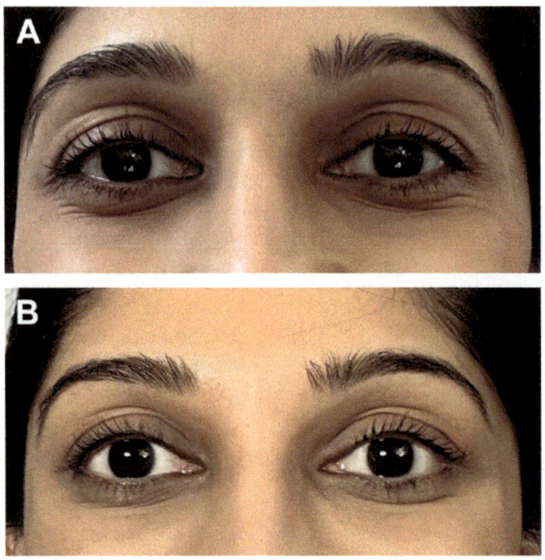

FIG. 4 A 35-year-old female received neurotoxin injections in the glabella, lateral crow's feet, lateral eyebrows, and 3 mm below the lash line in the mid-pupillary area, resulting in more open eyes and eyebrow lift. (**A**) Before and (**B**) after treatment.

Hyaluronic Acid

Hyaluronic acid (HA) injection into tear trough filler primarily addresses under-eye hollowing in patients with good skin elasticity and minimal eye bags.

Dermal Filler Complication

Filler complications include contour irregularities, Tyndall effect, or blue-gray dyschromia, nodules, filler migration, malar edema, and infection. Improper placement of filler can impede the drainage of lymphatic fluid, leading to prolonged swelling.

- Malar mounds can be defined as soft tissue swelling or lymphatic drainage issues, while festoons are drooping of skin and muscle with fat protrusion [41]. It is prudent to avoid the use of fillers in patients with a history of excessive swelling, malar mounds, or festoons, particularly if fluid accumulation is suspected due to compromised lymphatic drainage [42].
- Given the hydrophilicity of HA fillers, slightly underfilling and injecting in deeper anatomic planes such as periosteal in the tear trough, mid-cheek, or malar eminences may result in optimal outcomes. Most candidates for tear trough fillers also require mid-cheek augmentation, specifically targeting the medial sub-orbicularis oculi fat (SOOF). Therefore, it is advisable to treat the SOOF before addressing the tear trough (Fig. 5).
- To minimize the risk of soft tissue necrosis and vision loss from occlusion of ophthalmic and central retinal arteries complications, careful techniques such as slow injection of small aliquots of HA fillers into the tear trough, using Beckton Dickinson syringes with smaller needles for deep periosteum injection, or utilizing a 25 gauge blunt-tip cannula to prevent arterial penetration may be helpful [43].

Poly-L-lactic Acid

Poly-L-Lactic acid (PLLA) is a synthetic polymer that stimulates an inflammatory tissue response, leading to collagen deposition and dermal fibroplasia. While HA fillers offer immediate results and precise treatment for specific facial issues, PLLA provides broader volume expansion and collagen synthesis over time and may require multiple injection sessions spaced 4 to 6 weeks apart for optimal results. Although rarely used in the periocular region due to swelling and nodules, PLLA injection in the cheek can lead to malar augmentation and

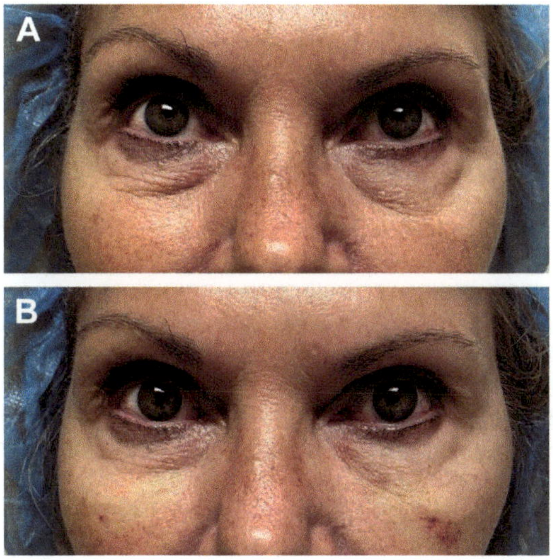

FIG. 5 Hyaluronic acid filler was injected into mid cheeks, suborbicularis oculi fat, and tear troughs. (**A**) Before and (**B**) after.

help bolster HA filler in the periorbital rejuvenation [44,45].

Calcium Hydroxyapatite

Like PLLA, calcium hydroxyapatite fillers (CaHA) are rarely used in the periorbital region due to the risk of nodule formation and irreversibility [45]. However, they can be effective in malar augmentation or in the nasojugal groove to help improve the appearance of the periorbital region [46].

REGENERATIVE MEDICINE

Limitation of Regenerative Medicine

While holding promise, regenerative medicine is constrained by limited data showing efficacy, attributed to small sample sizes in trials of periorbital rejuvenation. Lack of standardization in preparation and storage is another limitation, highlighting the need for more refined protocols and research for clinical use [47]. The FDA's guidelines for fat-based therapies focus mainly on adipocytes and do not fully address other associated significant cell types in the extracellular matrix [48].

Platelet rich plasma (PRP) and platelet-rich fibrin (PRF) are currently not FDA-approved for direct injection for periorbital rejuvenation, while the technologies to obtain them are FDA-approved [49].

Currently, the FDA has not approved polynucleotide and exosome products [50].

Autologous Fat Transfer

Fat grafts can not only treat volume loss but also promote tissue regeneration and neocollagenesis by enhancing vascularization and reducing fibrosis, primarily through the angiogenic, antifibrotic, and anti-inflammatory effects of adipose-derived mesenchymal stem cells [51]. This procedure involves harvesting fat from the patient's own body, making it a biocompatible choice for soft-tissue augmentation with near-permanent improved outcomes in the periorbital areas in treating tear trough deformity, dark circles, and periorbital rhytides from mid-face hollowing [52].

Fat grafts can be categorized based on particle size:

- Millifat (parcel size 2 – 2.4 mm)
- Microfat (1 – 1.2 mm)
- Nanofat (400 – 600 μm parcel size).

Microfat can effectively augment the upper and lower eyelids, while smaller nanofat injections may be suitable for thinner eyelid tissue, especially in mature skin [53]. Of note, disposable autologous fat tissue harvesting and transfer kits for macro, micro, and nanofat are FDA-approved for aesthetic body contouring and their use in periorbital rejuvenation would be considered off-label [54].

Platelet-Rich Concentrate

Platelet-rich concentrate is prepared by centrifuging a patient's blood to create an autologous solution of plasma containing a high concentration of growth factors, such as platelet-derived growth factors (PDGF), vascular endothelial growth factor, epithelial growth factor, and plasma proteins such as fibrin and fibronectin [51]. Often applied by injection, their side effects may include ecchymosis, pain, erythema, swelling, and, less commonly, a burning sensation [55].

- PRP releases a high concentration of PDGF within the first 15 minutes of use, followed by a significantly lower amount of release over up to 10 days. Clinical trials have evaluated the role of PRP in periocular texture improvement [56]. One study assessed the efficacy of a single PRP injection on crow's feet wrinkles and infraorbital dark circles. While a statistically significant improvement in infraorbital color homogeneity was observed, changes in stratum corneum hydration and wrinkle volume were not statistically significant [57]. Similarly, another clinical trial demonstrated notable improvement in dark circles after 3 monthly PRP sessions, with most patients seeing improvement after the third session, which persisted through a 6-month follow-up [58].

- PRF, a second-generation platelet concentrate, also containing growth factors, remains in a fluid state for approximately 15 minutes before solidifying into fibrin, requiring prompt utilization during the fluid state. Despite this constraint, PRF offers distinct advantages over PRP. Preparation is simpler, involving 1 short centrifugation step at a lower speed than for PRP. Unlike PRP, PRF preparation does not involve anticoagulants, making it suitable for individuals with hypersensitivity reactions. Furthermore, the PRF fibrin gel captures more leukocytes and platelets, leading to an increased release of cytokines and growth factors than PRP [59]. The fibrin structure also allows for a gradual and sustained release of these cytokines and growth factors over 10 days [60], consequently promoting sustained growth stimulation and tissue regeneration [61]. One study utilizing PRF specifically for periorbital rejuvenation, demonstrated improvement in periocular wrinkles, periorbital hyperpigmentation, and overall skin rejuvenation in 15 patients at 12-week follow-up, supporting the lasting effect of PRF [62]. Another study comparing PRF to PRP found that PRF more effectively volumizes tear trough hollows than PRP [63]. An advantage of PRF over HA fillers is that PRF provides more subtle results and does not carry long-term risks of migration, swelling, or edema.
- The author frequently employs PRF alone or in combination with other treatments, such as laser resurfacing and skin-tightening procedures for periorbital rejuvenation. For PRF alone, the protocol consists of 3 PRF treatments spaced 1 month apart, followed by maintenance sessions every 6 to 12 months (Fig. 6).

Polynucleotide

Extracted and purified from salmon trout germ cells, polynucleotides are sterilized DNA molecules used as injectable monotherapy or combined with HA or lasers such as CO2 lasers [64]. The viscoelasticity of the long DNA fragments in polynucleotide fillers serves as a temporary medium that allows for steady regeneration of the skin [65]. Polynucleotide fillers have been found to induce cellular migration and collagen synthesis from fibroblasts to facilitate skin regeneration and volume growth [66]. One or 2 mL(ml) of 15 mg/2 mL polynucleotide, applied in 3 to 4 sessions every 14 to 21 days, using a needle microdroplet in a linear retrograde fashion can improve skin hydration [64]. A study demonstrated a single injection of polynucleotide demonstrating a significant improvement in skin hydration in the periorbital region at week 16 [67].

Adverse effects of polynucleotide-based procedures were mild tenderness, erythema, scarring, or ecchymosis [64].

Exosomes

Exosomes are extracellular vesicles derived from stem cells and carry essential growth factors, proteins, mRNA, miRNA, and lipids [68]. Their capacity to be harnessed by epidermal keratinocytes to regulate cell functions, including proliferation, differentiation, and apoptosis, has led to their exploration for aesthetic application [68].

Exosomes may provide minimally invasive modalities for combating photoaging and rhytides [69]. Topical exosomes have been used alone or in combination with micro-needling, polydioxanone (PDO) threads, fractional ablative lasers, and energy-based

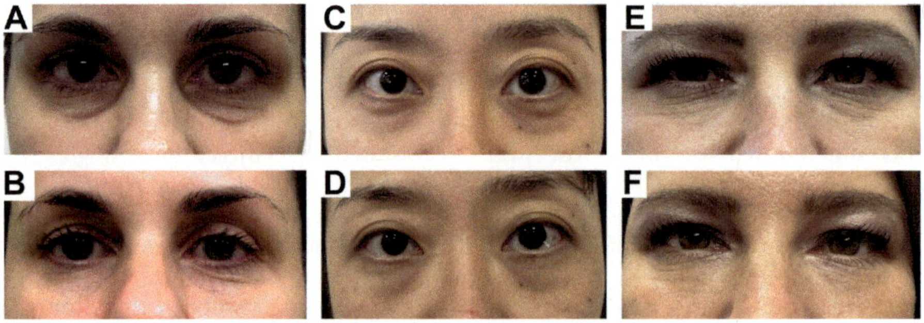

FIG. 6 Periorbital rejuvenation with PRF. (**A**) 52-year-old Caucasian female with severe inset eyes, hyperpigmentation, skin laxity, and dermatochalasis; (**B**) improved with 3 PRF and 3 fractional thermomechanical combination treatments. (**C**) 39-year-old Asian female with fat pad herniation and purplish hue of lower eyelids, (**D**) improved with 2 PRF treatments. (**E**) 43-year-old Caucasian female, with lower eyelid dermatochalasis and hyperpigmentation, (**F**) improved with 2 PRF treatments spaced 1 month apart.

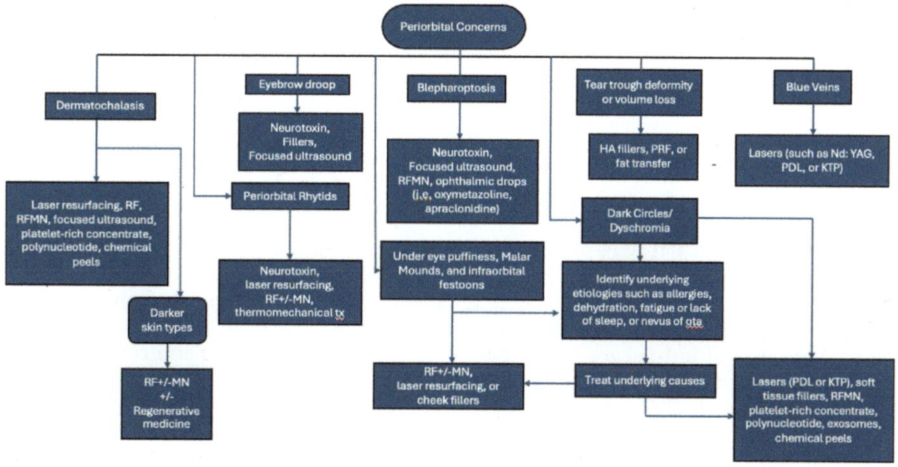

FIG. 7 Suggested management approach for non-surgical periorbital rejuvenation.

devices to reduce inflammation and stimulate collagen synthesis and angiogenesis in a relatively limited number of aesthetic practices [70–73].

SUMMARY

There are myriad minimally invasive procedures to utilize in periorbital rejuvenation, such as lasers and energy-based devices, regenerative medicine, fat grafts, fillers and toxins, and chemical peels. When offering such therapies, it is important to tailor them to specific needs while managing patient expectations (Fig. 7). To optimize efficacy and minimize side effects, providers should be adept in selecting therapies, whether used individually or in combination.

CLINICS CARE POINTS

- Fractional lasers utilize fractional photothermolysis to deliver energy in a grid-like pattern of micro-ablative columns, creating microthermal zones. This approach reduces the risk of side effects such as scarring and post-inflammatory hyperpigmentation, making it safer for darker skin tones.
- Ablative lasers are more effective than non-ablative lasers, and non-fractionated lasers are more effective than fractionated ones in skin rejuvenation. However, non-ablative and fractionated lasers have fewer side effects, offering a balance between efficacy and safety when employed in multiple treatments.
- Q-switched Nd:YAG lasers, with their short pulse duration, can effectively treat infraorbital blue veins by targeting melanin.
- While regenerative medicine has a potential role in periorbital rejuvenation, it is currently limited by small sample sizes, lack of standardization in preparation, and variability in storage conditions.

DISCLOSURE

The authors have nothing to disclose.

REFERENCES

[1] Glaser DA, Kurta A. Periorbital rejuvenation. Overview of nonsurgical treatment options. Facial Plast Surg Clin North Am 2016;24(2):145–52.

[2] Smith LD, Couch SM. Nonsurgical periorbital rejuvenation. Advances in Cosmetic Surgery 2019;2(1):107–19.

[3] El-Domyati M, Abd-El-Raheem T, Abdel-Wahab H, et al. Fractional versus ablative erbium:yttrium-aluminum-garnet laser resurfacing for facial rejuvenation: an objective evaluation. J Am Acad Dermatol 2013;68(1):103–12.

[4] Miller AD, Ortiz AE. Update on facial noninvasive skin tightening. Advances in Cosmetic Surgery 2022;5(1):145–55.

[5] Heitmiller K, Ring C, Saedi N, et al. Nonsurgical light and energy-based devices: utility in eyelid and periorbital surgery. Facial Plast Surg Clin North Am 2021;29(2):323–34.

[6] Sukal SA, Chapas AM, Bernstein LJ, et al. Eyelid tightening and improved eyelid aperture through nonablative fractional resurfacing. Dermatol Surg 2008;34(11):1454–8.

[7] Tsur Shenhav L, Shehade W, Muravnik G, et al. The safety and efficacy of a dual CO 2 and 1570-nm hybrid laser for

periorbital rejuvenation. Dermatol Surg 2023;49(5):479–82.
[8] Zelickson BD, Kilmer SL, Bernstein E, et al. Pulsed dye laser therapy for sun damaged skin. Lasers Surg Med 1999;25(3):229–36.
[9] Butler EG, McClellan SD, Ross EV. Split treatment of photodamaged skin with KTP 532 nm laser with 10 mm handpiece versus IPL: a cheek-to-cheek comparison. Lasers Surg Med 2006;38(2):124–8.
[10] Lee MWC. Combination 532-nm and 1064-nm lasers for noninvasive skin rejuvenation and toning. Arch Dermatol 2003;139(10):1265–76.
[11] Alavi S, Goodarzi A, Nilforoushzadeh MA, et al. Evaluation of efficacy and safety of low-fluence Q-switched 1064-nm laser in infra-orbital hyperpigmentation based on biometric parameters. J Lasers Med Sci 2022;13:e16.
[12] Lee TS, Kwek JWM, Ellis DAF. Treatment of periocular and temporal reticular veins with 1064-nm Nd:YAG Laser. J Cosmet Dermatol 2020;19(9):2306–12.
[13] Xu TH, Li YH, Chen JZS, et al. Treatment of infraorbital dark circles using 694 nm fractional Q-switched ruby laser. Lasers Med Sci 2016;31(9):1783–7.
[14] DiBernardo BE, Pozner JN. Intense pulsed light therapy for skin rejuvenation. Clin Plast Surg 2016;43(3):535–40.
[15] Barikbin B, Akbari Z, Vafaee R, et al. The efficacy of IPL in periorbital skin rejuvenation: an open-label study. J Lasers Med Sci 2019;10(Suppl 1):S64–7.
[16] Kołodziejczak A, Rotsztejn H. Efficacy of fractional laser, radiofrequency and IPL rejuvenation of periorbital region. Lasers Med Sci 2022;37(2):895–903.
[17] Tanzi EL, Alster TS. Single-pass carbon dioxide versus multiple-pass Er:YAG laser skin resurfacing: a comparison of postoperative wound healing and side-effect rates. Dermatol Surg 2003;29(1):80–4.
[18] Salameh F, Daniely D, Kauvar A, et al. Treatment of periorbital wrinkles using thermo-mechanical fractional injury therapy versus fractional non-ablative 1565 nm laser: a comparative prospective, randomized, double-arm, controlled study. Lasers Surg Med 2022;54(1):46–53.
[19] Safir M, Waizer I, Safir A, et al. Percutaneous delivery of liquid tetracycline using a thermal resurfacing drug delivery system for the treatment of festoons. Lasers Surg Med 2024;56(5):454–61.
[20] Fathi R, Pfeiffer M, Tsoukas M. Minimally invasive eyelid care in dermatology: medical, laser, and cosmetic therapies. Clin Dermatol 2015;33(2):207–16.
[21] Polder KD, Bruce S. Radiofrequency: thermage. Facial Plast Surg Clin North Am 2011;19(2):347–59.
[22] Fitzpatrick R, Geronemus R, Goldberg D, et al. Multicenter study of noninvasive radiofrequency for periorbital tissue tightening. Lasers Surg Med 2003;33(4):232–42.
[23] Key DJ, Boudreaux L. A proposed method for upper eyelid and infrabrow tightening using a transcutaneous temperature controlled radiofrequency device with opaque plastic eye shields. J Drugs Dermatol 2016;15(11):1302–5.
[24] Wu X, Cen Q, Zhu J, et al. Effectiveness and safety of nonablative fractional laser and infrared bipolar radiofrequency for treating periorbital wrinkles. J Cosmet Laser Ther 2022;24(6–8):91–7.
[25] Pak CS, Lee YK, Jeong JH, et al. Safety and efficacy of ulthera in the rejuvenation of aging lower eyelids: a pivotal clinical trial. Aesthetic Plast Surg 2014;38(5):861–8.
[26] Han HS, Park JW, Kim SY, et al. Safety and efficacy of high-intensity focused ultrasound for treatment of periorbital, perioral, and neck wrinkles: prospective open single-center single-arm confirmatory clinical trial. Dermatol Ther 2022;35(5):e15420.
[27] Pavicic T, Ballard JR, Bykovskaya T, et al. Microfocused ultrasound with visualization: consensus on safety and review of energy-based devices. J Cosmet Dermatol 2022;21(2):636–47.
[28] Lio ML, Chang CC, Chuang ADC, et al. Quantified facial rejuvenation utilizing high intense focus ultrasound with multiple penetrative depths. Clin Cosmet Investig Dermatol 2022;15:489–96.
[29] Park JY, Lin F, Suwanchinda A, et al. Customized treatment using microfocused ultrasound with visualization for optimized patient outcomes: a review of skin-tightening energy technologies and a pan-asian adaptation of the expert panel's gold standard consensus. J Clin Aesthet Dermatol 2021;14(5):E70–9.
[30] Hongcharu W, Boonchoo K, Gold MH. The efficacy and safety of the high-intensity parallel beam ultrasound device at the depth of 1.5 mm for skin tightening. J Cosmet Dermatol 2023;22(5):1488–94.
[31] Glover C, Richer V. Preventing eye injuries from light and laser-based dermatologic procedures: a practical review. J Cutan Med Surg 2023;27(5):509–15.
[32] Mainster MA, Stuck BE, Brown J. Assessment of alleged retinal laser injuries. Arch Ophthalmol 2004;122(8):1210–7.
[33] Nikalji N, Godse K, Sakhiya J, et al. Complications of medium depth and deep chemical peels. J Cutan Aesthet Surg 2012;5(4):254–60.
[34] Grimes PE. The safety and efficacy of salicylic acid chemical peels in darker racial-ethnic groups. Dermatol Surg 1999;25(1):18–22.
[35] Hevia O, Nemeth AJ, Taylor JR. Tretinoin accelerates healing after trichloroacetic acid chemical peel. Arch Dermatol 1991;127(5):678–82.
[36] Lee KC, Wambier CG, Soon SL, et al. Basic chemical peeling: superficial and medium-depth peels. J Am Acad Dermatol 2019;81(2):313–24.
[37] Solish N, Carruthers J, Kaufman Joely, et al. Overview of DaxibotulinumtoxinA for injection: a novel formulation of botulinum toxin type A. Drugs 2021;81:2091–101.
[38] Swift A, Green JB, Hernandez CA, et al. Tips and tricks for facial toxin injections with illustrated anatomy. Plast Reconstr Surg 2022;149(2):303E–12E.

[39] Wu WTL. Microbotox of the lower face and neck: evolution of a personal technique and its clinical effects. Plast Reconstr Surg 2015;136(5):92S–100S.
[40] Markey JD, White WM. Advances in nonsurgical periocular rejuvenation. Clin Plast Surg 2023;50(3):411–9.
[41] Lipp M, Weiss E. Nonsurgical treatments for infraorbital rejuvenation: a review. Dermatol Surg 2019;45(5): 700–10.
[42] Bravo BSF, Rocha CRM Da, de Bastos JT, et al. Comprehensive treatment of periorbital region with hyaluronic acid. J Clin Aesthet Dermatol 2015;8(6):30–5.
[43] Sharad J. Dermal fillers for the treatment of tear trough deformity: a review of anatomy, treatment techniques, and their outcomes. J Cutan Aesthet Surg 2012;5(4): 229–38.
[44] Schierle CF, Casas LA. Nonsurgical rejuvenation of the aging face with injectable poly-L-lactic acid for restoration of soft tissue volume. Aesthet Surg J 2011;31(1): 95–109.
[45] Trinh LN, Grond SE, Gupta A. Dermal fillers for tear trough rejuvenation. A Systematic Review 2021. https://doi.org/10.1055/s-0041-1731348.
[46] Corduff N. An alternative periorbital treatment option using calcium hydroxyapatite for hyperpigmentation associated with the tear trough deformity. Plast Reconstr Surg Glob Open 2020;8(2). https://doi.org/10.1097/GOX.0000000000002633.
[47] Zhang M, Park G, Zhou B, et al. Applications and efficacy of platelet-rich plasma in dermatology: a clinical review. J Cosmet Dermatol 2018;17(5):660–5.
[48] Jeyaraman M, Muthu S, Sharma S, et al. Nanofat: a therapeutic paradigm in regenerative medicine. World J Stem Cells 2021;13(11):1733–46.
[49] Dhurat R, Sukesh M. Principles and methods of preparation of platelet-rich plasma: a review and author's perspective. J Cutan Aesthet Surg 2014;7(4): 189–97.
[50] Rho NK, Han KH, Cho M, et al. A survey on the cosmetic use of injectable polynucleotide: the pattern of practice among Korean Dermatologists. J Cosmet Dermatol 2023. https://doi.org/10.1111/jocd.16125.
[51] Rigotti G, Marchi A, Sbarbati A. Adipose-derived mesenchymal stem cells: past, present, and future. Aesthetic Plast Surg 2009;33(3):271–3.
[52] Marten T, Elyassnia D. Periorbital fat grafting: a new paradigm for rejuvenation of the eyelids. Facial Plast Surg Clin North Am 2021;29(2):243–73.
[53] Tonnard P, Verpaele A, Peeters G, et al. Nanofat grafting: basic research and clinical applications. Plast Reconstr Surg 2013;132(4):1017–26.
[54] Raj S, Abu-Ghname A, Davis MJ, et al. Safety and regulation of fat grafting. Semin Plast Surg 2020;34(1): 59–64.
[55] Nofal E, Elkot R, Nofal A, et al. Evaluation of carboxytherapy and platelet-rich plasma in treatment of periorbital hyperpigmentation: a comparative clinical trial. J Cosmet Dermatol 2018;17(6):1000–7.
[56] Evans AG, Ivanic MG, Botros MA, et al. Rejuvenating the periorbital area using platelet-rich plasma: a systematic review and meta-analysis. Arch Dermatol Res 2021; 313(9):711–27.
[57] Mehryan P, Zartab H, Rajabi A, et al. Assessment of efficacy of platelet-rich plasma (PRP) on infraorbital dark circles and crow's feet wrinkles. J Cosmet Dermatol 2014;13(1):72–8.
[58] Al-Shami SH. Treatment of periorbital hyperpigmentation using platelet-rich plasma injections. J Dermatol Venereol 2014;3(5):87–94.
[59] Rizk HM, Sherif M, Al-Deen MS, et al. Comparative evaluation of Platelet Rich Plasma (PRP) versus Platelet Rich Fibrin (PRF) scaffolds in regenerative endodontic treatment of immature necrotic permanent maxillary central incisors: a double blinded randomized controlled trial Production and hosting by Elsevier. Saudi Dent J 2020; 32:224–31.
[60] Kobayashi E, Flückiger L, Fujioka-Kobayashi M, et al. Comparative release of growth factors from PRP, PRF, and advanced-PRF. Clin Oral Investig 2016;20(9): 2353–60.
[61] Diab NAF, Ibrahim ASM, Abdallah AM. Fluid platelet-rich fibrin (PRF) versus platelet-rich plasma (PRP) in the treatment of atrophic acne scars: a comparative study. Arch Dermatol Res 2023;315(5):1249–55.
[62] Ahmadi MR, Allah Golafshan H, Pezeshkian F, et al. Evaluation of the effect of platelet-rich fibrin matrix in the correction of periorbital wrinkles: an experimental clinical trial. Dermatol Pract Concept 2023;13(1). https://doi.org/10.5826/dpc.1301a50.
[63] Atsu N, Ekinci-Aslanoglu C, Kantarci-Demirkiran B, et al. The comparison of platelet-rich plasma versus injectable platelet rich fibrin in facial skin rejuvenation. Dermatol Ther 2023;2023(1). https://doi.org/10.1155/2023/3096698.
[64] Cavallini M, Bartoletti E, Maioli L, et al. Consensus report on the use of PN-HPT™ (polynucleotides highly purified technology) in aesthetic medicine. J Cosmet Dermatol 2020;20:922–8.
[65] Araco A, Araco F, Raichi M. Clinical efficacy and safety of polynucleotides highly purified technology (PN-HPT®) and cross-linked hyaluronic acid for moderate to severe nasolabial folds: a prospective, randomized, exploratory study. J Cosmet Dermatol 2023;22(1):146–55.
[66] Kim JH, Kwon TR, Lee SE, et al. Comparative evaluation of the effectiveness of novel hyaluronic acid-polynucleotide complex dermal filler. Sci Rep 2020;10(1):5127.
[67] Lee YJ, Kim HT, Lee YJ, et al. Comparison of the effects of polynucleotide and hyaluronic acid fillers on periocular rejuvenation: a randomized, double-blind, split-face trial. J Dermatolog Treat 2022;33(1):254–60.
[68] Xiong M, Zhang Q, Hu W, et al. Exosomes from adipose-derived stem cells: the emerging roles and applications in tissue regeneration of plastic and cosmetic surgery. Front Cell Dev Biol 2020;8. https://doi.org/10.3389/fcell.2020.574223.

[69] Hartman N, Loyal J, Fabi S. Update on exosomes in aesthetics. Dermatol Surg 2022;48(8):862–5.

[70] Kwon HH, Yang SH, Lee J, et al. Combination treatment with human adipose tissue stem cellderived exosomes and fractional co2 laser for acne scars: a 12-week prospective, double-blind, randomized, split-face study. Acta Derm Venereol 2020;100(18):1–8.

[71] Xiong M, Zhang Q, Hu W, et al. The novel mechanisms and applications of exosomes in dermatology and cutaneous medical aesthetics. Pharmacol Res 2021;166. https://doi.org/10.1016/j.phrs.2021.105490.

[72] D.I. Duncan, Combining PDO Threads with exosomes for microlifting, Cosmet Surg Times (2020) 1–16. Available at: https://www.intechopen.com/chapters/71782 (Accessed 1 November 2024).

[73] Chernoff G. The utilization of human placental mesenchymal stem cell derived exosomes in aging skin: an investigational pilot study. J Surg 2021;6(1336). https://doi.org/10.29011/2575-9760.001388.

Advances in Cosmetic Surgery 8 (2025) 49–60
ADVANCES IN COSMETIC SURGERY

The Challenging Facelift

John P. Fezza, MD*, Reed M. Fezza, MS
Department of Cosmetic Surgery, Center for Sight, Sarasota, FL, USA

KEYWORDS
• Full neck • Heavy neck • Subplatysmal fat • Obtuse neck • Cervicomental angle • Aging face • Face lift • Neck lift

KEY POINTS
- An obtuse neck can be challenging to rejuvenate in a facelift patient.
- Realistic expectations must be addressed prior to surgery.
- The causes if a challenging neck are multifactorial, inculding factors from the tissue layers of skin , muscle, fat and bone.

The lower face and neck exhibit some of the earliest and most telltale signs of aging with the start of jowls, loose neck skin, unwanted sub-mental fat deposits, and an obtuse profile. Five factors are critical in achieving an aesthetically pleasing neck including a defined lower mandibular border with no overhanging jowls, a subhyoid depression, visible thyroid cartilage, visible anterior border of the sternocleidomastoid muscle, and a cervicomental angle of approaching between 105 and 120° degrees [1]. Many patients seek correction of undesirable aging changes of the lower face and neck, as witnessed by an increase face and neck lift procedures in recent years [2]. The popularity of these procedures has been catapulted into the mainstream by both social media and the destigmatization of celebrities receiving elective surgery. This has created a unique challenge for surgeons as only the best and not the average results are shown on social media. The margin for error is small when performing an elective procedure such as a facelift and a full discussion of both the risks and benefits is critical. There are a myriad of factors that make some patients a challenging facelift candidate.

Meeting expectations is the most crucial aspect of performing any elective procedure. Understanding patient desires and pre-operatively discussing goals will enhance the chances of a successful outcome. Reviewing realistic outcomes are important prior to embarking with surgery. Many younger patients are heavily influenced by photographs that are altered by filters on social media, and these are often unobtainable results. Matching the correct procedure with the patient will ensure a more successful outcome. Also, some patients have body dysmorphic disorder and seek repetitive, unnecessary surgery in an attempt to reach an unattainable goal. These patients can be difficult, should be screened out, and counseled that surgery is not a good option.

The mantra of *first do no harm* should be foremost when assessing any patient for elective surgery. Preoperative screening for non-compliant patients is important and any potential patient that does not take surgery seriously, understands and accepts the risks, or will not comply to a standard post-operative plan should be avoided. A patient should agree to take 3 to 4 weeks post operatively off with restrictions including no exercise, heavy exertion, sun exposure, or nicotine use. Facelift is an elective surgery that is for a healthy patient, and any potential candidate should receive clearance from their doctor if their medical history dictates. Anesthesia risks should be discussed with surgical candidates and those with poor airways or sleep

*Corresponding author. Center for Sight, 2601 South Tamiami trail, Sarasota, FL 34239. *E-mail address:* jfezza@centerforsight.net

https://doi.org/10.1016/j.yacs.2024.11.001
www.advancesincosmeticsurgery.com
2542-4327/25/

apnea should be identified, and an anesthesia assessment performed prior to performing surgery to maximize safety.

Patients should discontinue all forms of nicotine use for 2 weeks prior and continue for 2 weeks after face and neck lift surgery. The author requires patients to sign a form that they will abstain from nicotine use, including vaping and smoking. This is done for patient safety and to improve healing and limit potential skin necrosis from nicotine-induced vascular compromise. Some authors feel a deep plane approach is safer in smokers as the flaps have a more robust, intact blood supple [3]. Recently marijuana use has increased with legalization in some states, and although it does not appear to affect healing with moderate use; there are concerns of intraoperative reactive airway secretions and even possible increased nicotine levels [4]. For this reason, marijuana use should be stopped prior to facelift surgery.

A thorough medical history is required to optimize a patient prior to surgery. All conditions that can impair healing should be considered and addressed. This includes blood sugar management in diabetic individuals to ensure an adequate healing response. If a delayed healing response is anticipated, then either deferring surgery or a more conservative approach with limited skin undermining is preferred. Any patient with potential for slow or delayed healing is encouraged to undergo post-operative hyperbaric oxygen treatments to enhance healing.

Cessation of blood thinners prior to surgery will also reduce the risk of a hematoma post operatively. Both antiplatelet and anticoagulant drugs should be stopped with guidance from a cardiologist if necessary. The recent inclusion of tranexamic acid, either intravenously or with local anesthesia, has proved beneficial in reducing bleeding, bruising and potentially decreasing the adverse event of a hematoma [5].

Blood pressure control is paramount in the healing phase to avoid an unwanted hematoma, and intraoperative blood pressure management may be required to limit bleeding. Pre-operative oral clonidine may be beneficial to lower blood pressure. Patients that are overweight should be counseled on weight loss, and surgery should be delayed until a desirable and acceptable weight is reached. This is done not only to ensure a safer procedure under anesthesia, but also a better long-term result. Significant or massive weight loss after surgery can lead to excess loose skin that does not recoil with a smaller facial shape [6,7]. Recently, injectable weight loss drugs, which limit gastric emptying, such as semaglutide, have gained wide acceptance and patients should be counseled to stop them 3 weeks prior to surgery to limit the risks under anesthesia such as aspiration and pneumonia [8].

Any patient that has undergone prior facial surgery, whether elective or reconstructive also poses an additional challenge to the facelift surgeon [9]. Prior anatomy has been altered and blood supply has the potential to be compromised, leading to poor healing [10,11]. Particular challenges are present in post-parotidectomy patients as the facial nerve has been manipulated, increasing a potential risk of motor nerve injury [12]. A thorough pre-operative examination incudes facial nerve function and any pre-existing palsies should be identified and identified prior to surgery. Obtaining prior surgical records is important in understanding what procedure was performed and if the tissue necessary to healing has been utilized or manipulated.

Patients who have undergone facial radiation for cancer can be poor candidates for facelift surgery as the blood supply necessary for healing has been compromised. The author prefers a deep plane approach in patients with radiation, as this avoids a thinner skin flap. The thicker deep plane flap incorporates a more substantial medial blood supply to enhance flap healing [13].

Gender is a factor in respect to creating challenges for facelifts. Male patients in general are more challenging for several reasons [14]. They have a larger body mass, require more drugs, and have larger heads necessitating more dissection. This requires more skin undermining, and the face and neck hairs of the beard have a significant blood supply. This causes more bleeding and a higher risk of hematoma. The author has experienced increased bleeding in male patients taking supplemental testosterone, and cessation of testosterone is recommendation 2 weeks prior to surgery. Popular male enhancement drugs, such as sildenafil, are arteriole dilators should be stopped 1 week prior to surgery to limit bleeding.

Many men have male pattern baldness, and some patients have alopecia and complete baldness, making scar camouflage more challenging [15]. (Fig. 1) A discussion about scar placement and scar visibility should be discussed with the patient in the surgical consult. Limiting skin tension on wounds, placing incisions in hidden creases around the ears and under the chin, as well as layered closure can be beneficial. Post-surgical scar modification may be necessary with laser skin resurfacing, 5-Flourouracil injections and silicone sheets, or gel. Keloid formers should be avoided, and hypertrophic scar formers should be identified pre-

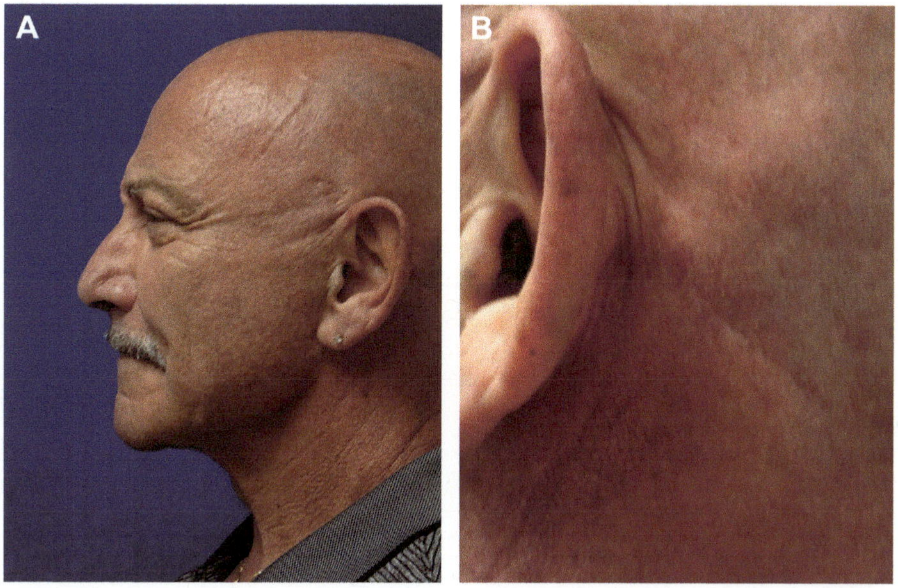

FIG. 1 (*A*) This bald man had good scar camouflage with his facelift, despite the lack of hair to conceal his wounds. (*B*) This is achieved with tensionless closure with incisions planned around natural skin lines and creases.

operatively and managed cautiously to achieve minimal scarring.

The treatment of the obtuse, full neck is particularly challenging, and a defined jawline and cervicomental angle often requires manipulation of the deeper, subplatysmal neck structures [16–19]. The causes of a full neck are multifactorial stemming from inadequate bone support, excess fat and skin and muscle laxity, and robust soft tissues (Figs. 2 and 3). Correction of the heavy neck must address all components contributing to the full neck, and intimate knowledge of anatomy and pathological aging changes of the face is crucial. An anatomically short, thick neck can be one cause of a full neck [20]. Short necks can stem from underlying vertically short, horizontally wide cervical bones, along with more robust soft tissues (Fig. 4). These patients are typically more endomorphic in their body habitus and are more difficult to correct surgically than thinner ectomorphic patients with long, lean necks. Patients with short, thick necks often have fuller faces, and buccal fat removal may be required to slim a round face.

Clinical examination of the lower face should include assessment of the facial shape on a front view. Skin tone and laxity in addition to the amount and location of facial and neck fat are contributing factors to facial shape and should be noted. Visual inspection and manual palpation are required to document the presence of a sub-mental skin crease or scars, platysma bands, and facial nerve function (Fig. 5).

The profile view is most valuable in showing patients aging changes with a blunted jaw angle and neck laxity. Examination of the sagittal view will reveal either a desirable straight shape, concave, or undesirable convex view with chin retrusion. There are many methods to assess chin projection, but Riedel's plane line is useful [21,22]. (Fig. 6) The chin should be in the same plane as a line that dropped from the upper lip to the lower lip. If the chin is behind this line, then retrogenia is present and a chin augmentation is needed to enhance the patient's profile and improve chin to neck balance. There are several ways to correct a retrusive chin, and these include osseous advancement surgery, anatomic alloplastic chin implants, or robust facial fillers. Most surgeons prefer the ease and permanent results of silicone implants, which can be easily placed and fixated in a subperiosteal plane to create a stronger jaw angle at the time of lower face rejuvenation (Fig. 7).

Additional anatomic factors, which may limit successful lower face correction, which can stem from skeletal support and bone configuration, as well as soft tissue such as fat and muscle considerations. Undesirable skeletal features in addition to microgenia include

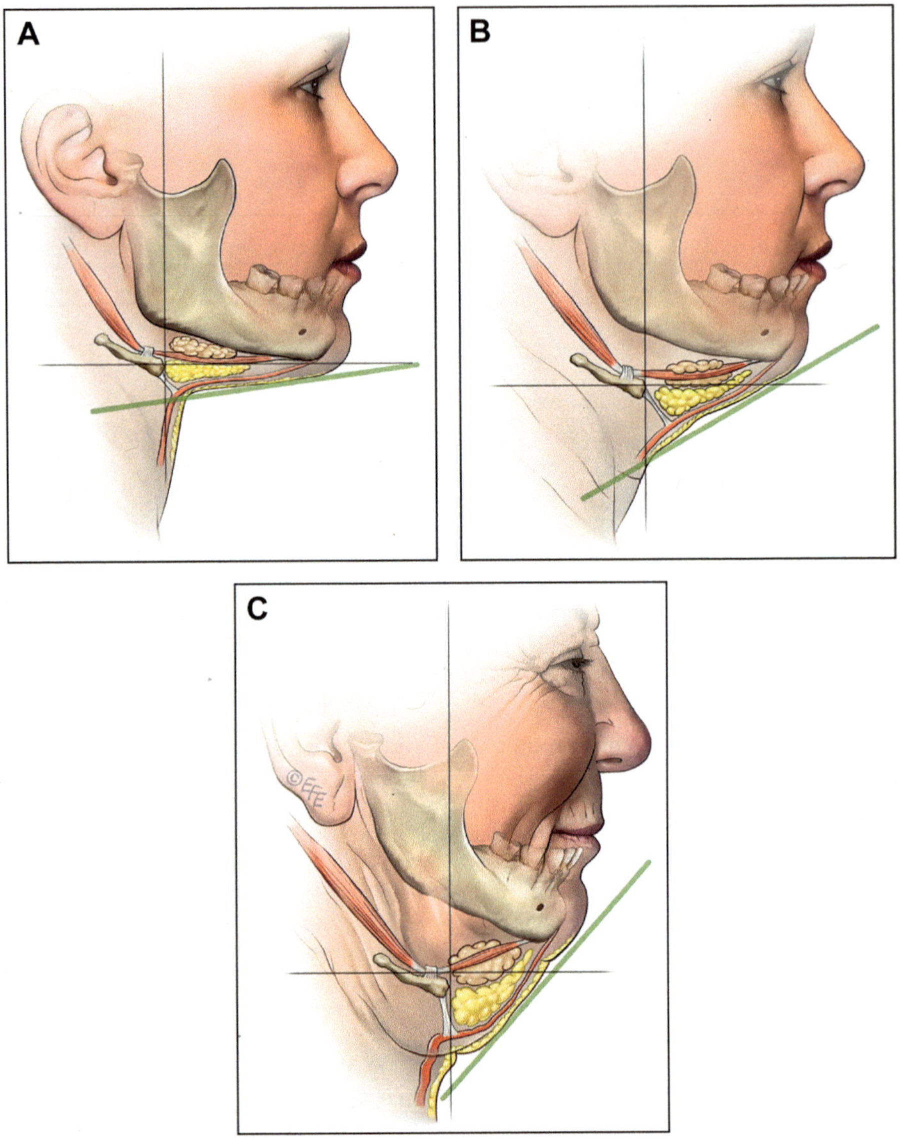

FIG. 2 (*A*) Ideal skeletal-soft tissue relation with well-defined jawline and optimal cervicomental angle. (*B*) A younger patient with a small mandible exhibits an imbalanced skeletal-soft tissue relation with obtuse cervicomental angle. (*C*) An older patient with imbalance due to atrophic skeletal support with lax hypertrophic subplatysmal volume, creating an obtuse cervicomental angle. The vertical line is the sagittal reference for position of the hyoid bone and shows the anterior displacement of soft tissue. The horizontal line is the axial reference for inferior displacement. The green oblique line demonstrates the change in the cervicomental angle. (Thomas Gerald O'Daniel, Optimizing Outcomes in Neck Lift Surgery, Aesthetic Surgery Journal, 41 (8), August 2021, 871–892, https://doi.org/10.1093/asj/sjab056.)

hyoid bone malposition, with a low or more anterior positioned hyoid bone (Fig. 8). This can blunt the cervicomental angle and limit the success of achieving a strong jawline and profile. Some authors have described repositioning the hyoid bone or recessing it by releasing the fascia on the anterior surface of the bone to allow the digastric muscle to recess the hyoid deeper and more posterior [23]. Fascial release to create setback of

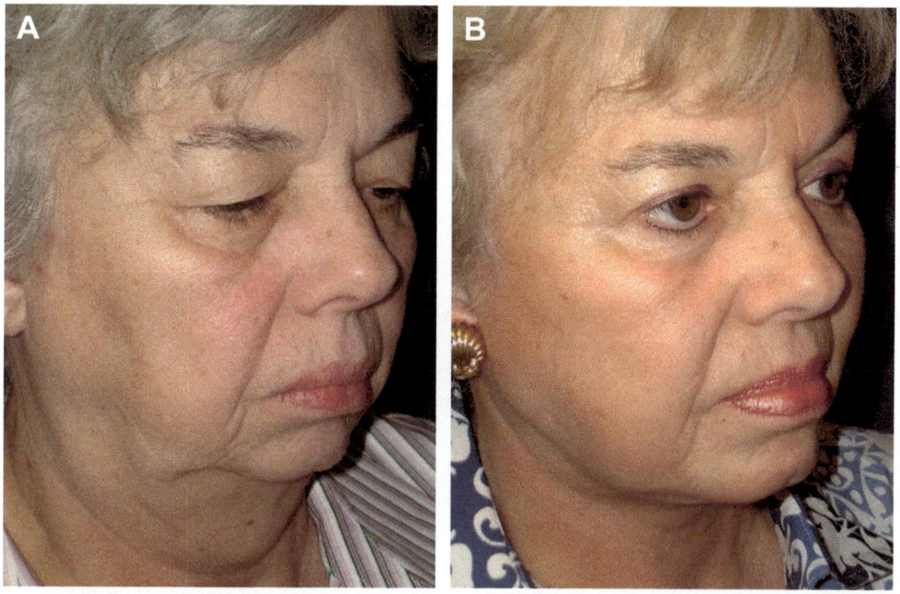

FIG. 3 (*A*) A before of a challenging patient with a full neck, obtuse angle, anterior hyoid bone, prominent submandibular glands, fat excess in pre-platysma and post-platysma regions and skin laxity. (*B*) Same patient after lower face and neck lift, chin implant, subplatysmal fat removal, shaving of the anterior portion of the digastric muscle, and midline platysmaplasty.

an anteriorly positioned hyoid bone, however, is beyond most surgeon's armamentarium. Others have described placing deep sutures from the overlying platysma muscle to the hyoid fascia below to further define an obtuse cervicomental angle [24].

A large or hypertrophied anterior digastric muscle can also limit achieving a desirable cerivco-mental angle. Debulking and shaving an anterior portion of the bulky muscle has been advocated to create a more defined submental region [25,26]. (Fig. 9) Others

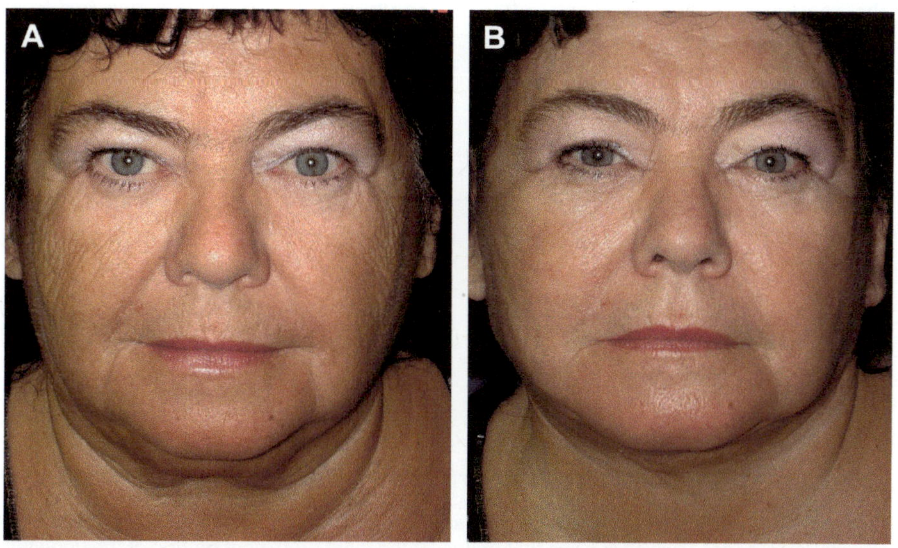

FIG. 4 (*A*) This before of a patient has a vertically short neck and horizontally wide. The challenge is achieving a sharp neck contour and definition when the jaw and chest are close together. (*B*) After facelift with subplatysmal fat removal and midline platysmaplasty.

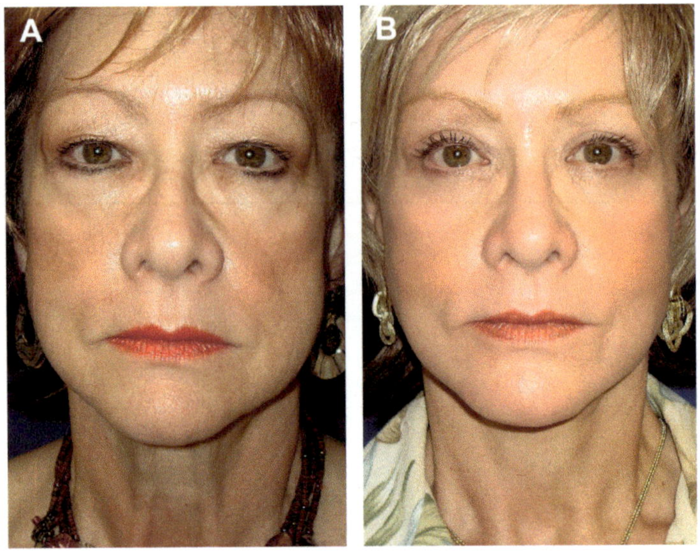

FIG. 5 (*A*) The platysma should be noted in the pre-operative examination and, as well as visually during surgery with direct exposure through a submental incision. This patient had significant visible bands on examination. (*B*) She underwent a facelift and midline platysma corset suture with improvement her neck contour.

have described plicating the anterior digastric muscles to achieve a more defined cervicomental angle, but the author often finds this unnecessary [23].

Ptotic or enlarged submandibular glands can also limit achieving a defined submental appearance and some surgeons debulk this salivary gland (Fig. 10). A submental incision is typically used to approach the glands and the posterior gland is kept intact [20,23,25,27,28]. Only the anterior portion of the gland is removed to mitigate against unwanted injury to the marginal mandibular branch of the facial nerve or facial artery. Many surgeons do not embrace gland resection due to complexity and risks, and a simpler surgical method of addressing an enlarged or ptotic gland is to suspend the gland or tighten the overlying platysma to support the gland in a more superior position [29]. Neuromodulator can be injected into the gland, which can shrink the gland non-surgically. This is a temporary solution, and reinjection is required to maintain results every 6 months.

Most commonly, surgeons focus on fat and platysma muscle modification to improve an obtuse neck. Fat is

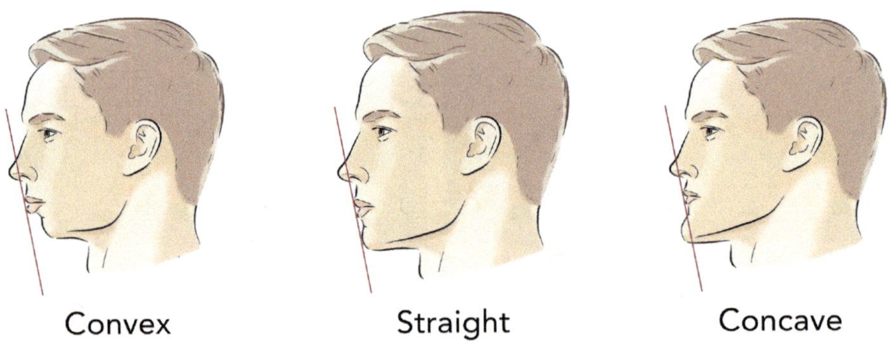

FIG. 6 There are 3 basic facial profiles, convex, straight, and concave. The lower face profile can be assessed with Reidel's Plane, which is a line that connects the most prominent portion of the upper and lower lips and touches the soft tissue menton. If the chin falls behind this line, it indicates that there is microgenia and chin augmentation is warranted.

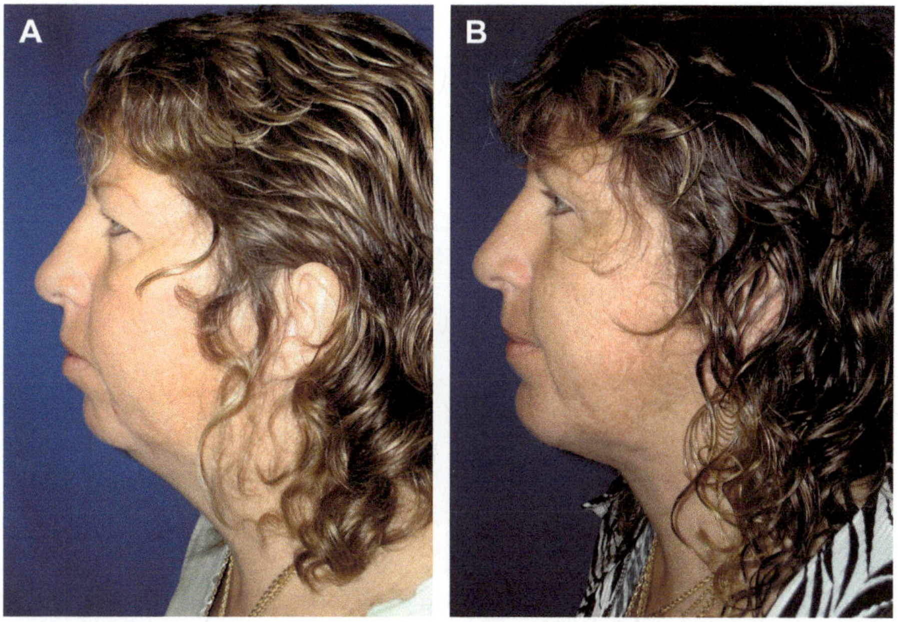

FIG. 7 (*A*) This before image of a patient with a challenging neck exhibited microgenia and underwent a facelift and a chin implant to improve her cervicomental region. (*B*) After facelift and chin implant.

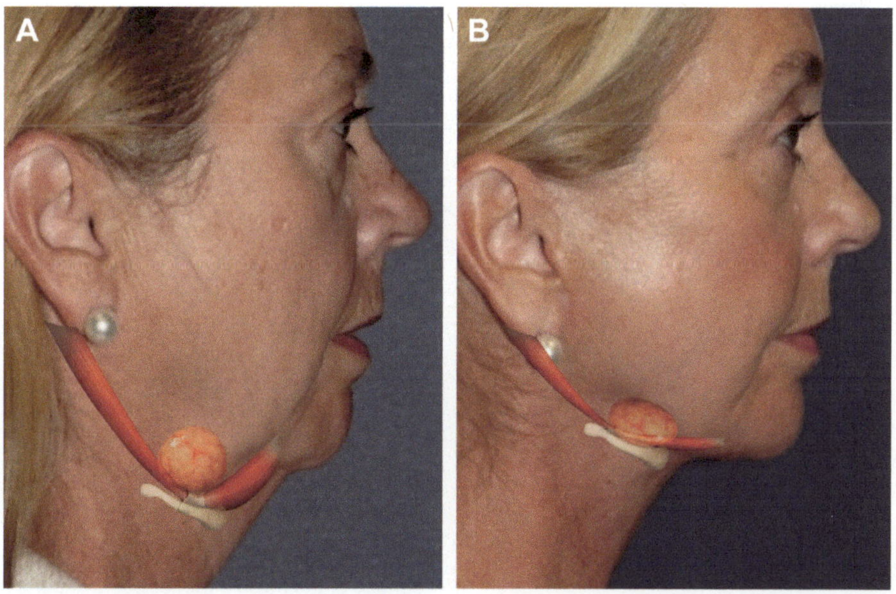

FIG. 8 (*A*) The overlay diagram shows enlarged submandibular glands, anterior digastric muscles, and malposition of the hyoid bone that contribute to an obtuse cervicomental angle in this 62-year-old female. (*B*) The overlay diagram shows the reduced submandibular gland and anterior digastric muscles with repositioning of the hyoid with the digastric plication 18 months after high superficial musculoaponeurotic system face-lift, microfat grafting, chin implant, and deep cervicoplasty. (Thomas Gerald O'Daniel, Optimizing Outcomes in Neck Lift Surgery, Aesthetic Surgery Journal, 41 (8), August 2021, 871–892, https://doi.org/10.1093/asj/sjab056.)

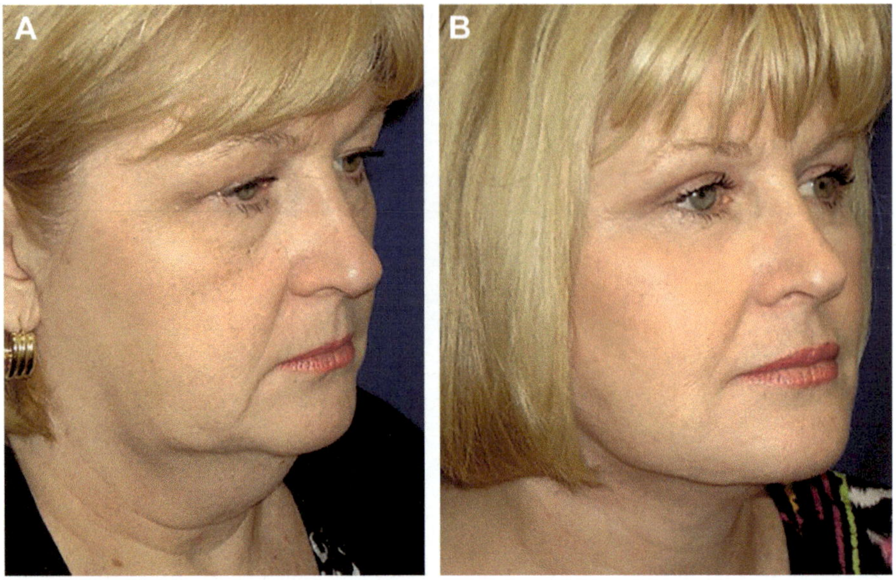

FIG. 9 (*A*) An anterior or low hyoid bone in addition to bulky anterior digastric muscles and large or ptotic submandibular glands can all contribute to an obtuse neck and poor cervicomental angle as seen in this patient. Conservative shaving of the anterior portion of the muscle debulks this fullness and can be accomplished through the incision in the mental crease, creating a more defined and smooth area under the chin. Glands can be resuspended, reduced, or even injected with a neuromodulator to improve jawline contour. Before facelift. (*B*) After facelift.

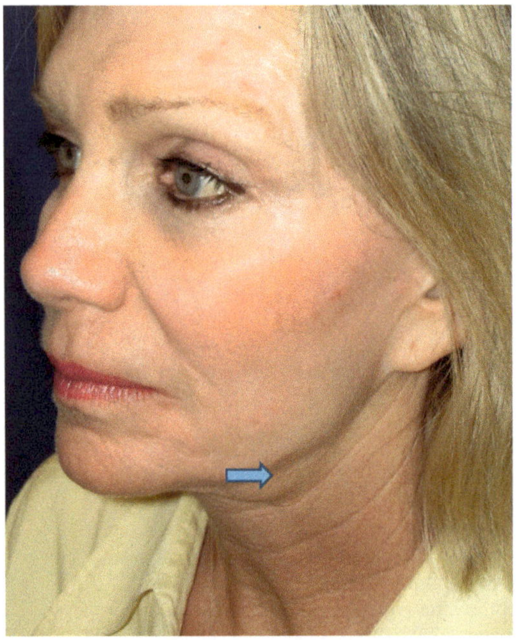

FIG. 10 Example of ptotic submandibular glands causing a bulge under the jawline.

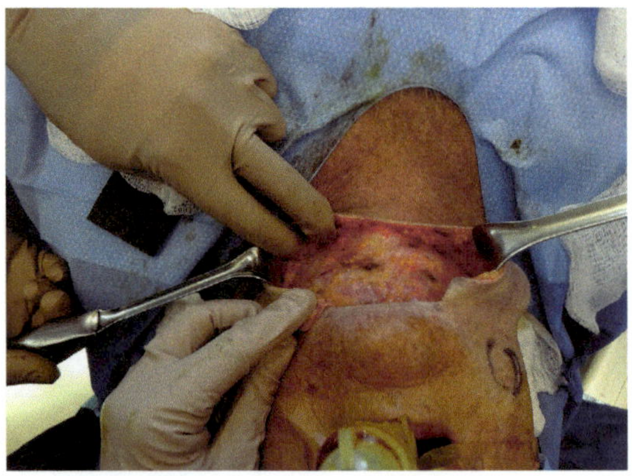

FIG. 11 Fat should be gently cleaned off the anterior surface of the muscle with scissors under direct visualization to allow accurate approximation of the midline muscle. This is in an intraoperative view an open neck during a w-plasty showing the platysma muscle and the decussation of the muscle at the hyoid bone prior to a corset suture of the bands If present, they should be sutured in the midline, except when they are very fine and the skin thin, in which cases the suture might be visible under the skin surface.

present in varying quantities in the subcutaneous, supra-platysma plane, or deeper in the sub-platysma zone. Various fatty deposits must be reduced, including not only the fat between the platysma muscle and skin but also below the platysma. Fat removal can be achieved with liposuction performed through a small, 2 mm submental incision in the submental crease. Fat reduction alone may be sufficient to restore desirable submental definition, particularly in patients under the age of 35 with good skin elasticity and tone. The author prefers direct fat excision over liposuction, as it is more precise. Direct fat debulking is performed though a 2 cm submental incision and this allows direct visualization of the fat and platysma muscle and is more accurate in fat debulking and preserving the thin underlying muscle from inadvertent liposuction trauma. Fat is easily removed with a facelift scissors peeling fat pearls off the underlying muscle (Fig. 11). This creates a clean platysma muscle and visualization of bands, which can be plicated if necessary. Jowl fat can also be sculpted with scissors under direct view from a lateral, pre-auricular incision. Conservative removal of jowl fat improves the jawline contour, but care should be taken to stay above the muscle layer to avoid weakness to the marginal mandibular area and unwanted lip paralysis.

Many heavy necks also have excess deep fat, which is located below the platysma muscle. This can be assessed prior to surgery by palpation, but direct visualization during surgery is most accurate. While pre-platysma fat can be suctioned, exploring below the platysma requires direct visualization because it is more vascular. To access this deep submental fat, the platysma muscle must be incised in the midline to expose to fat deep to the muscle. This oval shaped fat compartment can be robust and has 3 distinct compartments, central, medial, and lateral [30]. Selective removal of sub-platysma fat can further improve an obtuse jaw angle, and this deep fat should be removed carefully with scissors and meticulous bipolar cautery. Full central removal of this fat may occasionally be necessary to achieve a more defined jaw-neck angle [23,25]. (Fig. 12) The underlying mylohyoid muscle can be seen centrally with fat removal and dissections can be carried laterally below the 2 leaflets of the vertical platysma bands.

The platysma muscle should be addressed with a tightening procedure, either in the midline, laterally or both. The decision on how and where to manipulate the platysma is open to much debate. The author recommends an anterior platysma corset suture if there are bands noted on physical examination or seen during surgery through the submental view. An exception is if the bands are fine and the skin is thin, then an anterior platysma suture is not performed to limit creating a bulky suture line visible through the thin skin. If platysma bands are present, then the neck should be opened and explored under direct visualization through an incision in the submental crease. Platysma bands are identified, cleaned, and trimmed and sutures together in the midline with an anterior platysmaplasty using a running, locking 3-0 Vicryl suture (Fig. 13). The author's preferred method is to start superiorly at the top of the submental area and run the suture inferiorly to the

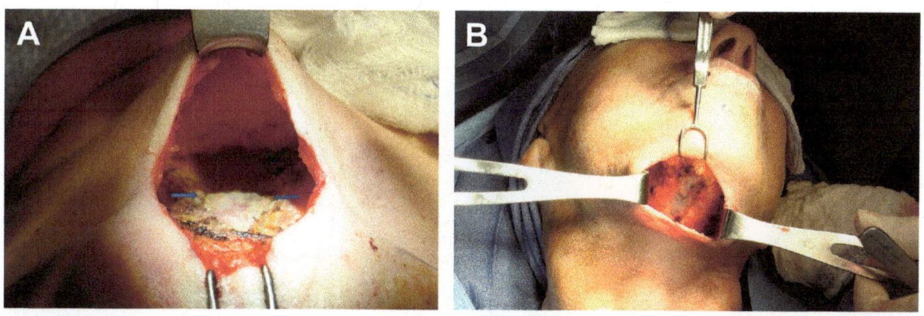

FIG. 12 (*A*) This view is from the submental incision exposing the cut edges of the platysma and area where the subplatysmal fat is located. The arrows indicate edges of platysma and debulked deep fat with exposure of the mylohyoid muscle. Subplatysma fat is oval shaped and has 3 parts: central, middle, and lateral. The platysma is opened in the midline to gain access, and careful removal can be conducted to create a sharper jaw angle. The fat is most prominent in the midline and is laced with blood vessels, necessitating diligent cautery. The platysma is sutured back over the reduced fat pocket in the midline with a running corset to create a smooth and youthful neck. (*B*) Anterior view of subplatysma fat reduction between the 2 medial defined edges of the platysma muscle in the midline.

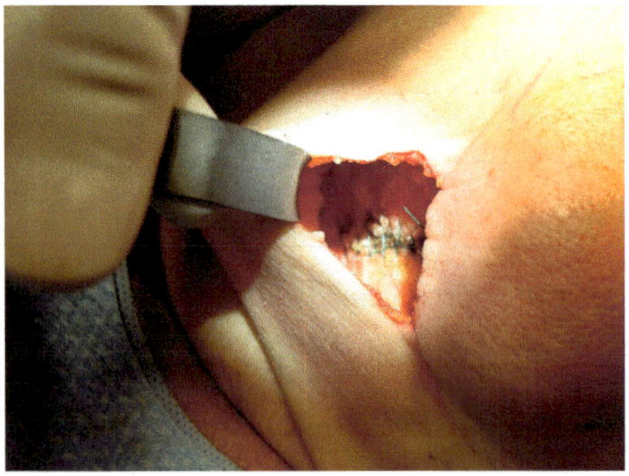

FIG. 13 The platysma is sutured in the midline with a running, locking 3-0 dissolvable suture, starting at the superior aspect from the submental incision.

thyroid cartilage and then return the suture superiorly back into the submental area, where it is tied off on itself. Small, 1 cm back cuts are placed with a cutting cautery at the lower edge of the platysma bands to help prevent band recurrence.

Lastly, skin texture and tone are critical factors in achieving an aesthetically pleasing face and neck lift result. Thick, sebaceous, elastic, and resilient skin with good recoil will yield a better result than those with thin, atrophic skin. Poor skin recoil to palpation, excessive laxity, and wrinkling can be challenging. Fine vertical neck wrinkles present at rest are a sign of poor skin tone, and the potential for relapse of loose neck skin after surgery. In more extreme cases, patients with excessively stretchy skin as seen in individuals with rare connective tissue disorders such as Ehlers-Danlos Syndrome should be counseled on the likelihood of recurrent skin laxity and can be poor candidates for cosmetic surgery. Excessive loose skin can be removed and re-draped; however, skin wrinkling and relapse of hanging skin must be discussed with the patient. Secondary tuck up surgeries performed within the first 2 years to remove lax sub-mental skin is a distinct possibility and should be addressed prior to surgery. These enhancement procedures are typically performed at a discounted price from the original surgery. If the submental skin redundancy is mild, a "T" crop surgery with direct skin removal can be used in the appropriate patient who is willing to accept a small anterior neck scar (Fig. 14).

An assessment of all the contributing factors allows the surgeon to best match the most appropriate procedure that will yield higher patient satisfaction. There are a wide variety of choices in rejuvenation of the jaw line, and this decision is based on anatomic knowledge, a thorough examination, and sound surgical principles, as well as an understanding of the typical aging changes anticipated at various milestones. Surgical corrections for obtuse lower face rejuvenation often involve anterior platysmaplasty, with sub-platysma fat removal for heavy necks. It is important to preserve facial fat while removing fat below the jaw line to restore a more defined cervico-mental angle. An aesthetically pleasing jaw angle can be achieved in challenging necks with conservative surgery addressing the various anatomic elements involving the bone, platysma, fat compartments, muscle, and skin (Fig. 15).

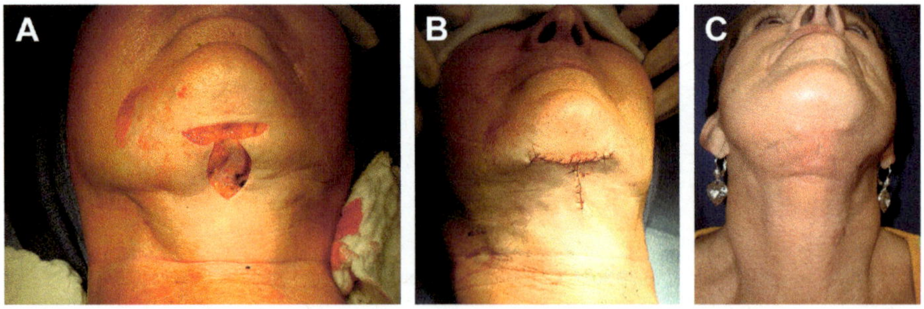

FIG. 14 (*A*) A "T-crop" excision can be an option to remove redundant skin under the chin in cases where there is residual sin laxity after a facelift. A T shape is marked starting in the submental crease and then a vertical portion is added to remove an ellipse of redundant skin. Excision of the skin allows easy access to the tissues in the submental region. The patient should be aware of a more visible scar. Direct exposure of the neck allows the surgeon a second opportunity to further tighten the platysma, shave the anterior digastric muscles, or remove residual fat. (*B*) Sutured T crop incision. (*C*) Final scar under chin from T crop.

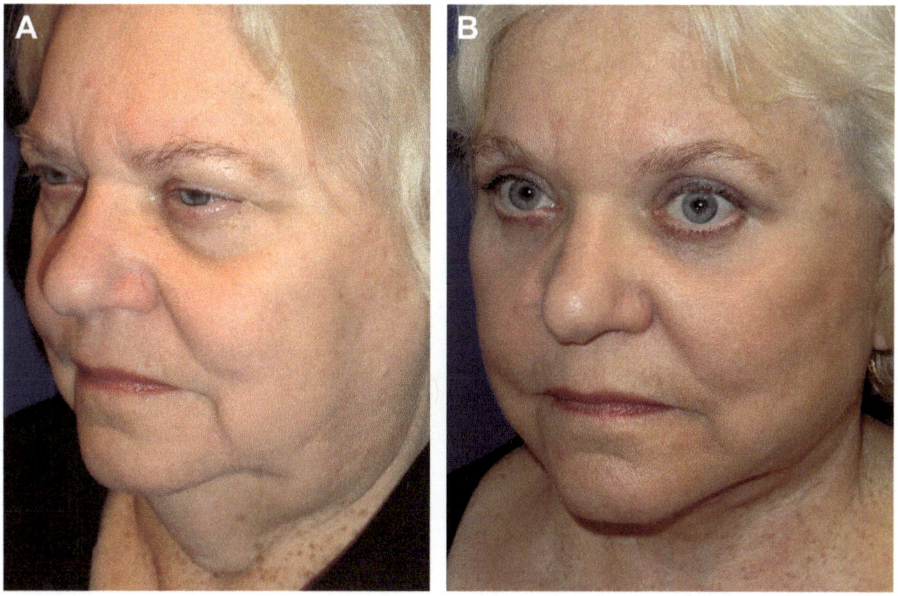

FIG. 15 (*A*) This challenging facelift patient had an obtuse neck. (*B*) She achieved a nice result by addressing all components of her full neck.

CLINICS CARE POINTS

Meeting expectations is the greatest challenge and a thorough assessment, and patient goals should be reviewed before surgery to match the best procedure to the patient's needs.

- The male facelift is more challenging due to several factors including larger heads, a robust blood supply to the beard causing more bleeding, and medicines which increase bleeding such as testosterone and sildenafil (Viagra).
- Nicotine and marijuana should be discontinued prior to surgery to enhance healing.
- Blood thinners should be stopped prior to surgery with the guidance of a clearance doctor, who also maximizes blood pressure.
- Weight loss drugs such as semaglutide should be stopped 3 weeks prior to surgery to improve gastric emptying and reduce pulmonary aspiration.
- An obtuse neck is a challenging facelift patient, and many anatomic structures need to be addressed during surgery. These include excess fat in both the pre- and sub-platysma planes, laxity of the platysma corrected with a midline platysma corset suture, heavy anterior digastric muscles shaved in select cases, and submandibular gland fulness identified. A low or anterior hyoid bone may also create an obtuse cervicomental angle and this can be improved with surgical maneuvers.
- Excessive skin laxity should be identified prior to surgery and the patients counseled of the potential for skin relapse under the chin and correct adjunctive procedures, such as a "T" crop.

DISCLOSURE

The authors have nothing to disclose.

REFERENCES

[1] Ellenbogen R, Karlin J. Visual criteria for success in restoring the youthful neck. Plast Reconstr Surg 1980; 66(6):826–37.
[2] ASPS (American Society of. Plastic Surgeons), Aesthetic plastic surgery stats. Aesthetic society procedural statistics 2023.
[3] Parikh S, Jacono A. Deep-plane face-lift as an alternative in the smoking patient. Arch Facial Plast Surg 2011; 13(4):283–5.
[4] Lu YH, Mahajan L, Rudy H. Patterns of marijuana use and nicotine exposure in patients seeking elective aesthetic procedures. Plast Reconstr Surg 2024;154(3): 478e–85e.

[5] Couto RA, Charafeddine A, Sinclair NR, et al. Local infiltration of tranexamic acid with local anesthetic reduces intraoperative facelift bleeding: a preliminary report. Aesthet Surg J 2020;40(6):587–93.
[6] Couto R, Charafeddine E, Zins J. Facelift in patients with massive weight loss. Clin Plast Surg 2019;46(4):559–71.
[7] Narasimhan K, Ramanadham S, Rohrich R. Face lifting in the massive weight loss patient: modifications of our technique for this population. Plast Reconstr Surg 2015;135(2):397–405.
[8] Fezza R, Rains B, Fezza T, et al. Emerging anesthesia risks with semaglutide. Plast Reconstr Surg Glob Open 2023;11(11):e5427.
[9] Skouras G, Skouras A, Skoura E. Revision and secondary facelift: problems frequently encountered. Plast Reconstr Surg Glob Open 2020;8(8):e2947.
[10] Wong AWJ, Fu-Chan W. Should we view the "Vessel-Depleted neck" as just a challenging neck? Plast Reconstr Surg 2024;154(3):628e–9e.
[11] Dibbs R, Chamata E, Ferry A, et al. Revision facelift and neck lift. Semin Plast Surg 2021;35(2):88–97.
[12] Cummins A, Surek C, Charafeddine A, et al. Facelift surgery following superficial parotidectomy: is it safe? Aesth Plast Surg 2020;44(2):354–8.
[13] Fezza J, Woodward J. Quantifying skin removal during a face-lift: does the approach matter? Dermatol Surg 2022;48(3):304–9.
[14] Foissac R, Colson T, Camuzard O, et al. Characteristics of the male facelift. Rev Laryngol Otol Rhinol (Bord) 2014;135(4–5):181–6.
[15] Connell B, Ana S. Male face lift. Aesthetic Surg J 2002;22(4):385–97.
[16] Fedok F, Chaikhoutdinov I, Garritano F. The difficult neck in facelifting. Facial Plast Surg 2014;30(4):438–50.
[17] Roy S, Buckingham E. The difficult neck in facelifting. Facial Plast Surg 2017;33(3):271–8.
[18] Smith R, Papel I. Difficult necks and unresolved problems in neck rejuvenation. Clin Plast Surg 2018;45(4):611–22.
[19] Marten T, Feldman J, Connell B, et al. Treatment of the full obtuse neck. Aesthetic Surg J 2005;25(4):387–97.
[20] Auersvald L, Auersvald A. The short neck: challenges and techniques. Facial Plast Surg 2022;38(6):650–67.
[21] Buschang PH, Fretty K, Campbell PM. Can commonly used profile planes be used to evaluate changes in lower lip position? Angle Orthod 2011;81(4):557–63.
[22] Guyuron B. Genioplasty. Plast Reconstruct Surg 2008;121(4):1–7.
[23] O'Daniel T. Optimizing outcomes in neck lift surgery. Aesthetic Surg J 2021;41(8):871–92.
[24] Le Louarn C. Hyo-neck lift evolution: neck lift with fixation of the platysma to the deep cervical fascia. Ann Chir Plast Esthet 2018;63(2):164–74.
[25] Feldman J. Neck lift my way; an update. Plast Reconstr Surg 2014;134(6):1173–83.
[26] Ramirez O. Cervicoplasty: nonexcisional anterior approach. Plast Reconstr Surg 1997;99(6):1576–85.
[27] Basaran K, Comert M. Ligasure-assisted submandibular gland excision in deep plane neck lift: review of 83 patients. Plast Reconstr Surg 2024. https://doi.org/10.1097/PRS.0000000000011419.
[28] Auersvald A, Auersvald LA. Innovative tactic in submandibular salivary gland partial resection. Plast Reconstr Surg Glob Open 2015;2(12):e274.
[29] Jacono A, Alemi S, Harmon AN. The effect of a novel platysma hammock flap during extended deep plane facelift on the signs of aging in the neck. Aesthet Surg J 2022;42(8):845–57.
[30] Rohrich R, Pessa J. The subplatysmal supramylohyoid fat. Plast Reconstr Surg 2010;126(2):589–95.

Advances in Cosmetic Surgery 8 (2025) 61–67
ADVANCES IN COSMETIC SURGERY

Chin Augmentation

Arianna Strome, MD[a], Alexa B. Steuer, MD, MPH[b], Susruthi Rajanala, MD[b], Jeffrey S. Dover, MD, FRCPC[b,c,d,*]

[a]The Ronald O. Perelman Department of Dermatology at NYU Langone Health, 240 East 38th Street 11th and 12th Floors, New York, NY 10016, USA; [b]Department of Dermatology, SkinCare Physicians, 1244 Boylston Street, Chestnut Hill, MA 02467, USA; [c]Department of Dermatology, Yale University School of Medicine, New Haven, CT, USA; [d]Department of Dermatology, Brown Medical School, Providence, RI, USA

KEYWORDS

• Chin augmentation • Dermal fillers • Hyaluronic acid fillers

KEY POINTS

- The appearance of the chin plays a key role in overall facial balance.
- Traditional procedures, such as chin implants, osseous genioplasties, and autologous grafting, may augment the appearance of the chin; however, they are invasive and associated with risks and down-time.
- Hyaluronic acid fillers are a safe and well-studied treatment to optimize chin dimensions and alignment.
- While injection techniques vary, most injectors target the pogonion, menton, and prejowl sulci for an overall positive augmented effect.

INTRODUCTION

The chin is one of the key features for overall facial appearance and symmetry [1]. Appearance of the chin, and its relationship to and proportionality with surrounding facial structures and to the neck are paramount to overall aesthetic balance [2]. Patients may present with concerns, for example, of a large nose, sagging neck, or jowls, failing to recognize the deficiency is lack of proportionality and alignment of the chin [1,3]. Herein, we will review the considerations and current practices for chin augmentation. We include a brief overview of surgical techniques such as alloplastic implants, autologous grafts, and osseous genioplasty and have focused on less invasive approaches, namely dermal fillers, for a more in-depth discussion of procedural technique.

Anatomic Considerations

The bony anatomy of the chin is defined by the underlying mandibular structure [4]. This provides the backbone for the anatomic planes of the chin, including projection, height, and width. The pogonion is the most anterior-projecting portion of the chin [3,5]. The height of the chin is defined by the menton, the most inferiorly projecting skeletal portion of the chin [3,5]. The midpoint between the pogonion and the menton is the gnathion [3]. The paragonion protrudes on the lateral sides of the pogonion and defines chin width [5]. These surface landmarks that define the chin compartment demarcate it from the jowl and submental compartments [3]. The muscles of the chin include the depressor anguli oris, depressor labii inferioris, and the centrally paired mentalis. The mental arteries serve as

*Corresponding author. SkinCare Physicians, 1244 Boylston Street, Suite 103, Chestnut Hill, MA 02467. *E-mail address:* jdover@skincarephysicians.net

https://doi.org/10.1016/j.yacs.2025.01.006 www.advancesincosmeticsurgery.com
2542-4327/25/

ABBREVIATIONS

3D	3-dimensional
ACRS	Allergan Chin Retrusion Scale
HA	hyaluronic acid

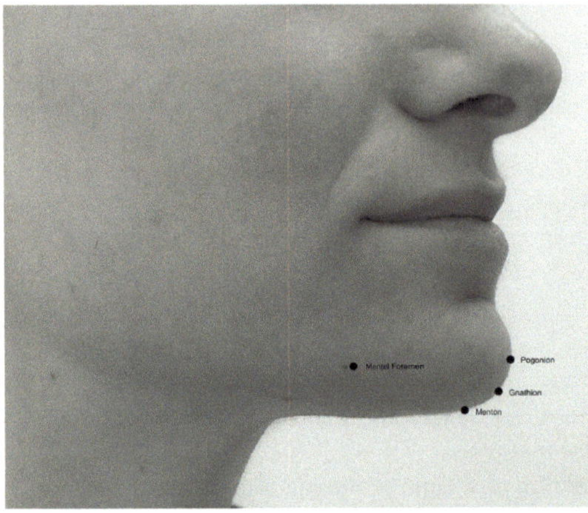

Anatomic Considerations in Chin Augmentation

the primary blood supply to the chin, exiting via the mental foramina on the lateral chin at the second bicuspid [3]. The inferior labial artery, labiomental artery, and submental artery also provide anastomotic arterial supply [3]. Finally, the inferior alveolar nerve which travels through the mandible and exits as the mental nerve provides the primary innervation to the chin and lower lip [1,3].

Options for Chin Augmentation

Alloplastic implant

Alloplastic surgical chin implantation has been cited as the most studied technique of chin augmentation [6]. It is well-suited for addressing inadequate chin projection; however, it is a suboptimal option for patients without adequate chin height or with chin asymmetry [1,7]. The procedure is safe and offers a permanent surgical option for chin augmentation [7,8]. Various materials may be used, available in different sizes and readily customizable to fit patient characteristics. For example, customized 3-dimensional (3D) printed implants are options to address mandibular asymmetries, though they may come at a higher financial burden. It is, nonetheless, an invasive surgical procedure, carrying risks of surgical intervention including hematomas, scar, hypergranulation for oral incisions, dehiscence, and infection [9,10]. Silicone implants, which are frequently used, can be associated with bone resorption, as well as dental erosion depending on its placement [6]. This may be obviated through fixation to the bone with a screw to prevent motion at the interface of the bone and implant. Over time, there is a low risk of malpositioning and displacement of the implant. Overall, however, when executed and secured properly, there is a very low complication rate for solid silicone implants.

Osseous genioplasty

Osseous genioplasty is a surgical technique that can address complex deformities of the chin, with the ability to augment all planes including projection, height, and width [11]. It affords a permanent solution to microgenia [11]. This procedure involves an osteotomy with intraoperative chin advancement and fixation with metal hardware in order to reapproximate the chin [11]. When compared with the alloplastic implant, an osseous genioplasty is a more invasive, complex technique with longer recovery time [1,6]. In addition to the invasiveness of this approach, the complexity of the procedure lends itself to being less commonly performed [1,6,11].

Autologous grafts

Autologous grafts may also be used in the correction of chin deformities. Bone grafts may be obtained for augmentation purposes if patients are undergoing an additional procedure. Fat grafting may be performed as a single intervention or adjunctive to an alloplastic implant or osseous genioplasty [6]. Fat grafting offers the ability to augment the chin in all 3 planes, however, patients with significant retrognathia are not good candidates. This is because excessive volume correction, for example, a projection change greater than 3 to 5 mm, can lead to chin ptosis [12]. The less invasive nature has increased attractiveness to patients; however, the procedure can fail to produce reliable outcomes due to variable graft survival [3,11,13]. In addition, a prospective study reported a 17.7% mean fat resorption rate at 6 months, regardless of what fat volume was injected [6,13]. Therefore, it is not a permanent solution and if used alone, will require patients to undergo repeated treatments over time.

Dermal fillers

According to the American Society for Plastic Surgery, surgical chin augmentations are down 38% compared with the year 2000 [3]. Although the reasons for this decline are multifaceted, in part, it is likely attributable to the increasing popularity of less invasive modalities, such as dermal fillers [3,5,6,14]. Dermal fillers are able to shape the chin in all 3 planes thus treating chin retraction, horizontal and height deficiencies, and asymmetry. While various dermal fillers are available, hyaluronic acid (HA) fillers are especially popular, as they offer the benefit of being a simple outpatient procedure, and reversibility in the event of complications or patient dissatisfaction. Furthermore, an added benefit of fillers is the ability to trial augmentation of the chin in a nonpermanent fashion to preliminarily assess the esthetic effect prior to a permanent implantation. Dermal fillers also often come at a lower financial burden to patients as compared with surgical interventions. While fillers are designed to last up to 2 years, in our experience chin filler often lasts much longer [6]. Filler injections are generally safe and well-tolerated, with adverse effects mainly limited to pain, redness, bruising, and swelling which subside within several days of the injections [14,15]. Severe reactions are rare and will be elaborated on further below.

TREATMENT SELECTION

Advantages and disadvantages exist for each of the options for chin augmentation. Ultimately, treatment selection is influenced by both the practitioner's evaluation of the patient, comfort with various procedures, and the patient's individual desire. Facial and plastic surgeons, for example, may be more accustomed to alloplastic chin implants, whereas dermatologists are more apt to recommend soft tissue fillers [16]. This, combined with a patient's tolerance for down-time and/or willingness to undergo a surgical procedure requiring general anesthesia, should be considered alongside the anatomic considerations and specific chin deformity when electing the appropriate augmentation technique [16].

PROCEDURAL TECHNIQUE: INJECTABLE FILLERS

Preoperative Planning

A full evaluation of the chin includes its relation to the nose, lips, teeth, and neck, as well as all components of skin and supporting skeletal, muscular, and soft-tissue structures [3,16]. Physical examination should include facial evaluation both at rest and in motion [3,16,17]. Photographs of at least 3 views should be obtained, including the profile bilaterally, oblique views bilaterally, and a frontal view [16,17]. The chin itself should be evaluated in all anatomic dimensions of projection, height, and width. There are several guidelines that can be used to evaluate ideal chin projection. The Gonzalez-Ulloa line, for example, is a vertical line that extends from the nasion downward, perpendicular to the Frankfurt plane (a line from the inferior orbital rim to the superior margin of the external auditory meatus) [4]. The ideal chin projection according to this evaluation should meet or fall just short of this line [3,4]. A simpler method describes that for men, the chin pogonion projection should be in line with the lower lip vermillion border, whereas in women, it should be 1 to 2 mm behind the lower lip vermillion border [2,3]. With regard to width, the ideal proportions for women are in line with the width of the medial canthi, and for men are in line with the oral commissures [3]. Regarding chin height, the ideal facial alignment should be divided into equal thirds: hairline to nasion, nasion to subnasale, and subnasale to menton [2,3].

In addition to anatomic considerations, a detailed history, including clinical history, past trauma, orthodontic treatment, or oral surgery is essential. History of any prior injectable treatments and response to treatments should also be elicited [3,17]. Clinicians should also inquire about any upcoming dental procedures or procedures that may have occurred in the preceding week, as some recommend postponing injections to minimum 1 week, and sometimes 2 weeks, from any dental procedures.

Prep and Patient Positioning

Prior to injection, any makeup should be removed. Topical anesthetic cream may be applied, if the patient desires, 30 to 40 minutes prior to injection; however, is not a necessity for all patients. A semirecumbent position may be comfortable for patients, as well as provide a posterior support for the head throughout the procedure, in order to minimize movement. The areas to be injected should then be carefully cleansed with an antiseptic solution (such as chlorhexidine or isopropyl alcohol).

Procedural Approach

The selection of the filler used should allow for both structural support but also appear natural with muscular contraction [18]. An ideal filler for the chin has a high G prime (G′) to improve shape in 3D proportions but also flexibility to conform to facial movement [2,16–18]. G refers to the firmness or elasticity of the filler, and products with higher G′ tend to recoil to their original shape, which allows for structural integrity in this location [19]. Currently, the Food and Drug Administation (FDA) has approved 2 dermal fillers for use in the chin—Juvederm Voluma XC (Allergan plc, Dublin, Ireland) and Restylane Defyne (Galderma, Uppsala, Sweden) [20].

There are many different approaches to chin augmentation with filler, and ultimately, the injector's preference and practices will influence product selection, as well as injection technique. Centrally, filler injections into the chin are performed in a layer deep to the mentalis muscle, usually with a bolus technique using a needle, as opposed to a cannula. Several smaller supraperiosteal depots injected lateral to the midline to both round out the chin, as well as create a smooth transition are also commonly performed [2,3]. The prejowl sulcus can be addressed with subdermal fanning of the filler, either with a needle and massage, or with cannula [3,5,17,18,21–23]. Manual molding frequently throughout the procedure for further shaping of the area being treated is often recommended [17,24]. Care should be taken to avoid the mental foramen, through which the mental nerve, artery, and vein traverse, which can be found approximately 1.5 cm superior to the mandibular border in line with the first and second premolar [24]. In addition, when injecting in the peri-jowl region or on the mandibular body, care should be taken to avoid the facial artery [17,22]. One must be mindful that the facial artery crosses the inferior border of the mandible anterior to the insertion of the masseter, running deep and branching into the superior and inferior labial arteries [3,17,22]. In the area of the lateral jawline, it can be avoided by injecting in a subdermal plane [22].

Immediate Postprocedural Care

While injecting and immediately afterward, it is important to observe the color of the skin. Indications of an abnormal reaction might include sudden pain, local blanching, or livedo. In any of these instances, injections should be stopped for rapid reassessment and intervention. Otherwise, firm pressure, with a folded gauze and flat palm, may be applied to the injection area to control any mild local, pinpoint bleeding. Cold compresses may be applied for pain relief and to minimize bruising [5]. Patients should be made aware that bruising and swelling may occur, in addition to a sensation of soreness in the area, sometimes pronounced with mastication when injecting on or near the jawline. This will typically resolve within several days to 1 week.

CLINICAL RESULTS IN THE LITERATURE

There is a relative paucity of comparative evidence between the various modalities of chin augmentation, and among the different injectable fillers. A recent systematic literature review examining studies of HA filler for chin augmentation found overall high patient satisfaction among 917 patients included across all studies, with a relatively low complication rate [14].

Vanaman and colleagues described their experience with high-viscosity HA dermal fillers (Restylane Lyft; Galderma SA, Lausanne, Switzerland; Juvederm Voluma XC, Allergan, Inc, Parsippany-Troy Hills, NJ, USA), in addition to calcium hydroxyapatite fillers (Radiesse (+), Merz North America, Inc, Raleigh, NC, USA) in a review of chin augmentation [3]. Their techniques employed no more than 1 to 2 mL of filler total with supraperiosteal injections performed with a needle in the midline, several smaller supraperiosteal depots lateral to the midline to round out the chin. Cannula was employed if softening of the prejowl sulcus was necessary [3].

One study aimed to assess the use of a chin and jawline grid as a guide to nonsurgical treatment with a high G′, high cohesivity filler. In addition to the grid guideline, this study employed cannula technique among 30 patients, injecting 0.1 to 1.5 mL of filler in the chin apex, 0.3 to 0.7 mL to the labiodental sulcus, and 0.1 to 1.5 mL along the jawline. Ninety-six percent of patients rated their appearance after treatment as "much improved" or "very much improved" [22].

In another international study, Chen and colleagues employed a stepwise specified injection technique using a high elasticity HA injectable for chin augmentation. In this retrospective study among 326 patients, HA filler was first injected supraperiostially at the paragonion close to the inferior border of the mandible and roughly perpendicular to the nasal alar or medial canthus with a 27-gauge needle [5]. This was followed by needle bolus at the pogonion. Finally, a 25-gauge, 3-cm cannula, and fanning technique were used at the junction of the pogonion, menton, and paragonion to increase volume and smoothen [5]. Similarly, for individuals with a prejowl sulcus, a cannula was used to inject filler for softening. In this study, with a mean injection volume of 1.85 mL of HA filler, the shape and contour of the chin was significantly improved in all patients with durable improvement at 6-month follow-up by the authors.

Beer and colleagues aimed to assess the effectiveness and safety of VYC 20-L (Juvederm Voluma XC; Allergan plc, Dublin, Ireland) to address volume deficit and retrusion in the chin and prejowl sulci using an evaluator-blinded delayed treatment-controlled study design [23]. Assessments were performed at 6 months and 12 months, including both treatment-blinded investigator and participant assessments and self-assessments. 27G one-half-inch needles were used for supraperiosteal and/or subcutaneous injections into the pogonion, menton, and prejowl sulci, along with 25G 1.5 inch cannulas in the menton and prejowl sulci. Almost all patients (99.3%) were treated at the pogonion, 77.8% at the menton, and 87.5% at the prejowl sulci, with an average treatment volume of 2.6 mL for initial treatment, and 1.4 mL for follow-up treatment. Injection volumes were similar among treatment and nontreatment participants. Participants were deemed responders if they had at least a 1-point improvement in their Allergan Chin Retrusion Scale (ACRS) score, which was observed in 56.3% of the treatment group at 6 months (P=.0019). The evaluating investigators rated 91.2% of participants as "improved" or "much improved" in the treatment group at 6 months with durable results at 12 months. Approximately 87% of participants in the treatment group rated themselves as "improved" or "much improved" at 6 months [23].

Marcus and colleagues employed similar methods to assess Restylane Defyne (Galderma, Uppsala, Sweden) for augmentation and correction of chin retrusion [18]. In this randomized, evaluator-blinded, parallel group, nontreatment-controlled study across 11 centers, 107 patients with mild to moderate chin retrusion were treated, with 33 nontreatment controls. Follow-ups were performed at 3 days, 12, 24, 36, and 48 weeks after treatment. Injections were performed using a 27G one-half inch needle with the investigator's chosen technique. Responders were participants with a greater than 1-point improvement from baseline on the Galderma Chin Retrusion Scale and esthetic improvement was also assessed using the Global Aesthetic Improvement Scale by evaluators and patients alike. The mean total volume injected was 3.6 mL including initial treatment and 4-week touch up. Injections at both the pogonion and the surrounding areas were performed using both serial puncture and/or linear retrograde, and specifically at the pogonion, supraperiosteal depot technique was used, with a mean treatment volume of 1.67 mL. Eighty-one percent of the treatment group were rated responders at 12 weeks (P<.001), with high patient satisfaction rates. Ninety-six percent of treatment participants remained improved at 48 weeks. [18].

A prospective, single-blinded, randomized controlled study across 10 international sites was performed to assess the safety and effectiveness of VYC-25L (Juvederm Volux; Allergan plc, Dublin, Ireland) in restoring and creating facial volume in subjects with chin retrusion [21]. Treatments were performed using a 27G 13 mm needle according to investigator's evaluation and technique. Subjects were seen at 1, 3, 6, 9, and 12 months for safety and effectiveness visits and 3 and 14 days for safety visits. Here, the primary effectiveness was determined through computer-facilitated programmed image analysis comparing the mean change from baseline between treatment and controls in the glabella-subnasale-pogonion angle. Secondary effectiveness was esthetic improvement as rated by investigators and subjects using the Global Aesthetic Improvement Scale (GAIS) as well as 3 Facial Appearance, Quality of Life, and Adverse Events (FACE-Q) scales. Among 90 subjects in the treatment group and 29 subjects in the control group, treatment characteristics were similar with nearly all receiving initial treatment at the pogonion, mentum, and prejowl sulci and 76% receiving treatment at the sublabial crease. Treatment volumes were also similar in both groups with 2.28 mL in the treatment group on average at initial treatment, and 1 mL at 1-month touch-up on average. The mean change in the glabella-subnasale-pogonion angle was 2.12° in the treatment group compared with −0.38° in the control group at month 3, and this gradually declined over time in both groups but remained 1.28° at 12 months for the treatment group. Over 90% of subjects had improved/much improved GAIS scores and responses on FACE-Q Satisfaction and Psychological Well-Being Scales [21].

Overall, while comparative studies are lacking, published data show safety and efficacy of high G′ filler targeting the pogonion, menton, and pre-jowl sulci to smoothen the chin and improve retrusion. Further large-scale and comparative trials are needed to help further guide technique and product selection.

POTENTIAL COMPLICATIONS AND MANAGEMENT

Common complications encountered with dermal fillers include injection site reactions such as bruising, swelling, pain, and erythema [3,5,14]. Across these studies in the literature, the majority of patients experienced mild to moderate injection site reactions immediately following the injection, such as some tenderness at the site, and less frequently erythema or swelling [5,18,21–23]. A minority of patients experienced asymmetry following filler injections, which can be addressed through filler correction of asymmetry and/or neurotoxin injections into the mentalis. This may improve the esthetic appearance and also the longevity of the filler [5]. Treatment-related adverse events, such as delayed nodules, and more rarely infection, have been cited in a handful of patients [21,23]. When present, hyaluronidase can be used for delayed-onset nodules and as shown improvement [21].

Serious complications are rare; however, the most severe potential risk of injections is vascular compromise either secondary to intra-arterial injection, injection-related edema, or arterial compression [25]. Although exceedingly rare, it has been reported to occur on several occasions [12,26–28]. Risk of vascular compromise can be mitigated by periosteal injections and careful consideration of the anatomy, particularly near the mental foramen, while the chin is not considered a high risk area traditionally, there can be considerable variation and anastomoses in this region and prompt recognition and management of occlusion are essential [26]. This should be addressed with the injection of the area with ample hyaluronidase, and simultaneous massage, warm compresses, and possibly topical nitroglycerin [5,25]. The patient should be continuously assessed until the color and pain improves in the region, as repeat cycles of hyaluronidase injections, massage, and topical therapies may be necessary. It may be beneficial to have the patient remain in the office for at least 30 minutes to be re-evaluated and confirmed safe by the physician before they leave [5].

SUMMARY

Chin augmentation can be accomplished by a variety of surgical and minimally invasive techniques. HA fillers are a safe and well-studied treatment to optimize chin dimensions and alignment. Providers should select a high G′ and high cohesivity filler to provide appropriate structural support to the region. While injection techniques can vary, most injectors target the pogonion, menton, and prejowl sulci to create shape and balance and inject more deeply centrally and more superficially in the subcutaneous region moving more laterally. Chin filler injections can be performed safely with careful consideration of the location and depth of vessels, but swift recognition and management of potential vascular occlusion is also critical. Future research can help elucidate optimal filler choice and injection strategies to minimize occlusion risk.

CLINICS CARE POINTS

- Optimizing chin shape and structure plays a key role in facial balance, symmetry, and youthfulness. While several invasive techniques can help to augment the chin, hyaluronic acid fillers are a minimally invasive and low risk treatment option.
- Proper anatomic evaluation and assessment of chin position is crucial for procedural planning. High G′ and high cohesivity fillers such as Restylane Lyft, Defyne or Contour, and Juvederm Voluma or Volux offer the necessary firmness and structure needed to support the chin.
- Chin filler treatments are tolerated well overall, with swelling and bruising being the most common adverse events. While rare, vascular occlusion must be promptly identified and managed.
- While clinical studies evaluating filler overall show efficacy and high treatment satisfaction, further large-scale comparative studies are needed to elucidate product choice and ideal treatment techniques to enhance esthetic outcome and minimize risks.

DISCLOSURE

Dr J.S. Dover is a consultant to Revance, AbbVie and Galderma and the SkinCare Physicians research department has had research funded by AbbVie, Revance, and Galderma.

REFERENCES

[1] Sykes JM, Fitzgerald R. Choosing the best procedure to augment the chin: is anything better than an implant? Facial Plast Surg 2016;32:507–12.
[2] Sykes JM, Suárez GA. Chin advancement, augmentation, and reduction as adjuncts to rhinoplasty. Clin Plast Surg 2016;43:295–306.
[3] Vanaman Wilson MJ, Jones IT, Butterwick K, et al. Role of nonsurgical chin augmentation in full face rejuvenation: a review and our experience. Dermatol Surg 2018;44:985–93.
[4] González-Ulloa M, Stevens E. The role of chin correction in profileplasty. Plast Reconstr Surg 1968;41:477–86.
[5] Chen B, Ma L, Wang J. Chin augmentation with hyaluronic acid: an injection technique based on anatomical morphology. Dermatol Surg 2022;48:747–51.
[6] Oranges CM, Grufman V, di Summa PG, et al. Chin augmentation techniques: a systematic review. Plast Reconstr Surg 2023;151:758e–71e.
[7] Newberry CI, Mobley SR. Chin augmentation using silastic implants. Facial Plast Surg 2019;35:149–57.
[8] Liao CD, Rodriguez E, Zhao K, et al. Complications following alloplastic chin augmentation: a systematic review of implant materials and surgical techniques. Ann Plast Surg 2023;90:S515–20.
[9] White JB, Dufresne CR. Management and avoidance of complications in chin augmentation. Aesthet Surg J 2011;31:634–42.
[10] Sharma EM, Smith KD. Facial implants. In: StatPearls. Treasure Island (FL): StatPearls Publishing LLC.; 2024.
[11] Chan D, Ducic Y. A simplified, reliable approach for advancement genioplasty. JAMA Facial Plast Surg 2016; 18:114–8.

[12] Wang Q, Guo X, Wang J. Autogenous fat grafting for chin augmentation: a preliminarily clinical study of cosmetic outcome. J Craniofac Surg 2015;26:e625–7.

[13] Basile FV, Basile AR. Prospective controlled study of chin augmentation by means of fat grafting. Plast Reconstr Surg 2017;140:1133–41.

[14] Ou Y, Wu M, Liu D, et al. Nonsurgical chin augmentation using hyaluronic acid: a systematic review of technique, satisfaction, and complications. Aesthetic Plast Surg 2023;47:1560–7.

[15] Guo Y, Wang J, Wei W, et al. Treatment of chin retrusion with botulinum toxin plus hyaluronic acid filler in comparison with hyaluronic acid filler alone: a randomized, evaluator-blinded, controlled study. Aesthet Surg J 2024; 44:537–44.

[16] Chin OY, Sykes JM. Optimizing the chin and jawline appearance: does surgery or injection make sense? Facial Plast Surg 2019;35:164–71.

[17] Braz A, Eduardo CCP. Reshaping the lower face using injectable fillers. Indian J Plast Surg 2020;53:207–18.

[18] Marcus K, Moradi A, Kaufman-Janette J, et al. A randomized trial to assess effectiveness and safety of a hyaluronic acid filler for chin augmentation and correction of chin retrusion. Plast Reconstr Surg 2022;150:1240e–8e.

[19] Fagien S, Bertucci V, von Grote E, et al. Rheologic and physicochemical properties used to differentiate injectable hyaluronic acid filler products. Plast Reconstr Surg 2019;143: 707e–20e.

[20] USFDA Administration, Available at: https://www.accessdata.fda.gov/scripts/cdrh/devicesatfda/index.cfmstart_search=1&Search_Term=lmh&Approval_Date_From=&Approval_Date_To=&sort=approvaldatedesc&PAGENUM=10.

[21] Ogilvie P, Sattler G, Gaymans F, et al. Safe, effective chin and jaw restoration with VYC-25L hyaluronic acid injectable gel. Dermatol Surg 2019;45:1294–303.

[22] Bertossi D, Robiony M, Lazzarotto A, et al. Nonsurgical redefinition of the chin and jawline of younger adults with a hyaluronic acid filler: results evaluated with a grid system approach. Aesthet Surg J 2021;41:1068–76.

[23] Beer K, Kaufman-Janette J, Bank D, et al. Safe and effective chin augmentation with the hyaluronic acid injectable filler, VYC-20L. Dermatol Surg 2021;47:80–5.

[24] Moradi A, Shirazi A, David R. Nonsurgical chin and jawline augmentation using calcium hydroxylapatite and hyaluronic acid fillers. Facial Plast Surg 2019;35: 140–8.

[25] Cohen JL, Biesman BS, Dayan SH, et al. Treatment of hyaluronic acid filler-induced impending necrosis with hyaluronidase: consensus recommendations. Aesthet Surg J 2015;35:844–9.

[26] Yuan JT, Chang TW, Yu SS, et al. Mental artery occlusion from poly-L-lactic acid injection at the lateral chin. Dermatol Surg 2017;43:1402–5.

[27] Fang M, Rahman E, Kapoor KM. Managing complications of submental artery involvement after hyaluronic acid filler injection in chin region. Plast Reconstr Surg Glob Open 2018;6:e1789.

[28] Yang Y, Zhou G, Chen K, et al. Super-selective intra-arterial dissolution therapy for lingual artery occlusion resulting due to the use of hyaluronic acid for chin augmentation: the first reported case. J Cosmet Dermatol 2022;21: 3358–61.

Advances in Cosmetic Surgery 8 (2025) 69–76
ADVANCES IN COSMETIC SURGERY

Lasers and Lights for Acne

Alexa B. Steuer, MD MPH[a], Susruthi Rajanala, MD[a], Nazanin Saedi, MD[b,c], Jeffrey S. Dover, MD, FRCPC[a,d,e,*]
[a]SkinCare Physicians, Chestnut Hill, MA, USA; [b]Department of Dermatology, Thomas Jefferson University, PA, USA; [c]Dermatology Associates of Plymouth Meeting, Plymouth Meeting, PA, USA; [d]Department of Dermatology, Yale University School of Medicine, New Haven, CT, USA; [e]Department of Dermatology, Brown University Medical School, Providence, RI, USA

KEYWORDS
• Acne • Light therapy • Laser therapy • 1726 nm laser

KEY POINTS
- Light and laser therapies for acne represent viable independent and adjunctive treatment options, for those in whom topical and systemic therapies have been inadequate or are otherwise intolerable or contraindicated.
- There are several forms of light therapy and lasers that have shown effectiveness in treating active acne through targeting *Cutibacterium acnes*, the sebaceous glands, or both.
- To maximize safety and efficacy, knowledge of appropriate laser science and parameters, in addition to careful patient evaluation and selection, is essential.

INTRODUCTION: INNOVATIVE MODALITIES FOR THE TREATMENT OF ACTIVE ACNE

Acne vulgaris is the most common skin condition in the United States, affecting 85% of individuals aged 12 to 24 and approximately 50% of adults [1,2]. In addition to the physical manifestations, it is a condition that carries with it significant psychosocial morbidity [3,4]. The pathogenesis is multifactorial, involving increased sebum production, proliferation of *Cutibacterium acnes*, inflammation, and hypercornification of the pilosebaceous unit [5].

Standard treatments for acne include topical and systemic medications, employed in an escalating manner tailored to the level of disease activity. These may include topical retinoids, benzoyl peroxide, topical antimicrobials, in addition to systemic antimicrobials, hormonal therapy, and retinoids. Patients with moderate-to-severe acne that persists despite standard therapy and/or those who may have contraindications or intolerances to systemics, such as isotretinoin, light-based therapies, photodynamic therapy (PDT), and lasers, have been used [2,3].

Light and laser therapies may be divided based on their ability to target *C acnes*, the sebaceous gland, or both [4]. Light therapies, such as red light and blue light, or the combination of the two, tend to involve specific porphyrins that selectively absorb various wavelengths of light, subsequently causing bacterial destruction. In addition to *C acnes*, destruction of the sebaceous glands occurs through this same principle during PDT. The efficacy of lasers, however, is based on the theory of selective photothermolysis, whereby brief pulses of optical radiation are selectively absorbed by a target chromophore with preferential absorption of a specific wavelength [6]. This causes selective tissue injury of the target chromophore, while sparing surrounding structures [6].

*Corresponding author. SkinCare Physicians, 1244 Boylston Street, Suite 103, Chestnut Hill, MA 02467. *E-mail address:* jdover@skincarephysicians.net

https://doi.org/10.1016/j.yacs.2024.12.001 **www.advancesincosmeticsurgery.com**
2542-4327/25/

ABBREVIATIONS	
ALA	aminolevulinic acid
FDA	Food and Drug Administration
FST	Fitzpatrick skin type
IGA	Investigator Global Assessment
IPL	intense pulsed light
KTP	potassium titanyl phosphate
MAL	methyl aminolevulnate
Nd:YAG	neodymium-doped yttrium aluminum garnet
PDL	pulsed dye laser
PDT	photodynamic therapy

Several lasers have been used with variable success in the treatment of active acne, including fractionated carbon dioxide (CO_2), potassium titanyl phosphate (KTP), infrared, pulsed dye laser (PDL), neodymium-doped yttrium aluminum garnet (Nd:YAG), diode, Erbium glass, and Alexandrite lasers [3]. The pain associated with some of these treatments and variable effectiveness is a barrier for many of these devices. This occurs due to their lack of selectivity and the absorption of light by water [7]. Through study of the absorption spectrum of sebum, it was determined that 1726 nm exhibited 1.2 times the optical absorption in sebaceous glands as compared to water [8]. Light absorbed at this wavelength selectively destroyed sebaceous glands alone, while sparing the surrounding epidermis [2,8]. More recently, 1726 nanometer (nm) lasers have been approved by the US Food and Drug Administration (FDA) for the treatment of moderate-to-severe acne.

Herein, the authors outline the procedural techniques and data for these newly approved 1726 nm lasers. They also provide a brief overview of other light and laser therapies for acne.

PROCEDURAL TECHNIQUE

Preoperative Planning

Prior to any procedure, it is important for the clinician to engage in a detailed discussion of the risks, benefits, side effects, and possible outcomes for the procedure. Traditionally, lasers and light therapies have been considered for patients with moderate-to-severe acne after topical and oral medication failure. It is especially important in these patients to set expectations, as many patients do see improvement, but there are still some who do not [4]. In addition, multiple treatments are almost always required, necessitating consideration from a logistical as well as financial perspective. After thorough discussion, the patient should sign an informed consent documenting that this pretreatment discussion occurred, and he/she consents to proceed. A series of standardized pretreatment and posttreatment photographs should be taken for assessment, ideally including frontal, 45° and 90° angles at baseline, pretreatment, and follow-up using consistent camera settings.

The choice of device depends on both availability to the practitioner and patient characteristics. Factors to consider when selecting a device include the patient's Fitzpatrick skin type (FST), the area affected by active acne, and the presence or absence of acne scarring. For example, for a patient with a lighter skin type and involvement of the back, light-based therapies that can target a larger surface area more efficiently might be selected. With regard to 1726 nm lasers, the 2 devices that are currently FDA-approved are the AviClear Laser System (Cutera, Inc.) and the Accure Laser System (Accure Acne Inc.) [5]. To date, there are no studies that directly compare the AviClear and Accure lasers. The AviClear device is a 1726 nm diode laser that uses a 3 mm spot size and contact cooling [5]. The Accure device is a 1726 nm fiber laser with forced air cooling that employs an infrared camera for continuous epidermal temperature monitoring, in order to allow for treatment to a peak epidermal temperature (40–46°C) as an objective clinical endpoint [5]. Both devices are FDA approved to treat acne in all skin types. The Accure device notably has 2 modes that differ in that one utilizes injectable anesthesia (the "Standard Mode"), while the other (the "Boost Mode") utilizes topical anesthesia and a proprietary pulsing method [5].

Preparation and Patient Positioning

The patient should lie in a comfortable position for the treatment, ideally slightly supine so that the clinician may readily access all areas of the face. The area should be cleansed with an antiseptic agent (ie, alcohol or chlorhexidine). For the 1726 nm lasers, degreasing with acetone should also be performed [1,2]. In the experience of the authors, a brief period (3–5 minutes) of water-moistened gauze is applied to the face in order to cool the area prior to lasing. The area should be dried prior to beginning the administration of laser pulses. All standard laser safety precautions should be in place (including eye shields for the patient, goggles for the clinicians, and closed-door examination room with signage indicating lasing in process).

In terms of selection of laser parameters, the studies that have been performed with the AviClear laser employ a fixed 3.1 mm spot size, with fluences ranging from 10 to 60 J/cm^2 and a pulse duration ranging from 10 to 60 ms [1,2]. In one study including patients FST II-VI, an average fluence of 20.5 J/cm^2 and 22.8 J/cm^2 for single and double pulse, respectively, was used, with a maximum pulse duration of 50 ms. [2].

Procedural Approach

Once laser parameters are chosen, the patient is in the appropriate position, and all safety precautions are in place, laser pulses should be administered using the appropriate settings. Unlike other lasers, there is no visible clinical endpoint with the 1726 nm lasers. AviClear treats to a target fluence and Accure treats to a target epidermal temperature, both correlating to sebaceous gland destruction [5]. Laser pulses are administered with the tip in full contact with the skin for the duration of the pulse, as well as the precooling and postcooling. Pulses are administered by treating one area and moving on immediately to the next adjacent area until the whole face is treated, without any double pulses. A single pass over the entire face represents one treatment. The duration of each treatment is approximately 30 minutes [5].

Immediate Post-Procedural Care

There are no necessary interventions immediately post-procedurally. Cold compresses or gel packs may be applied for comfort. Avoidance of heat sources (such as hot tubs or saunas) for 1 to 2 days after treatment is recommended, as well as limiting exercise on the day of treatment to avoid generating heat in the skin. Skin irritants like retinols, benzoyl peroxide, and salicylic acids should be avoided for approximately 1 week before and after treatment. Gentle skin care should be emphasized, with use of a gentle skin cleanser and moisturizer 1 to 2 times daily for approximately 3 to 5 days after treatment. Of paramount importance is sun protection. Sunscreen, ideally a mineral-based sunscreen with SPF 30 or higher, may be applied immediately after treatment and should be applied daily, in addition to avoidance of direct sun exposure. This is especially important in the week or 2 after treatment given the vulnerability of the skin after laser treatments.

CLINICAL RESULTS IN THE LITERATURE

This section details the variety of laser and light-based devices used for management of acne and is supported by a comprehensive literature review. It should be noted that while there is sufficient literature supporting use of each of the devices discussed, large-scale comparative and consensus data are limited given variation in study protocols, treatment regimens, and lack of standardized outcome measures for acne improvement [9,10].

Lights

Photodynamic therapy

PDT is the oldest light-based acne treatment and as such has the greatest body of supportive evidence, especially for patients who are nonresponders or have a contraindication to isotretinoin [11]. PDT involves application of a photosensitizer (such as topical aminolevulinic acid [ALA] or methyl aminolevulnate [MAL]) that is then photoactivated, resulting in singlet oxygen and free radical damage that is toxic to *C acnes* and sebaceous glands [4,12]. Hongcharu and colleagues demonstrated the effectiveness of topical ALA plus red light PDT in 22 subjects who received treatment on the back at 4 sites, including ALA plus red light, ALA alone, light alone, and untreated control [12]. They demonstrated both histologic changes in pilosebaceous units as well as decreased bacterial porphyrin fluorescence, sebum production, and acne in association with ALA PDT. These results, however, were achieved with significant side effects. Edema, erythema, and pain were common. Crusting and hyperpigmentation occurred, and in individuals who received multiple PDT treatments, over half had long-lasting hyperpigmentation at 20 weeks after treatment [12].

While various laser and light sources can be used as photosensitizers, a recent systematic review suggested that visible red light and intense pulsed light (IPL) treatments following a 1 hour incubation time are most efficacious [13]. A pilot study assessed utility of PDL-based PDT, using a 7.0 to 7.5 J/cm^2 fluence, 10 ms pulse duration, and 10 mm spot size. All 14 patients in the PDL-PDT treatment group cleared completely over a mean of 3 treatment sessions, compared to a mean of 32% lesion clearance in the PDL-only group and 20% lesion clearance in the standard of care group (topical therapies, oral antibiotics, and oral contraceptives) [14]. The most frequent adverse event and treatment limitation of PDT were patient discomfort. While MAL has been reported to be less painful compared to ALA, a recent study showed no significant difference in reduction of acne lesions for MAL-sensitized PDT versus red-light-only PDT [15].

PDT, and in particular ALA PDT, is an effective treatment of active acne; however, the side effect profile makes it a challenging modality for patients to tolerate throughout and immediately following the treatment. In addition, there are significant long-term side effects, including post-inflammatory hyperpigmentation, that require careful consideration prior to use in patients already prone to this adverse effect. Controlled trials are essential to prove efficacy with more gentle approaches affording this treatment the ability to be more widely applicable.

Red and blue light

LED red and blue light therapy have been FDA-approved for acne treatment since 2009 and work by destroying *C acnes* and activating cytokine release for an anti-inflammatory effect [4]. A recent review article comprising 38 studies found that overall 92% of patients experienced at least partial improvement in active acne lesions with visible light, with a minimal adverse event profile including mild skin irritation and erythema [16]. A randomized trial of 28 patients comparing the efficacy of red light versus blue light for mild-to-moderate acne found no significant difference in reduction of acne lesions between the 2 treatment groups, though the red light group had fewer adverse events (notably the red light group had no instances of hyperpigmentation) [17]. While twice-weekly regimens are standard for visible light therapy, a recent comparative study showed both once and twice weekly treatment protocols was equally effective at reducing inflammatory lesions [18]. Controlled trials, however, are lacking and the demonstrated utility of these treatments would benefit from comparison of red and/or blue light therapy to no-treatment controls to provide further insight.

Intense pulsed light

IPL devices emit polychromatic light, and the different wavelengths target various aspects of acne pathogenesis—namely destruction of sebaceous glands and reduction of *C acnes* colonization—ultimately leading to reduction of inflammatory acne lesions. Zdrada and colleagues assessed various skin properties in 27 patients following 4 weekly IPL treatments and found that sebum production decreased through IPL, while skin hydration and pigmentation remained unaffected [19]. A recent meta-analysis, though limited by variation in study protocol and patient selection, showed that IPL treatments were non-superior to PDL and Nd:YAG treatments. In addition, IPL had lower efficiency among darker FSTs with higher risk of adverse events [20]. Like other laser and light treatments, IPL can also be used as an adjunct to topical or oral therapies. A trial by Qu and colleagues compared use of minocycline along versus minocycline with a series of 3 IPL treatments. Results showed significantly improved inflammatory lesion count and decreased erythema in the combination treatment group [21]. Overall, while IPL is well tolerated and efficacious, providers should exercise caution in patients with darker skin tones.

Lasers

Pulsed dye laser

PDLs exert a multimodal therapeutic effect on acne lesions. The 595 nm infrared wavelength targets the vascular component of inflammatory lesions and may also exhibit an anti-inflammatory effect by activation of cytokines [4]. A prospective study of 41 adults with mild-to-moderate inflammatory acne assessed utility of low fluence PDL treatments (1.5–3 J/cm^2, 3 ms pulse duration, 5 mm spot size). Subjects were randomized to 4 sessions of PDL versus sham treatment. Results showed significantly greater reduction in active acne lesions in the treatment group, with greatest improvement after the first treatment [22]. Furthermore, PDL has effectiveness in adult female acne, whereby lesion count reduced anywhere from 49% to 92%, with an added benefit of improvement in erythematous acne scars [23]. A randomized study of 46 acne patients compared low-dose isotretinoin (0.25 mg/kg/day) versus standard-dose isotretinoin (0.5 mg/kg/day) plus 5 sessions of PDL (4.5–5.5 J/cm^2, 3 ms pulse duration, 10 mm spot size). Results showed significantly greater improvement in acne lesions in the PDL group versus standard of care, with fewer rebound flares and adverse effects [24]. Compared to IPL, PDL may also exert a more lasting effect on acne lesions. A split-face study by Choi and colleagues treated 20 patients at 2 week intervals for a total of 4 sessions (8–10 J/cm^2 fluence, 40 ms pulse duration, 10 mm spot size for PDL; 530–750 nm, 7.5–8.3 J/cm^2, 2.5 ms pulse duration, 2 passes for IPL). While both devices lead to initial improvement, the IPL-treated side showed significant rebound, while the PDL-treated side had lasting improvement in acne, with an average lesion count of 14% of baseline at the conclusion of the study [25]. Overall, through likely a multifactorial mechanism, PDL may be an effective modality for active acne, with little down time. Further studies are needed to determine how PDL compares to other treatments, as well as the parameters for this to be safely employed in darker skinned individuals.

Potassium titanyl phosphate

Similar to PDL, KTP lasers also target vasculature, sebaceous glands, and reduce *C acnes* counts [9]. Baugh and

Kucaba published a randomized split-faced study comparing KTP treatments (4 twice-weekly treatments; 12 J/cm^2 fluence, 30–40 ms pulse width, 50% overlap) to contact cooling only. While there was a statistically significant improvement in Michaelsson acne severity scores for the treated side at 1 week posttreatment, this effect was not sustainable at 4 weeks after the final treatment (patient satisfaction with treatment, however, remained high at this interval) [26]. A follow-up trial by Yilmaz and colleagues noted no significant difference in improvement of Michaelsson acne severity scores in once-weekly compared to twice-weekly regimens (5–12 J/cm^2, 20–40 ms pulse duration, 4 mm spot size) [27]. Taken together, this suggests that KTP lasers, in addition to IPL and PDL, are highly effective for erythema that may occur following acne. However, for KTP, the data for active acne treatment are limited.

Neodymium-doped yttrium aluminum garnet

While 1064 nm Nd:YAG lasers traditionally have been used for acne scar treatment, several studies support their role in treating active acne lesions. Gold and colleagues treated 100 patients with 650 ms Nd:YAG laser (28–64 J/cm^2 fluence, 2–3 mm spot size, pulse stacking with 5–15 pulses per lesion). Immediate improvement was noted in inflammatory lesions, and patients reported high satisfaction and found pain levels tolerable [28]. Bakus and colleagues treated 20 patients with moderate-to-severe inflammatory acne with 8 treatments of long-pulse Nd:YAG laser followed immediately by treatment with Q-switched Nd:YAG laser. At a minimum of 12 month follow-up, patients showed an 81% reduction in acne lesions, with 60% of patients having 90% or greater reduction, with no side effects other than transient erythema [29]. A recent randomized study compared use of long-pulse 1064 nm Nd:YAG with IPL treatment of active acne. Thirty patients were randomized into 2 groups and received 3 treatment spaced 2 weeks apart (settings of 40–50 J/cm^2 fluence, 40 ms pulse duration, 7 mm spot size for Nd:YAG, 7 J/cm^2 fluence, and 3 ms pulse width for IPL). Results showed significant improvement of overall lesions in the Nd:YAG group but not in the IPL-treated group. Furthermore, patients in the Nd:YAG group had more improvement in non-inflammatory lesions compared to inflammatory (P=.099), along with fewer rebound flares compared to the IPL group [30]. Another recent trial compared efficacy of Nd:YAG with PDL for inflammatory acne in a split-face design. Thirty-four patients received 3 treatments at 2 week intervals (8.5 J/cm^2 fluence, 10 ms pulse duration, 7 mm spot size for PDL, 30 J/cm^2 fluence, 5 ms pulse duration, and 7 mm spot size for Nd:YAG). Both sides were treated with a single pass and 10% overlap. Results showed no significant difference in reduction of acne lesions between the 2 treated sides; however, patients preferred Nd:YAG treatment due to fewer adverse events including erythema and swelling [31]. Case reports and smaller studies suggest that Nd:YAG lasers can successfully treat active acne with minimal side effects; however, controlled studies examining this modality are lacking.

A 650 microsecond pulsed Nd:YAG (Aerolase) has been shown to be effective for treating active acne. In a recent study, 23 patients (FST I-VI) with mild-to-severe acne received 5 treatments, 2 weeks apart and were followed 30 days and 90 days after the last treatment. The median percent reduction in lesion count was 48.15% after one treatment and 83.72% after treatment 3, and remained at 86.67% at 90 days. These treatments were well tolerated, and adverse events were not observed. Larger clinical trials with longer follow-ups are needed to evaluate the long-term efficacy of the device for acne.

Ablative lasers

While ablative resurfacing lasers are more commonly used in the treatment of acne scars than active acne lesions, the literature does support the use of fractional ablative lasers to target and destroy sebaceous glands, ultimately improving acne. A recent randomized split-face study compared use of fractional CO_2 (0.74 J/cm^2, 11.9% density) versus Nd:YAG laser (30–35 J/cm^2, 20 ms pulse frequency, 10 mm spot size) for inflammatory acne, with 4 treatment sessions spaced every 2 weeks. Results showed significantly greater improvement in Global Acne Severity scale for the lesions treated with CO_2 laser compared to Nd:YAG, with greater reported patient satisfaction [32]. A case series of 3 patients with treatment-resistant acne showed improvement with fractional Erbium:YAG laser resurfacing. Patients were treated every 3 months with the following settings: 3.5 mJ/cm^2, 1.5 ms pulse duration, and 5 Hz. Results showed significant improvement in Investigator Global Assessment (IGA) score in all patients, with all 3 scoring IGA 0 to 1 (clear to almost clear) at 3 month follow-up [33]. Although ablative modalities may be effective in achieving reduction in inflammatory lesion count, this treatment is aggressive and is of limited clinical practicality, especially with other less invasive and less risky treatment options available.

1726 nm lasers

Goldberg and colleagues studied the AviClear device in 17 patients and performed 3 treatments, spaced up to 7 weeks apart. Patients experienced a statistically significant reduction in inflammatory lesion count of 52% to 56% 4 to 12 weeks following treatment. At 24 months posttreatment, patients had a 97% reduction in inflammatory lesion count [1]. This was achieved without significant pain (mean of 4.9 out of 10 in discomfort score), with no use of topical anesthetic. Alexiades and colleagues treated a larger patient population of 104 individuals, FST II-VI, with 3 AviClear laser treatments, spaced approximately 1 month apart [2]. A greater than 50% reduction in active inflammatory lesions was seen in 32.6% of patients at 4 weeks, 79.8% of patients at 12 weeks, and 87.3% at 26 weeks. In comparison to baseline, with no subjects clear or almost clear, 36% and 41.8% were clear or almost clear at 12 week and 26 week follow-up, respectively. Patients tolerated the procedure with minimal discomfort and no topical anesthetic and there were no serious adverse events [2].

There are several institutional review board-approved clinical trials of the Accure laser. Preliminary and unpublished data demonstrated an 80% reduction in acne lesions among 12 patients noted 12 weeks after the fourth monthly treatment [5]. In 30 patients treated with the Standard Mode, all participants experienced a 50% reduction in acne lesions at 4, 8, 12, and 24 weeks after 4 monthly treatments, and a 90% decrease at 12 months. Side effects were similar to the AviClear laser, including erythema, edema, brief acne flares, and rarely dryness or crusting [5].

The newly approved 1726 nm lasers have demonstrated effectiveness in 2 controlled trials for the treatment of active acne. Further clinical experience and larger controlled trials will be beneficial to underscore the clinical utility of these devices.

POTENTIAL COMPLICATIONS/RISKS

When deciding which laser or light-based treatment to use, the practitioner must not only consider how to achieve the desired effects, but also be aware of potential side effects associated with general laser use, such as erythema, blistering, and burns. Patient tolerability is also a factor to consider, along with skin type and treatment area.

With both laser and light-based therapies, erythema has been cited as a commonly observed side effect. Light-based therapies, such as PDT, may also be associated with pain. In addition to these side effects, various lasers including CO_2, PDL, and Nd:YAG lasers have been shown to cause transient post-inflammatory hyperpigmentation, while infrared lasers and PDL may cause edema [9]. These side effects can be mitigated by tailoring appropriate energy setting and treatment procedures to achieve the desired outcome at minimal risk.

With regard to 1726 nm lasers, 2 studies including 17 and 104 participants, respectively, found mild erythema and edema to occur in nearly all patients [1,2]. Both typically resolved within hours to 3 days after the treatment [1,2]. In the smaller study, a minority of patients (29%, n = 5) experienced blistering in small areas of the treatment field, subsequently followed by scabbing, hyperpigmentation, and scarring. There was significant improvement by 3 months after the occurrence of all of these adverse effects, without intervention [1]. Among 104 patients who underwent treatment with a 1726 nm laser for acne, there was no incidence of vesiculation, blistering, scarring, or hyperpigmentation [2]. An acneiform flare-up occurred in 44% of patients; however, this was temporary, lasting 2 to 3 days prior to clearing [2].

SUMMARY

Lasers and light therapies can be highly effective in the treatment of active acne. Either as a monotherapy or in conjunction with various topicals and/or systemics, the data that are available highlight that these treatment modalities hold promise. Although the studies available have various limitations, including relatively small study sizes and a relative lack of directly comparative data between modalities, there is evidence to support a variety of light and laser therapies, many of which, such as PDT or PDL, have been utilized for other dermatologic indications for many years. It is important to carefully consider the patient's level of disease severity and skin type when selecting a device for treatment. While future studies may further elucidate long-term efficacy and side effect profile, the newly FDA-approved 1726 nm lasers show promising results for the effective treatment of acne across all skin types.

CLINICS CARE POINTS

- For patients with acne in whom compliance with topical medications poses an issue, or who cannot tolerate/prefer to avoid systemic medications, laser and light therapies should be considered.
- Light therapies, such as red and blue light therapy, tend to target *C acnes* and can be effective in

reducing inflammatory lesion count. PDT causes damage to *C acnes*, as well as sebaceous glands, and has proven effectiveness in improving acne. Side effects, however, are common, including pain, erythema, and edema, and long-term side effects, such as hyperpigmentation. IPL has also proven to be efficacious; however, clinicians should exercise caution regarding this modality in darker skin types.

- The newly FDA-approved 1726 nm lasers selectively target and destroy sebaceous glands and appear to be effective for the treatment of mild-to-severe inflammatory acne. They demonstrated a significant reduction in inflammatory lesion count in a manner that was generally very well tolerated by patients of all FSTs. Among lasers for active acne, these devices, in the authors' experience, may have the highest utility. Our clinical understanding will benefit from future larger studies and broader clinical experience.
- Several studies have demonstrated the ability of various lasers, namely PDL, KTP, fractionally ablative lasers, and Nd:YAG lasers to improve acne with durable results. Further studies including comparison to commonly used medical therapies for acne, as well as larger sample sizes, are needed.

DISCLOSURE

Drs Rajanala and Steuer have no disclosures. Dr Dover receives research funding from Cutera. Dr Saedi receives research funding from Aerolase.

REFERENCES

[1] Goldberg D, Kothare A, Doucette M, et al. Selective photothermolysis with a novel 1726 nm laser beam: a safe and effective solution for acne vulgaris. J Cosmet Dermatol 2023;22:486–96.
[2] Alexiades M, Kothare A, Goldberg D, et al. Novel 1726 nm laser demonstrates durable therapeutic outcomes and tolerability for moderate-to-severe acne across skin types. J Am Acad Dermatol 2023;89:703–10.
[3] Li MK, Liu C, Hsu JTS. The use of lasers and light devices in acne management: an update. Am J Clin Dermatol 2021;22:785–800.
[4] Mariwalla K, Rohrer TE. Use of lasers and light-based therapies for treatment of acne vulgaris. Laser Surg Med 2005;37:333–42.
[5] Bittar J, Hooper P, Dover JS. 1726 nm lasers for the treatment of acne vulgaris. Skin Therapy Lett 2024;29:5–7.
[6] Anderson RR, Parrish JA. Selective photothermolysis: precise microsurgery by selective absorption of pulsed radiation. Science 1983;220:524–7.
[7] Scopelliti MG, Kothare A, Karavitis M. A novel 1726-nm laser system for safe and effective treatment of acne vulgaris. Lasers Med Sci 2022;37:3639–47.
[8] Sakamoto FH, Doukas AG, Farinelli WA, et al. Selective photothermolysis to target sebaceous glands: theoretical estimation of parameters and preliminary results using a free electron laser. Laser Surg Med 2012;44:175–83.
[9] Goldberg DJ, Andriessen A, Bhatia AC, et al. Treatment of mild to severe acne with 1726 nm laser: a safe alternative to traditional acne therapies. J Cosmet Dermatol 2023;22:3026–32.
[10] Barbaric J, Abbott R, Posadzki P, et al. Light therapies for acne. Cochrane Database Syst Rev 2016;9:Cd007917.
[11] Riddle CC, Terrell SN, Menser MB, et al. A review of photodynamic therapy (PDT) for the treatment of acne vulgaris. J Drugs Dermatol 2009;8:1010–9.
[12] Hongcharu W, Taylor CR, Chang Y, et al. Topical ALA-photodynamic therapy for the treatment of acne vulgaris. J Invest Dermatol 2000;115:183–92.
[13] Boen M, Brownell J, Patel P, et al. The role of photodynamic therapy in acne: an evidence-based review. Am J Clin Dermatol 2017;18:311–21.
[14] Alexiades-Armenakas M. Long-pulsed dye laser-mediated photodynamic therapy combined with topical therapy for mild to severe comedonal, inflammatory, or cystic acne. J Drugs Dermatol 2006;5:45–55.
[15] Wojewoda K, Gillstedt M, Tovi J, et al. Optimizing treatment of acne with photodynamic therapy (PDT) to achieve long-term remission and reduce side effects. A prospective randomized controlled trial. J Photochem Photobiol, B 2021;223:112299.
[16] Akuffo-Addo E, Ramsay K, Mohsen S, et al. Visible light in the treatment of acne vulgaris. J Cutan Med Surg 2024;12034754241265697.
[17] Li J, Li J, Zhang L, et al. Comparison of red light and blue light therapies for mild-to-moderate acne vulgaris: a randomized controlled clinical study. Photodermatol Photoimmunol Photomed 2022;38:459–64.
[18] Nitayavardhana S, Manuskiatti W, Cembrano KAG, et al. A comparative study between once-weekly and alternating twice-weekly regimen using blue (470 nm) and red (640 nm) light combination LED phototherapy for moderate-to-severe acne vulgaris. Laser Surg Med 2021;53:1080–5.
[19] Zdrada J, Stolecka-Warzecha A, Odrzywołek W, et al. Impact of IPL treatments on parameters of acne skin. J Cosmet Dermatol 2022;21:2015–20.
[20] Lu L, Shi M, Chen Z. Efficacy of IPL therapy for the treatment of acne vulgaris: a meta-analysis. J Cosmet Dermatol 2020;19:2596–605.
[21] Qu H, Wang Y, Yang F, et al. A randomized, controlled trial of intense pulsed light in combination with minocycline hydrochloride for the treatment of inflammatory acne vulgaris. J Cosmet Dermatol 2022;21:3386–92.
[22] Seaton ED, Charakida A, Mouser PE, et al. Pulsed-dye laser treatment for inflammatory acne vulgaris: randomised controlled trial. Lancet 2003;362:1347–52.
[23] Communication P. Arielle Kauvar, MD. Controversies and conversations 2023;Vancouver, Canada.

[24] Ibrahim SM, Farag A, Hegazy R, et al. Combined low-dose isotretinoin and pulsed dye laser versus standard-dose isotretinoin in the treatment of inflammatory acne. Laser Surg Med 2021;53:603–9.
[25] Choi YS, Suh HS, Yoon MY, et al. Intense pulsed light vs. pulsed-dye laser in the treatment of facial acne: a randomized split-face trial. J Eur Acad Dermatol Venereol 2010;24:773–80.
[26] Baugh WP, Kucaba WD. Nonablative phototherapy for acne vulgaris using the KTP 532 nm laser. Dermatol Surg 2005;31:1290–6.
[27] Yilmaz O, Senturk N, Yuksel EP, et al. Evaluation of 532-nm KTP laser treatment efficacy on acne vulgaris with once and twice weekly applications. J Cosmet Laser Ther 2011;13:303–7.
[28] Gold MH, Goldberg DJ, Nestor MS. Current treatments of acne: medications, lights, lasers, and a novel 650-μs 1064-nm Nd: YAG laser. J Cosmet Dermatol 2017;16: 303–18.
[29] Bakus AD, Yaghmai D, Massa MC, et al. Sustained benefit after treatment of acne vulgaris using only a novel combination of long-pulsed and Q-switched 1064-nm Nd: YAG lasers. Dermatol Surg 2018;44:1402–10.
[30] Monib KME, Hussein MS. Nd:YAG laser vs IPL in inflammatory and noninflammatory acne lesion treatment. J Cosmet Dermatol 2020;19:2325–32.
[31] Chalermsuwiwattanakan N, Rojhirunsakool S, Kamanamool N, et al. The comparative study of efficacy between 1064-nm long-pulsed Nd:YAG laser and 595-nm pulsed dye laser for the treatment of acne vulgaris. J Cosmet Dermatol 2021;20:2108–15.
[32] Hammoda TM, Ahmed NA, Hamdino M. Fractional CO(2) laser versus 1064-nm long-pulsed Nd:YAG laser for inflammatory acne vulgaris treatment: a randomized clinical trial. Lasers Med Sci 2023;38:187.
[33] Guida S, Lippolis N, Giovani M, et al. Ablative fractional erbium:YAG laser resurfacing: a treatment option for acne. Dermatol Pract Concept 2022;12:e2022024.

Advances in Cosmetic Surgery 8 (2025) 77–85
ADVANCES IN COSMETIC SURGERY

Exosomes

What Is Going on?

Milan Minesh Hirpara, BA, Megan Nguyen, BA, Natasha Mesinkovska, MD, PhD*
Department of Dermatology, University of California, Irvine, 843 Health Sciences Road, Hewitt Hall 1001, Irvine, CA 92697, USA

KEYWORDS
• Exosomes • Extracellular vesicles • Regenerative medicine • Aesthetics • Wound healing • Pigmentation • Hair growth

KEY POINTS

- Exosomes, small extracellular vesicles, show potential in aesthetic medicine due to their role in cell communication and regeneration.
- The source of exosomes (eg, stem cells, blood, and adipose tissue) impacts therapeutic potential and safety.
- Current challenges include standardized exosome production, purity, and regulatory hurdles for clinical use.
- Despite promising preclinical results, there is need for rigorous clinical trials to confirm efficacy and safety.
- Food and Drug Administration (FDA) approval remains a major barrier, as exosome-based therapies currently lack regulatory clarity.

INTRODUCTION

Exosomes are nanoscale, endosomal extracellular vesicles (EVs) known for their role in facilitating intercellular communication. EVs are broadly classified into 3 main categories: exosomes (30–150 nm), microvesicles (100–1000 nm), and apoptotic bodies (50–5000 nm) (Fig. 1) [1]. These vesicles serve as carriers for a wide array of lipids, proteins, and nucleic acids, enabling the precise delivery of biological signals to recipient cells. Exosomes have drawn the greatest interest among EVs due to their small size and biocompatibility, elevating their potential as therapeutic agents.

The formation of exosomes begins with the invagination of the plasma membrane, resulting in the development of early endosomes that mature into multivesicular bodies (MVBs). These MVBs release exosomes into the extracellular space through fusion with the plasma membrane. Encased in a protective lipid bilayer, exosomes transport a specialized cargo of proteins and nucleic acids that have been recognized to be reflective of their cell of origin (Fig. 2). Moreover, MVB and exosome formation and release are primarily regulated through the endosomal sorting complexes required for transport (ESCRT) pathway, although ESCRT-independent pathways have also been proposed [1]. Therefore, ESCRT pathway proteins such as Alix, TSG101, HSC70, and HSP90β are expected to be found in exosomes regardless of their origin cell [1].

The biological function of exosomes is closely tied to their cellular source and determined by their cargo composition and downstream effects. Exosomes derived from mesenchymal stem cells (MSCs), keratinocytes, immune cells, endothelial cells, and platelets have distinct biochemical signatures and applications. For example, MSC-derived exosomes from sources such as adipose tissue, bone marrow, and umbilical cord are used to facilitate wound healing. Meanwhile, exosomes

*Corresponding author. *E-mail address:* natashadermatology@gmail.com

https://doi.org/10.1016/j.yacs.2024.12.005 **www.advancesincosmeticsurgery.com**
2542-4327/25/

ABBREVIATIONS

AA	alopecia areata
ADSC-Exos	adipose stem cell-derived exosomes
AGA	androgenetic alopecia
DPC-Exos	DPC-derived exosomes
DPCs	dermal papilla cells
ESCRT	endosomal sorting complexes required for transport
EVs	extracellular vesicles
HACS	human adipose tissue stem cell-derived exosome solution
HPE	human platelet extract
IL	interleukin
MITF	microphthalmia-associated transcription factor
MMP	matrix metalloproteinases
MSCs	mesenchymal stem cells
MVBs	multivesicular bodies
PI3K/AKT	phosphatidylinositol 3-kinase/ protein kinase B
PRP	platelet-rich plasma
TGF-β1	transforming growth factor beta-1
TNF-α	tumor necrosis factor alpha
TYR	tyrosinase
UCB-MSCs	umbilical cord blood mesenchymal stem cells

originating from endothelial cells are typically involved in angiogenesis signaling [1].

The process of isolating and purifying exosomes remains a technical challenge due to the heterogeneity of the exosome source. Several techniques are available for exosome isolation, including ultracentrifugation, ultrafiltration, polymer precipitation, and microfluidics-based methods (Fig. 3). Among these, ultracentrifugation is the most widely used approach as it separates exosomes based on size and density [1]. However, this method is time-consuming, costly, and may compromise the structural integrity of the vesicles. The choice of isolation technique must be tailored to the source of exosomes to ensure optimal recovery and preservation of functionality.

Despite these challenges, exosomes have emerged as valuable tools in therapeutic research and clinical applications. There is evidence that MSC-derived exosomes exhibit cardioprotective effects by improving cardiac function and lowering oxidative stress in myocardial ischemia-reperfusion models [2]. Similarly, exosomes from macrophages can enhance immune responses by presenting MHC class II molecules to activate antigen-specific T cells, currently evaluated for applications in infectious diseases such as tuberculosis [3].

The potential of exosomes in dermatology and in aesthetic medicine is only beginning to be explored. Emerging evidence highlights their role in key areas such as wound healing, skin rejuvenation, pigmentation modulation, and hair growth (Fig. 4). A critical evaluation of these applications centers on the underlying mechanisms of exosome function and reported

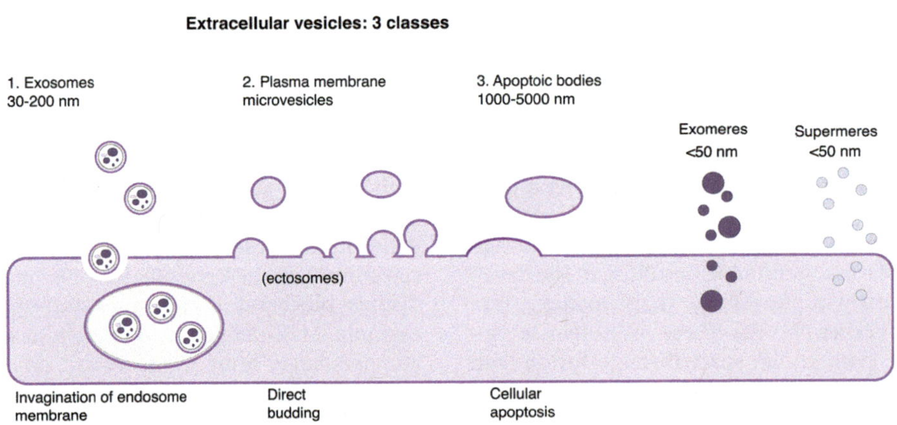

FIG. 1 Classification and biogenesis of EVs. Exosomes (30–150 nm) are formed through invagination of endosomal membranes, microvesicles (100–1000 nm), by direct budding of the plasma membrane, and apoptotic bodies (50–5000 nm) from cellular apoptosis. Smaller nanovesicle subtypes include exomeres (<50 nm) and supermeres (30–80 nm).

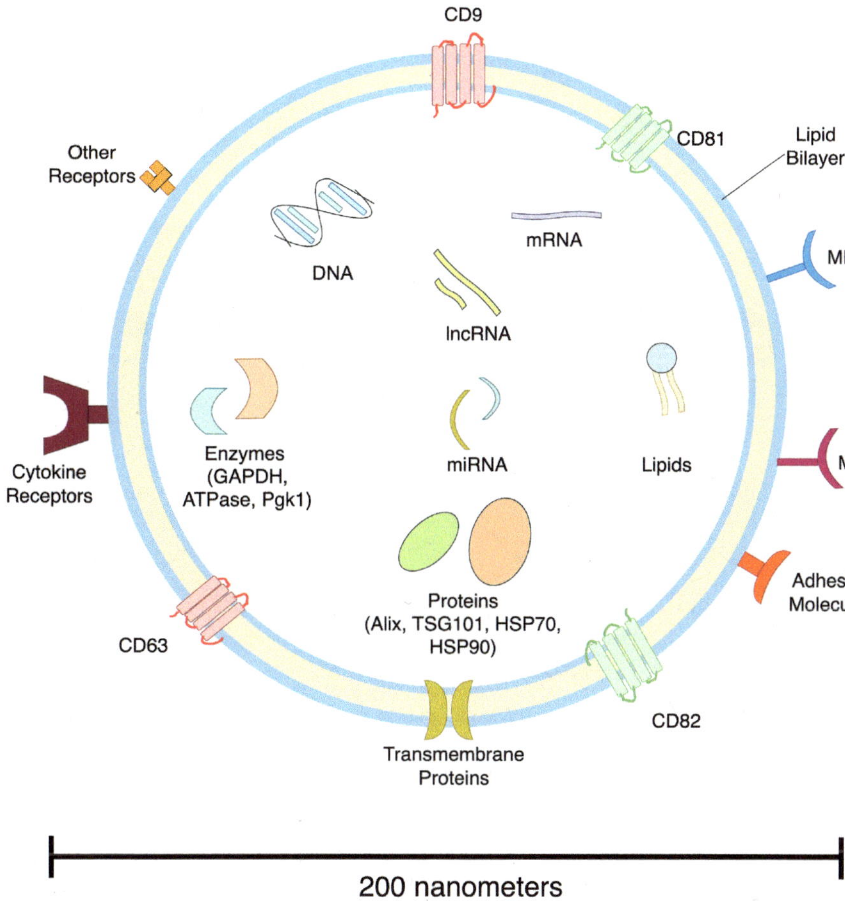

FIG. 2 Structural composition and molecular cargo of exosomes. The lipid bilayer-enclosed nanovesicles, containing diverse biomolecules derived from their parent cells. Key surface markers facilitate intercellular communication and antigen presentation. Contents of these nanovesicles include nucleic acids, lipids, enzymes, and biogenesis-associated proteins (ALIX, TSG101).

outcomes. Through their ability to mediate cellular communication and deliver targeted signals, exosomes hold the potential for many aesthetic therapeutic strategies. The current published data may have inherent biases favoring positive outcomes, emphasizing the need for more robust and substantiated clinical evidence to validate their efficacy and safety.

CLINICAL APPLICATIONS

Healing and Scar Remodeling

Wound healing is a dynamic and complex biological process involving multiple overlapping phases: inflammation, proliferation, and remodeling. Effective repair requires the coordination of diverse cell types, including keratinocytes, fibroblasts, inflammatory and endothelial cells, which collectively contribute to re-epithelialization, angiogenesis, and remodeling. Exosomes have emerged as promising therapeutic agents in wound healing due to their applicability in mediating intercellular communication.

In vitro and animal studies

Over 50 studies have explored exosome roles in dermal wound healing in rodent models [4]. The primary source of exosomes in these studies were mesenchymal stem cells (40%) or umbilical stem cells (10%), but other sources include human platelet-rich plasma (PRP), human umbilical vein endothelial cells, fibroblasts, keratinocytes, and macrophages. The most common isolation technique reported was ultracentrifugation and the most common method of

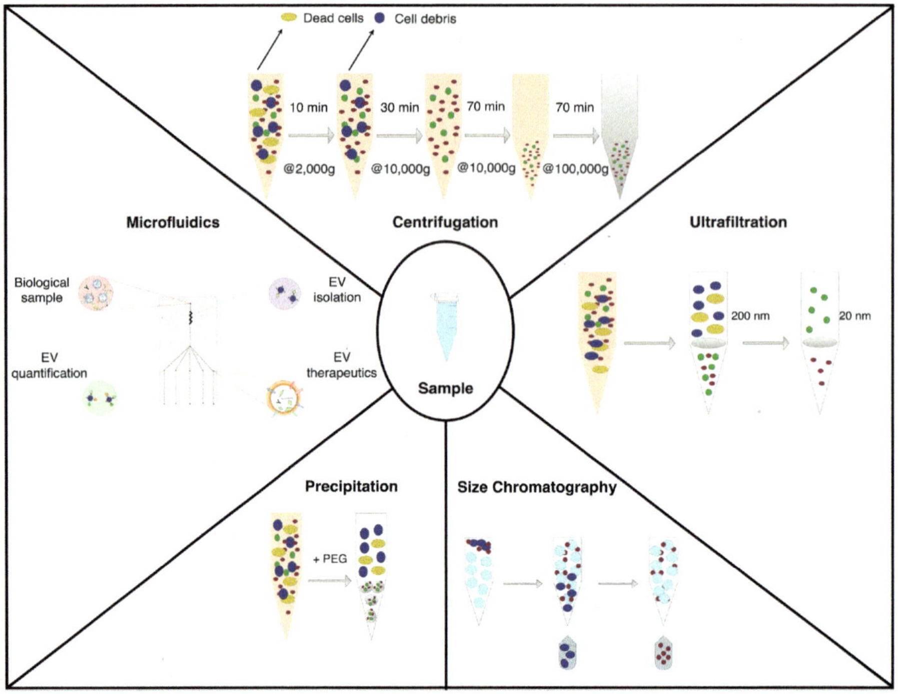

FIG. 3 Overview of common techniques for EV isolation and purification from biological samples. In the centrifugation method, dead cells and debris are sequentially removed through low-speed centrifugation, followed by high-speed ultracentrifugation to pellet EVs. *Ultrafiltration* employs membranes with specific pore sizes to separate particles and isolate EVs based on size. *Microfluidics* enables precise EV isolation, quantification through integrated microchannels and sorting techniques. *Size-exclusion chromatography* separates EVs by passing the sample through a porous matrix, allowing fractionation based on size. *Polyethylene glycol-based precipitation*, often combined with centrifugation, facilitates enrichment by aggregating EVs for separation.

administration was subcutaneous injection. Despite the heterogeneity of molecular cargo across studies, exosomes were found to have therapeutic properties and aid in cutaneous wound healing, regardless of the model, mode of administration, exosome concentration, the number of administrations, or the source of exosomes. Exosome cargo varied with most published studies focusing on microRNA-21 (miR-21). The proposed mechanisms by which miR-21 influences wound healing is by stimulating angiogenesis and activating the phosphatidylinositol 3-kinase/protein kinase B (PI3K/AKT) pathway. Overall, exosome administration has shown to significantly improve wound closure in 81% of mice studies, enhance vascularity in 50%, and promote collagen deposition and wound-bed viability. Other reported outcomes included increased fibroblast proliferation, improved collagen maturation, and reduced scarring [4]. Similarly, in diabetic wound healing studies, stem cell derived exosomes are primarily used, but sources such as menstrual blood and bovine milk have been studied [5]. Published evidence indicates that exosome therapy can improve diabetic wound healing rates, neovascular density, re-epithelialization, collagen deposition, and scar width. Additionally, analyses of inflammatory markers have demonstrated decreased levels of interleukin (IL)-6, IL-1β, and tumor necrosis factor alpha (TNF-α) [6].

In scar remodeling, adipose stem cell-derived exosomes (ADSC-Exos) have demonstrated notable efficacy in the treatment of keloids by enhancing mitochondrial autophagy via modulation of the phosphoinositide 3-kinase/protein kinase B/mechanistic target of rapamycin (PI3K/AKT/mTOR) pathway [7]. ADSC-Exos with noncoding ribonucleic acid (RNAs), particularly miR-194, significantly reduced hypertrophic scarring by downregulating transforming growth

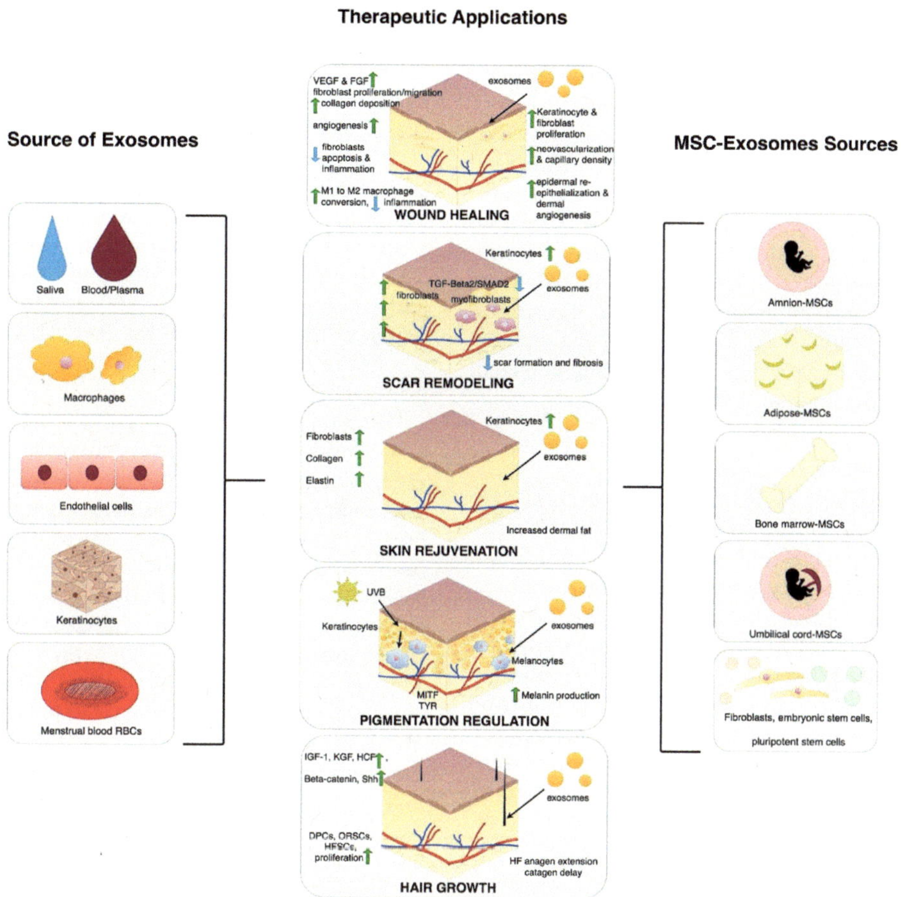

FIG. 4 Sources and therapeutic applications of exosomes. The individual columns illustrate exosome sources, aesthetic therapeutic applications, and MSC-exosome sources.

factor beta-1 (TGF-β1) expression, thereby affecting aberrant fibroblast proliferation and collagen synthesis [8].

Clinical studies

ADSC-Exos have been studied as adjuvant therapy for atrophic acne scars treated with fractional CO_2 laser. In a randomized, split-face study including 25 patients the ADSC-Exos treated side reported better scar reduction compared to untreated controls (32.5% vs 19.9%), reduced posttreatment erythema, and supposedly shorter recovery times (4.1 days vs 4.3 days). There were no exosome specific adverse effects reported in this series [5].

In a double-blind, placebo-controlled clinical study assessed the safety and potential therapeutic effects of platelet-derived exosomes in healthy participants (n = 11). Participants were subjected to wounds from a 4 mm punch biopsy on inner arms, with 1 site treated with exosomes (100 μg) and the other with isotonic solution. Both the treatment and placebo groups achieved complete wound closure within an average of 22.8 ± 8.7 days, and all wounds were fully healed by day 30. No serious adverse events were noted [9].

A phase II clinical trial consisting of 32 participants investigated the topical application of 10% secretome gel derived from human umbilical cord mesenchymal stem cells(UCB-MSCs) for treating chronic ulcers caused by diabetes (5 participants) and leprosy (27 participants). The study demonstrated significant reductions in wound length (from 2.41 cm to 1.65 cm), width (from 1.83 cm to 1.19 cm), and area (from 6.69 cm^2 to 4.00 cm^2) 1 month after treatment with no adverse effects reported [10].

Skin Rejuvenation

Skin aging is a multifaceted process driven by both intrinsic factors, such as genetics and metabolic processes, and extrinsic factors, including ultraviolet radiation. These factors collectively cause structural and functional changes in the skin, particularly within the extracellular matrix. Photodamage plays a significant role in skin aging by fragmenting collagen, reducing its production, and accumulating abnormal elastin and degraded collagen, which contribute to wrinkles, loss of firmness, and uneven skin texture. Exosomes are increasingly emphasized as promising therapeutic agents to mitigate these effects by promoting collagen synthesis and reducing matrix degradation.

In vitro and animal studies

In vitro studies on human dermal fibroblasts show that exosomes from human umbilical cord blood mesenchymal stem cells (UCB-MSCs) can induce fibroblast migration and increase expression of collagen I, fibronectin and elastin, while reducing matrix metalloproteinases (MMP)-1 levels [11]. Similarly, in animal studies, ADSC-Exos were shown to increase type I collagen and decrease type III collagen and MMP 1/3 [12]. In animal models of photoaging, subcutaneous injection of ADSC-Exos preserved the thickness of the epidermis and dermis following ultraviolet B (UVB)-radiation [12]. Exosomes derived from three-dimensional (3D) spheroid-cultured human fibroblasts demonstrated superior efficacy to monolayer fibroblast and MSC demonstrating more collagen synthesis, reduced inflammation, and better mitigation from UVB-photoaging in mice [13]. The mechanism involved downregulation of TNF-α and upregulation of TGF-β, which enhanced type I procollagen production and reduced MMP-1 expression. Exosomes derived from embryonic stem cells, such as those containing mmu-miR-291a-3p, were shown to inhibit cellular senescence in human fibroblasts by targeting the TGF-β pathway, restoring telomere length, and reducing deoxyribonucleic acid (DNA) damage [14].

Clinical studies

There are several studies demonstrating some evidence of exosomes improving aging features. In a 12-week randomized, split-face study with 28 participants (20 F, 8 M; skin type III-IV; age 54.0 ± 7.8 (43–66) years), human adipose tissue stem cell-derived exosome solution (HACS) applied before microneedling (1 mm) significantly reduced wrinkles (12.4% vs 6.6%, $P \leq .031$), increased elasticity (11.3% vs a 3.3%, $P = .002$), increased hydration (6.5% vs 4.5%, $P = .037$), and reduced melanin index (9.9% vs 1.0%, $P = .044$) compared to control. Histopathological findings revealed enhanced collagen and elastic fiber density, further demonstrating the superior efficacy of the HACS treatment [15].

In a randomized, double-blind, placebo-controlled study with 40 patients (30 F, 10 M; age 32–76 years; 22 white and 18 nonwhite), a topically applied human placental MSC exosomes group (n = 20) showed significant improvements in skin tone, clarity, vascularity, and wrinkle reduction ($P < .0001$) with 75% reporting being *extremely satisfied* by day 120, compared to 0% in the control group, and no adverse reactions reported [16].

Human platelet extract (HPE) is an allogeneic exosome product derived from leukocyte-reduced apheresed platelet. A clinical trial on the safety and tolerability of HPE with 56 participants (48 F 8 M; age 54 ± 11 (40–80) years; skin types I-IV) with mild to moderate global face wrinkles demonstrated statistically significant improvement in overall skin health score after 6-week use. There was a notable reduction in erythema area by −2.39 ($P = .005$), brown spot fractional area by −0.0161 ($P \leq .0001$), and wrinkle fractional area across facial regions by 0.01 to 0.04 ($P \leq .0023$). Luminosity scores increased by 5.42 ($P \leq .0001$), and color evenness improved by 0.071 ($P \leq .0001$) Skin texture, radiance, and firmness improved on average 0.3, 0.4, and 0.1 points, respectively There was no visible improvement in skin sagginess [17].

Pigmentation Control

Exosomes have the potential to modulate pigmentation by regulating melanin synthesis and enhancing melanosome degradation, offering therapeutic promise for conditions like melasma and hyperpigmentation.

In vitro and animal studies

Keratinocyte-derived exosomes with miR-675 and miR-330-5p can inhibit melanogenesis by directly targeting microphthalmia-associated transcription factor (MITF). MITF is a pivotal transcription factor that governs the expression of tyrosinase (TYR) and other proteins essential for melanin production [18]. Similar mechanism of MITF downregulation has been described with miR-181a-5p Exo from human amniotic MSC [19]. Exosomes containing miR-199a can increase melanosome degradation through autophagy activation [19]. Interestingly, exosomes derived from hypertrophic scar fibroblasts significantly reduced the mRNA and protein expression of pigmentation-related factors, including paired box-3 (Pax3), sex-determining region Y-related high mobility group-box-10 (Sox10), MITF, TYR, and TYR-related proteins [20].

Clinical studies

Clinical studies evaluating the efficacy of exosomes in pigmentation control are limited. One open-label study including 12 female participants (46.64 ± 13.05 year old) with Fitzpatrick types II-IV with moderate-to-severe facial hyperpigmentation evaluated the efficacy of rose stem-cell-derived exosomes combined with microneedling. By week 12, participants exhibited a 13% reduction in superficial pigmentation, a 16% reduction in deep pigmentation, a 7.34% reduction in redness, and a 6.3% improvement in skin quality, with no major adverse events reported. Psychometric scores for life quality also significantly improved [21].

Hair Growth

The use of exosomes in hair growth regulation and as therapy for alopecia is still in nascent stages.

In vitro and animal studies

Most current evidence derived from in vitro and animal studies centers on regulation of the hair follicle growth cycle by dermal papilla cells (DPCs) [22]. DPC-derived exosomes (DPC-Exos) have shown the most promise primarily by enhancing Wnt/β-catenin signaling, a critical pathway for hair growth and regeneration. In animal studies, DPC-Exos can stimulate the early onset of anagen phase, delay the catagen, and upregulate key signaling molecules such as sonic hedgehog, keratinocyte growth factors, and β-catenin [22].

ADSC-Exos also demonstrate potential in promoting hair growth by mitigating dihydrotestosterone effects, primarily by downregulating TGF-β1 signaling and through targeting small mother against decapentaplegic family member 3 (SMAD3) (miR-122-5p) [23]. When compared to PRP exosomes, ADSC-Exos are found to support hair growth by increasing proliferation of human DPCs, dermal thickness, and hair bulb size [23].

Clinical studies

Exosome-based therapies are a promising avenue for treating androgenetic alopecia (AGA), alopecia areata (AA), and hair disorders. The strength of clinical evidence remains limited as most trials are industry-sponsored, lack transparency and scientific rigor. Many reports combine exosome injections with adjunctive hair procedures such as microneedling and lasers, both of which independently benefit hair growth, complicating the interpretation of exosome-specific effects.

In AGA, foreskin-derived MSC exosomes scalp injections of 30 AGA patients (30 M; age 22–65 years; hair loss III-VI, Norwood-Hamilton). After 12 weeks, a statistically significant increase in hair density was observed, with no adverse events reported [24]. Similarly, ADSC-Exos delivered via microneedling to 39 patients with male and female pattern hair loss showed marked improvements in hair density and thickness after 12 weekly sessions [25]. Aside from microneedling-related discomfort, no exosome-related adverse effects were noted. Multiple sessions of ADSC-Exos scalp therapy with microneedling (n = 30; AGA; 16 F 14 M; age 47 ± 7.58) significantly increased hair density, with mild, temporary scalp redness and tingling [22]. Recent comparative study positions exosomes superiorly to PRP treatments, with better outcomes in hair regrowth after fewer sessions and maintained results for up to 28 months, with no serious adverse events in either group.

Exosome-based therapies have also been trialed for AA. Rose stem cell-derived exosomes applied through electroporation in one AA patient improved hair density and reduced hair loss after 12 sessions without adverse events. A combination of rose stem cell exosomes with fractional picosecond laser treatments in another patient with AA and poliosis circumscripta, yielded additional benefits, with restored hair growth and pigmentation in affected areas [26].

MSC exosomes have shown potential in treating acquired trichorrhexis nodosa, a hair shaft disorder characterized by fragility and breakage. In a case series involving 3 patients, monthly scalp injections of MSC exosomes led to improvement in hair density, length, pigmentation, and cuticle recovery. These results were sustained at 1-year follow-up, as confirmed by photographic documentation, dermoscopy, and scanning electron microscopy [27].

LIMITATIONS

Exosome-based therapies hold significant promise in aesthetic and regenerative medicine; however, multiple barriers exist that must be addressed before their widespread use and commercialization. The primary limitation lies in the lack of standardization in exosome production, which affects the consistency and reliability of therapeutic outcomes. Variability in source material, isolation techniques, and purification methods introduces biological heterogeneity, leading to inconsistencies in exosome yield, content, and quality. Additionally, storage conditions and the absence of regulatory oversight in exosome preparation contribute to uncertainties regarding the purity and functional integrity of marketed exosome products.

Another major concern is the limited clinical evidence supporting exosome efficacy and safety in humans. Exosomes present unique theoretic risks, including their potential to carry oncogenic material from donor cells, modulate immune responses or encapsulate pathogens such as prions and viruses. Achieving targeted delivery to specific tissues remains a technical hurdle, as exosomes can circulate systemically and interact with off-target cells, potentially leading to unintended organ effects. Questions also remain about the duration of exosome activity in the body, with concerns regarding implications for prolonged or delayed effects.

While preclinical studies and early-phase trials report promising results, clinical data remain sparse, and lack robust design, appropriate controls, standardized dosages, and long-term follow-ups. The safety profile of exosomes in aesthetic use is not fully understood. While topical exosome applications are generally considered safe, adverse events such as granulomas, necrosis, and anaphylaxis have been reported in cases with adjunct skin barrier disruption [28,29]. Additionally, the FDA has warned the use of exosome products following a report of five patients in Nebraska experiencing serious adverse events including bacteremia after the use of exosome product derived from C-sectioned placentas [30].

Currently, the only one FDA-approved stem cell-based product contains hematopoietic progenitor cells derived from cord blood, indicated for limited use in patients with hematologic disorders or malignancies. No exosome-based products have received FDA approval yet. The FDA has addressed misleading claims by some clinics suggesting that these products are not subject to regulatory provisions for drugs and biological products, stating such claims are "simply untrue." However, stem cell-derived therapies can be offered in clinical trials under an Investigational New Drug application—a clinical investigation plan reviewed and approved by the FDA. Addressing limitations will require well-designed clinical trials, stringent manufacturing standards, and comprehensive regulatory frameworks to ensure the safety, efficacy, and scalability of exosome-based therapies.

SUMMARY

Exosome-based therapies represent a potentially transformative innovation in aesthetic and regenerative medicine, with applications spanning wound healing, skin rejuvenation, pigmentation regulation, and hair growth. Evidence from preclinical and clinical studies highlights their capacity to facilitate cellular communication, collagen synthesis, regulate melanogenesis, and modulate inflammation, yielding encouraging outcomes. However, challenges remain, particularly regarding standardization and variability in isolation techniques, underscoring the need for rigorous investigation to ensure optimal efficacy and safety. Advancing this field will require greater transparency about exosome composition and the role of adjunctive therapies. While the promise of exosome-based treatments is significant, further large-scale, independent, and well-designed studies are essential to validate their clinical effectiveness and elucidate mechanisms of action.

CLINICS CARE POINTS

- The support for the use of exosomes in human cutaneous applications is limited.
- There is evidence for application of exosomes in wound healing and scar remodeling from animal models, and the limited human trials support potential for enhanced recovery time and scar remodeling.
- In esthetics, exosomes have been shown to enhance outcomes including wrinkle reduction, hydration, hyperpigmentation control, and hair growth, usually when combined with adjunct therapies, such as microneedling.
- Be cautious when selecting and using exosome products, as variability in source and preparation methods can lead to inconsistent formulations. Always prioritize products that meet stringent quality and safety standards.
- All patients considering exosome-based treatments should be thoroughly educated about associated risks, potential side effects, and the current lack of FDA approval for these therapies.

DISCLOSURES

The authors have nothing to disclose.

REFERENCES

[1] Doyle LM, Wang MZ. Overview of extracellular vesicles, their origin, composition, purpose, and methods for exosome isolation and analysis. Cells 2019;8(7):727.

[2] Lai RC, Arslan F, Lee MM, et al. Exosome secreted by MSC reduces myocardial ischemia/reperfusion injury. Stem Cell Res 2010;4(3):214–22.

[3] Cheng Y, Schorey JS. Exosomes carrying mycobacterial antigens can protect mice against Mycobacterium tuberculosis infection. Eur J Immunol 2013;43(12):3279–90.
[4] Prasai A, Jay JW, Jupiter D, et al. Role of exosomes in dermal wound healing: a systematic review. J Invest Dermatol 2022;142(3 Pt A):662–78.e8.
[5] Kwon HH, Yang SH, Lee J, et al. Combination treatment with human adipose tissue stem cell-derived exosomes and fractional CO2 laser for acne scars: a 12-week prospective, double-blind, randomized, split-face study. Acta Derm Venereol 2020;100(18).
[6] Qiao Z, Wang X, Zhao H, et al. The effectiveness of cell-derived exosome therapy for diabetic wound: a systematic review and meta-analysis. Ageing Res Rev 2023;85:101858.
[7] Liu C, Khairullina L, Qin Y, et al. Adipose stem cell exosomes promote mitochondrial autophagy through the PI3K/AKT/mTOR pathway to alleviate keloids. Stem Cell Res Ther 2024;15(1):305.
[8] Xu Z, Tian Y, Hao L. Exosomal miR-194 from adipose-derived stem cells impedes hypertrophic scar formation through targeting TGF-β1. Mol Med Rep 2024;30(6):216.
[9] Johnson J, Law SQK, Shojaee M, et al. First-in-human clinical trial of allogeneic, platelet-derived extracellular vesicles as a potential therapeutic for delayed wound healing. J Extracell Vesicles 2023;12(7):e12332.
[10] Tan ST, Aisyah PB, Firmansyah Y, et al. Effectiveness of secretome from human umbilical cord mesenchymal stem cells in gel (10% SM-hUCMSC gel) for chronic wounds (diabetic and trophic ulcer) – phase 2 clinical trial. J Multidiscip Healthc 2023;16:1763–77.
[11] Kim YJ, Yoo SM, Park HH, et al. Exosomes derived from human umbilical cord blood mesenchymal stem cells stimulates rejuvenation of human skin. Biochem Biophys Res Commun 2017;493(2):1102–8.
[12] Liang JX, Liao X, Li SH, et al. Antiaging properties of exosomes from adipose-derived mesenchymal stem cells in photoaged rat skin. BioMed Res Int 2020;2020:6406395.
[13] Hu S, Li Z, Cores J, et al. Needle-free injection of exosomes derived from human dermal fibroblast spheroids ameliorates skin photoaging. ACS Nano 2019;13(10):11273–82.
[14] Bae YU, Son Y, Kim CH, et al. Embryonic stem cell-derived mmu-miR-291a-3p inhibits cellular senescence in human dermal fibroblasts through the TGF-β receptor 2 pathway. J Gerontol A Biol Sci Med Sci 2019;74(9):1359–67.
[15] Park GH, Kwon HH, Seok J, et al. Efficacy of combined treatment with human adipose tissue stem cell-derived exosome-containing solution and microneedling for facial skin aging: a 12-week prospective, randomized, split-face study. J Cosmet Dermatol 2023;22(12):3418–26.
[16] Chernoff G. The utilization of human placental mesenchymal stem cell derived exosomes in aging skin: an investigational pilot study. J Surg 2021;6:1388.
[17] Proffer SL, Paradise CR, DeGrazia E, et al. Efficacy and tolerability of topical platelet exosomes for skin rejuvenation: six-week results. Aesthet Surg J 2022;42(10):1185–93.
[18] Kim NH, Choi SH, Kim CH, et al. Reduced MiR-675 in exosome in H19 RNA-related melanogenesis via MITF as a direct target. J Invest Dermatol 2014;134(4):1075–82.
[19] Wang XY, Guan XH, Yu ZP, et al. Human amniotic stem cells-derived exosmal miR-181a-5p and miR-199a inhibit melanogenesis and promote melanosome degradation in skin hyperpigmentation, respectively. Stem Cell Res Ther 2021;12(1):501.
[20] Cui HS, Joo SY, Cho YS, et al. Exosomes derived from hypertrophic scar fibroblasts suppress melanogenesis in normal human epidermal melanocytes. Int J Mol Sci 2024;25(13):7236.
[21] Theodorakopoulou E, Aguilera SB, Duncan DI. A New therapeutic approach with rose stem-cell-derived exosomes and non-thermal microneedling for the treatment of facial pigmentation. Aesthet Surg J Open Forum 2024;6.
[22] Lee E, Choi MS, Cho BS, et al. The efficacy of adipose stem cell-derived exosomes in hair regeneration based on a preclinical and clinical study. Int J Dermatol 2024;63(9):1212–20.
[23] Cheng M, Ma C, Chen HD, et al. The roles of exosomes in regulating hair follicle growth. Clin Cosmet Invest Dermatol 2024;17:1603–12.
[24] Ersan M, Ozer E, Akin O, et al. Effectiveness of exosome treatment in androgenetic alopecia: outcomes of a prospective study. Aesthetic Plast Surg 2024;48(21):4262–71.
[25] Park BS, Choi HI, Huh G, et al. Effects of exosome from adipose-derived stem cell on hair loss: a retrospective analysis of 39 patients. J Cosmet Dermatol 2022;21(5):2282–4.
[26] Lueangarun S, Cho BS, Tempark T. Hair repigmentation of poliosis circumscripta in androgenetic alopecia patient treated with exosomes and fractional picosecond laser. J Cosmet Dermatol 2024;23(6):2307–11.
[27] Chen X, Pang J, Li J, et al. Mesenchymal stem cell exosomes therapy for acquired trichorrhexis nodosa: a case series. J Cosmet Dermatol 2024.
[28] Tawanwongsri W, Vachiramon V. Skin necrosis after intradermal injection of lyophilized exosome: a case report and a review of the literature. J Cosmet Dermatol 2024;23(5):1597–603.
[29] Zhuang J, Chen Y, Hu J. Treatment of anaphylaxis after injection of stem cell exosomes with 5-fluorouracil and triamcinolone acetonide. J Craniofac Surg 2023;34(2):e198–9.
[30] Fiore K. FDA Warns Exosome Maker for Marketing outside its IND — agency also raises concern about a potentially contaminated product batch. MedPage Today 2024. Available at: https://www.medpagetoday.com/special-reports/exclusives/108371. Accessed December 4, 2024.

Advances in Cosmetic Surgery 8 (2025) 87–96
ADVANCES IN COSMETIC SURGERY

Combining Non-ablative Resurfacing with Radiofrequency Microneedling for Acne Scarring

Kathleen Coerdt, MD[a], Susruthi Rajanala, MD[b], Alexa B. Steuer, MD, MPH[b], Jeffrey S. Dover, MD, FRCPC[b,c,*]
[a]Department of Dermatology, Cleveland Clinic Foundation, A60, 9500 Euclid Avenue, Cleveland, OH 44195, USA; [b]Department of Dermatology, SkinCare Physicians, Suite 103, 1244 Boylston Street, Chestnut Hill, MA 02467, USA; [c]Department of Dermatology, Yale University School of Medicine, New Haven, CT, USA

KEYWORDS
• Acne scarring • Non-ablative fractional laser • Ablative fractional laser • Radiofrequency microneedling
• Energy-based devices • Non-ablative resurfacing

KEY POINTS

- Most patients suffer from a combination of acne scar types, so a multifaceted approach to treatment is generally recommended to optimize outcomes.
- Ablative lasers are generally regarded as the gold standard for facial resurfacing; however, the downtime and side effect profile limit their use in clinical practice.
- Both non-ablative fractional lasers (NAFL) and microneedling with radiofrequency (MNRF) show significant and similar improvements in acne scaring.
- Combining NAFL and MNRF leverages distinct mechanisms of action, aiming to improve the efficacy of treatment for acne scarring.
- Combined NAFL+MNRF treatment shows significant improvement in acne scarring, though further studies are needed to clarify the difference in efficacy between combined treatment and monotherapy.

INTRODUCTION: NATURE OF THE PROBLEM

Acne vulgaris is one of the most common inflammatory skin disorders, affecting an estimated 95% to 100% of adolescent boys and 83% to 85% of adolescent girls, often continuing into adulthood [1,2]. Acne scarring—a frequent and often permanent consequence—impacts up to 95% of individuals with acne vulgaris [2–4]. Scarring varies from mild to severe, with approximately 30% of patients presenting with more severe forms.

Acne scarring can cause a substantial physical and psychological burden. Numerous studies have highlighted the emotional toll of acne scars, with patients reporting higher rates of anxiety, depression, and diminished self-esteem [1,4–6]. Profound psychosocial consequences can influence self-confidence, social interactions, relationships, academic performance, and professional life (Fig. 1) [2]. Given the high incidence of acne scarring, as well as the detrimental impact on patient quality of life, effective treatment options are critical.

Acne vulgaris induces chronic cutaneous inflammation, which disrupts the balance between matrix degradation and collagen synthesis, leading to the formation of scars [2].

*Corresponding author. Department of Dermatology, SkinCare Physicians, Suite 103, 1244 Boylston Street, Chestnut Hill, MA 02467. *E-mail address:* jdover@skincarephysicians.net

https://doi.org/10.1016/j.yacs.2024.12.002
www.advancesincosmeticsurgery.com
2542-4327/25/

ABBREVIATIONS

AFL	ablative fractional lasers
ECCA	échelle d'évaluation clinique des cicatrices d'acné
MNRF	microneedling with radiofrequency
NAFL	non-ablative fractional lasers

Acne scars can be broadly categorized into hypertrophic or atrophic types.

- Hypertrophic: result from excessive collagen production and can develop into keloidal or raised scars.
- Atrophic: result from insufficient collagen deposition and can develop into 3 subtypes of scars.

Atrophic scars are more common, accounting for 80% to 90% of acne-related scarring [1,2]. They are further subclassified into ice pick (V-shaped), boxcar (U-shaped), and rolling (M-shaped) scars, each with distinct morphologies and treatment challenges (Fig. 2) [1]. In most patients, a combination of these scar types is present, requiring a multifaceted approach to treatment.

Atrophic subtypes.

a. Ice pick: most common type (60%–70%)
   i. Narrow and deep
   ii. Least responsive to treatment
b. Boxcar: second most common type (20%–30%)
   i. Broad and shallow (can be deep)
   ii. Most responsive to treatment
c. Rolling type: least common type (15%–25%)
   i. Wave-like or undulating appearance due to fibrous septa tethering the overlying skin to the fascia
   ii. Moderately responsive to treatment

A wide range of therapeutic options is available for addressing acne scars, including: non-surgical techniques such as dermal fillers, chemical peels, dermabrasion, microneedling, and platelet-rich plasma injections; surgical procedures such as subcision, punch excision, punch grafting, punch elevation, and elliptical excision; and energy-based devices, such as ablative fractional laser (AFL), non-ablative fractional laser (NAFL), and microneedling with radiofrequency (MNRF) [1–4,7–9]. Among these, energy-based devices have become central to treatment of acne scarring and are increasingly recognized as first-line treatments.

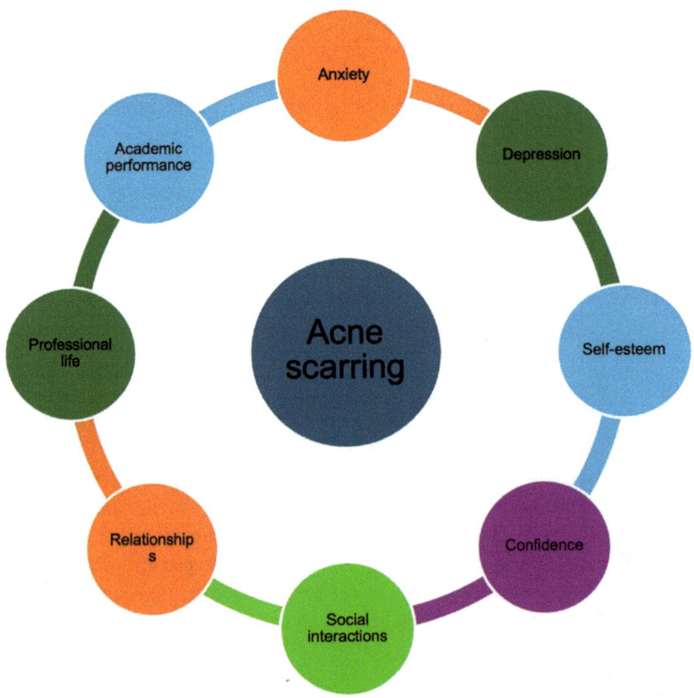

FIG. 1 Psychosocial impacts of acne scarring on patients. (*Adapted from* Salameh F, Shumaker PR, Goodman GJ, et al. Energy-based devices for the treatment of Acne Scars: 2022 International consensus recommendations. Lasers Surg Med 2022;54:10–26.)

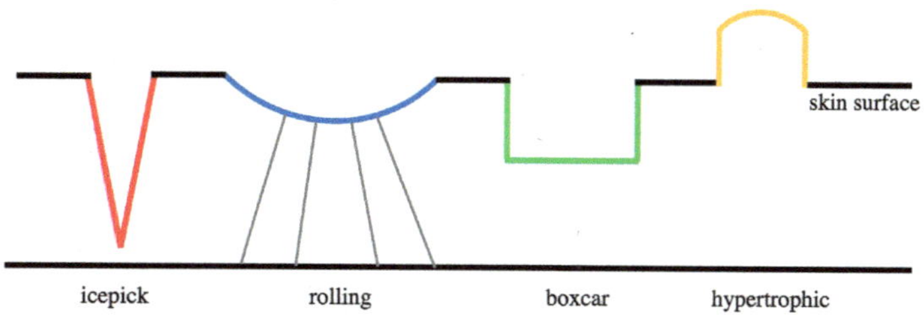

FIG. 2 Types of acne scars. (*Adapted from* Jacob CI, Dover JS, Kaminer MS. Acne scarring: a classification system and review of treatment options. J Am Acad Dermatol 2001;45:109-17.)

Ablative non-fractional lasers and AFL, such as carbon dioxide and erbium lasers, are considered the gold standard for resurfacing. Ablative lasers deliver a wavelength of light that vaporizes the epidermis and dermis, with the dermal penetration depending on the depth and energy selected by the clinician [10]. AFL utilizes fractional thermolysis to create microthermal treatment zones with this wavelength of light, with the interspersed untreated epidermis and dermis helping to reduce downtime and speed re-epithelialization [10]. Ablative non-fractional lasers, AFL, and, more recently, combination AFL + MNRF have been described in the literature for the treatment of acne scarring [8,10–12]. While they can offer significant improvements in acne scarring, the longer recovery times and higher risk of complications with ablative lasers limit their use [10,12]. In contrast, NAFL and MNRF are less aggressive, offering enhanced patient tolerance, shorter recovery periods, and a more favorable safety profile, making them increasingly popular in clinical practice.

This article aims to explore the therapeutic potential of combining NAFL and MNRF in the treatment of acne scarring. We will review the clinical outcomes associated with this combination therapy, discuss the benefits and risks, and offer practical considerations for integrating these treatments into real-world clinical practice. Ultimately, we seek to provide an evidence-based framework to optimize therapeutic outcomes, improving both the aesthetic results and the quality-of-life for individuals affected by this common and often emotionally burdensome condition.

BACKGROUND: MONOTHERAPY EFFICACY

Non-ablative Fractional Laser

NAFL operate through the principle of fractional photothermolysis, in which microscopic columns of thermal energy are delivered to the epidermis and/or dermis with preservation of the stratum corneum [13]. This stimulates fibroblasts, leading to neocollagenesis and neoelastogenesis (Fig. 3A). The depth and density of the laser's thermal columns can be adjusted, providing clinicians with precise control over energy delivery to the dermis.

Extensive research supports the efficacy of NAFL in improving acne scarring [14–19].

- Alster and colleagues [14] demonstrated a 51% to 71% improvement in acne scarring after 3 monthly treatments with a 1550-nm erbium-doped fiber NAFL.
- In a randomized controlled trial, Hedelund and colleagues [15] showed a significant improvement in acne scarring for patients after 3 monthly treatments with a 1540-nm NAFL ($P = .0313$).
- Bencini and colleagues [16] evaluated 87 patients with moderate-to-severe acne scarring, treating them with 6 sessions of a 1540-nm erbium glass fiber NAFL at 3-week intervals. Six months post-treatment, 92% (80/87) of patients demonstrated marked improvement, while 8% (7/87) of patients showed moderate improvement.

These findings have been corroborated in subsequent studies, solidifying NAFL as an efficacious treatment of acne scarring [17–19].

Radiofrequency Microneedling

MNRF is a procedure in which microneedles penetrate the epidermis with minimal damage and deliver controlled electromagnetic radiation to the dermis, creating thermal injuries in the dermis [3,9]. This activates fibroblasts, stimulates the release of growth factors, and promotes both neocollagenesis and neoelastogenesis (Fig. 3B) [3,5,12]. The ability to adjust the depth of needle penetration allows for tailored treatments, enabling clinicians to target various layers of the dermis depending the severity and type of scarring [3].

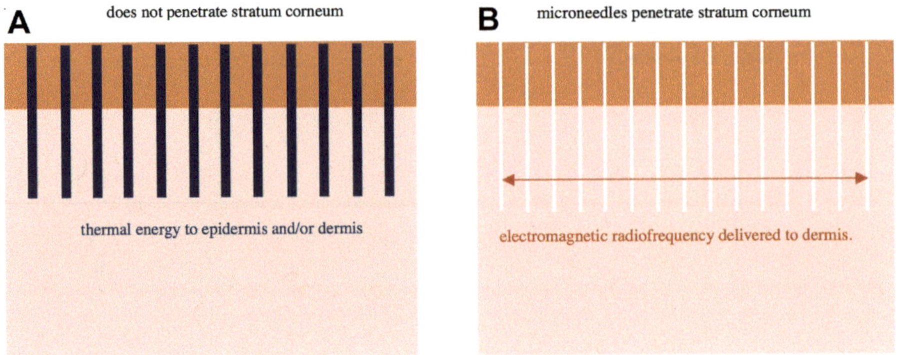

FIG. 3 Schematic of the mechanism of action (MOA) of non-ablative fractional laser (NAFL) and microneedling with radiofrequency (MNRF). (**A**) Schematic of MOA of NAFL in which microscopic columns of thermal energy are delivered to the epidermis and/or dermis while not penetrating the stratum corneum. (**B**) Schematic of the MOA of MNRF in which microneedles penetrate the epidermis and deliver controlled electromagnetic radiation to the dermis. (*Data from* Refs. [3,5,12].)

Similarly to NAFL, MNRF has been shown to be effective for the treatment of acne scarring.

- Cho and colleagues evaluated the efficacy of bipolar MNRF in patients with mild to moderate acne scarring, observing improvement in over 70% of patients after 2 monthly treatments ($P<.05$) [20].
- A retrospective study by Chandrashekar and colleagues investigated the efficacy of MNRF in patients with acne scarring with 4 sessions at 6-week intervals [21]. Notably, 85.71% of patients with Grade 4 scars showed an improvement of 2 grades, 80.64% of patients with Grade 4 and Grade 3 scars improved by 2 grades, and 76.47% of patients with Grade 3 scars improved by 2 grades.

Further studies have reinforced these findings, demonstrating MNRF as an effective modality for acne scarring [9,22,23].

Non-ablative Fractional Laser Monotherapy Versus Microneedling with Radiofrequency Monotherapy

When comparing NAFL and MNRF head-to-head for the treatment of acne scarring, studies have demonstrated comparable efficacy between the 2 modalities:

- Rongsaard & Rummaneethorn conducted a randomized, split-face trial involving 20 patients, treating one side of the face with a 1550-nm NAFL and the other with MNRF at 4-week intervals for 3 sessions. Both groups showed significant improvements on a grading scale ranging from 0 to 4, with NAFL yielding a mean improvement of 2.86 ± 0.42 on the grading scale ($P<.001$) and MNRF achieving a mean improvement of 2.70 ± 0.37 ($P<.001$). However, there was no statistically significant difference in efficacy between the 2 treatment modalities [24].
- Chae and colleagues led a trial in which 40 patients were randomized to receive either NAFL or MNRF at 4-week intervals for 3 sessions. Acne scarring was graded using the échelle d'évaluation clinique des cicatrices d'acné (ECCA) score, showing a mean improvement of 25% in the NAFL group ($P<.01$) and 18.6% in the MNRF ($P<.01$). While NAFL demonstrated a larger reduction in scar severity, the difference between the groups was not significant ($P>.05$). When evaluating an improvement by scar type subgroups, there was not a significant difference between the 2 treatments ($P>.05$) [4].

SURGICAL TECHNIQUE

Pre-operative Planning

Ideal candidates for combination treatment with NAFL and MNRF are those with moderate to severe acne scarring [3,6]. As with any procedure, pre-treatment consultation is crucial and should include a thorough discussion regarding treatment protocol, risks, benefits, alternatives, and expected results. It is important to counsel patients regarding realistic expectations for improvement, and that multiple treatment sessions are often needed, especially for deeper atrophic acne scars. Patients should also be aware of potential downtime prior to scheduling the procedure. After consultation, patients should provide written informed consent. Prior to treatment, baseline photographs should be taken of the treatment area (direct anterior view, 45-degree oblique views, and 90-degree side views), and photos should be repeated at each visit to monitor improvement. Typically, NAFL and MNRF are performed together at the same visit, but for patients who have a risk of prolonged healing or are prone to hyperpigmentation, then these 2 treatments may be spaced out and alternated at 2 to 4 week intervals, though patients should be aware that this approach will result in a longer total treatment time and slower or reduced improvement [3].

In our practice, we use the 1550-nm erbium doped-fiber laser (Fraxel, Solta Medical; Bothwell, WA) for NAFL treatment. For MNRF, we employ Legend Pro (Lumenis Be Ltd; Yokneam, Israel), the Morpheus 8 (InMode; Irvine, CA), and the Genius (Lutronic; Billerica, MA). For patients with higher Fitzpatrick skin types, use of insulated tips and bipolar electrodes will prevent epidermal heating and protect against hyperpigmentation. We recommend treating first with NAFL followed by MNRF- we employ laser settings of 50 to 70 J/cm^2, treatment level 8, with 8 passes, with decreased energy, density, and/or treatment level for skin of color. MNRF settings are detailed further below in the Procedural Approach section.

Preparation and Patient Positioning

Prior to treatment, the provider should apply an even layer of topical numbing ointment (30% compounded lidocaine ointment) for 45 to 60 minutes to the treatment area to ensure patient comfort. The skin should then be cleansed with gauze followed by alcohol to degrease and sanitize the skin. The patient should be positioned supine, and each device should be positioned close enough for the hand piece to easily reach all areas to be treated. Standard laser safety protocols should be employed, including appropriate signage on the examination room door and eye protection for both patient and clinician. Prior to MNRF, clinician should also confirm there is no pacemaker in place.

Procedural Approach

For NAFL treatment, we recommend treating the whole face to avoid a treatment demarcation line, while MNRF can be limited to the area of scarring. For NAFL, we treat by unit of the face to allow for clinician comfort and accuracy, starting with the cheeks, followed by the chin and upper lip, nose, and ending with the forehead. In each sub-region, the laser handpiece should be directed along the skin in a single back and forth motion, with 50% overlap between each row; this pattern should be repeated perpendicularly in the same treatment sub-region, to yield a total of 8 passes. Clinical endpoint is mild erythema and edema.

For MNRF, for Legend Pro, we pretreat with pure glycerin and pre-heat the target area with the TriPollar tip to a temperature of 100 to 102°F. The area is then treated with a single pass with a 7x7mm, 0.2 mm depth trifractional tip, followed by a second pass with a 6x6mm, 1.0 mm depth tip. Of note, given the pre-heating in the protocol, we do not recommend use of topical numbing if the Legend Pro is being used given risk of burn due to decreased temperature sensation. For the Morpheus 8 device, we use the 24-pin tip and perform 3 passes with decreased depth and energy with each subsequent pass, noted below (Table 1). For the Genius device, we perform 2 passes using the M49 tip, with passes and energy noted below (Table 2). For patients with Fitzpatrick skin types V and VI, energy settings should be decreased by at least 25%.

For MNRF devices, the handpiece should be held perpendicularly to the skin with mild pressure to avoid over-penetration of the needles and should be held in full contact of the skin for the entirety of the pulse, with no overlapping pulses to avoid overtreating. Clinical endpoint is mild pinpoint bleeding. The clinician should also assess patient pain level intermittently throughout the treatment.

Immediate Post-Procedural Care

Post MNRF, skin should be cleansed with wet gauze, and mild pressure may be applied to stop any pinpoint bleeding. Topical vitamin C serum may then be applied as the micro-channels in the treated skin will enhance topical absorption [25]. Following this, direct application of ice packs can help with post procedure discomfort. For 3 to 5 days post treatment, patients

TABLE 1
Recommended Treatment Settings for the Morpheus8 Microneedling with Radiofrequency Device

	Depth	Energy Level
First pass	3 mm	25
Second pass	2 mm	20
Third pass	1 mm	15

TABLE 2
Recommended Treatment Settings for the Genius Microneedling with Radiofrequency Device

	Depth	Energy Level	Pulse Duration
First pass	2 mm	10W	200 ms
Second pass	1.5 mm	8W	200 ms

should avoid harsh or abrasive topicals such as scrubs, chemical exfoliants, and retinols and instead use a gentle cleanser and emollient moisturizer until healed. Sun protection is crucial post treatment, with use of sunscreen with SPF 30 or higher (mineral based sunscreens are typically gentler over treated skin), and sun avoidance behaviors. Patients should be counseled that their skin may be pink and feel tight or rough for about 5 days post procedure, though they can resume makeup if desired after 2 days.

CLINICAL RESULTS IN THE LITERATURE: COMBINATION THERAPY

Combination Non-ablative Fractional Lasers + Microneedling with Radiofrequency for Acne Scarring

A multimodal treatment approach is often considered for acne scarring, given that most patients present with a combination of scar types [3]. A recent consensus study found that 95% of experts recommend combining treatment modalities for optimal results [2,3]. Combining NAFL and MNRF has been proposed as a strategy, leveraging the distinct mechanisms of action of each device [9].

Initial studies on the combined use of NAFL and MNRF have shown promising results, with notable improvements in scarring, as well as minimal adverse effects (Table 3). Sharad and colleagues examined 18 patients with moderate-to-severe atrophic scarring. Patients received alternating treatments with a 1565-nm erbium glass NAFL and MNRF at 4-week intervals for 8 sessions, resulting in a total of 4 NAFL and 4 MNRF treatments. At 12-month follow-up, 6 patients (33.3%) experienced a 3-grade improvement in scarring, 11 patients (61.1%) had a 2-grade improvement, and 1 patient (5.6%) showed a 1-grade improvement. The study demonstrated a significant median improvement in acne scarring ($P<.001$). Boxcar and rolling scars showed the most improvement, whereas ice pick scars showed the least improvement, consistent with previous studies on acne scar treatment [6].

Take Home Point: An alternating NAFL + MNRF treatment regimen at 4-week intervals showed significant improvement in acne scarring ($P<.001$).

Clinical Practice Point: Alternating NAFL + MNRF is a safe and effective treatment regimen to improve acne scarring.

Two additional studies compared a combination NAFL + MNRF regimen to NAFL monotherapy. Kwon and colleagues conducted a prospective, split-face study with 26 subjects [26]. The participants received 3 sessions of 1550-nm erbium glass NAFL on one side of the face and NAFL followed by MNRF on the other side at 4-week intervals. Both treatments demonstrated significant improvements in ECCA score ($P<.01$), with the combination therapy showing a significantly greater improvement compared to NAFL monotherapy ($P<.05$). Subgroup analyses demonstrated more improvement for those with moderate-to-severe acne scarring, and the combination regimen was superior to NAFL monotherapy only in those patients with moderate-to-high baseline severity in acne scarring ($P<.05$). Interestingly, histologic analysis of pre-treatment and post-treatment skin biopsies revealed greater increases in the interstitial fibers throughout the dermis in the combination therapy group, as well as increased expression of TGF-beta, a key regulator of fibroblast activity and collagen production [5].

Take Home Point: Both NAFL monotherapy and NAFL + MNRF combination therapy showed significant improvements in acne scarring ($P<.01$); however, combination therapy was superior to monotherapy in patients with moderate-to-severe acne scarring ($P<.05$).

Clinical Practice Point: Combination NAFL + MNRF therapy may be more useful in those with moderate-to-severe acne scarring than NAFL monotherapy.

Hartmann and colleagues conducted a study comparing 1550-nm NAFL monotherapy to alternating NAFL + MNRF in a prospective, double-blinded, split-face trial of 20 patients with moderate-to-severe acne scarring. Four sessions at 4-week intervals were completed; monotherapy patients received 4 NAFL treatments and

TABLE 3
Summary of Published Studies Assessing Combination Therapy with Non-ablative Fractional Lasers and Microneedling with Radiofrequency

Author	Study Type	Treatment	Regimen	FST	Follow-up	Results
Sharad [6], 2022	Retrospective analysis	Alternating NAFL + MNRF	Q4wk x 8 mo	III-V	12 mo	NAFL + MNRF: *P*<.001
Kwon et al [5], 2018	Split-face, prospective clinical trial	NAFL vs combination NAFL + MNRF	Q4wk x 3 mo	III, IV	5 mo	NAFL: *P*<.01 NAFL + MNRF: *P*<.01 NAFL + NMRF vs NAFL: *P*<.01
Hartmann et al [3], 2024	Split-face, prospective clinical trial	NAFL vs alternating NAFL + MNRF	Q4wk x 4 mo	II-IV[a]	6 mo	NAFL: *P*<.001 NAFL + MNRF: *P*<.001 NAFL vs alternating NAFL + MNRF: *P*>.05

[a] Lower fluence and lower density chosen for darker Fitzpatrick skin types.

alternating patients received 2 NAFL and 2 MNRF treatments. Both treatment regimens demonstrated significant improvements in global ECCA scores, with 55% and 53% improvement, respectively (both $P<.001$). There were no statistically significant differences between the 2 treatment sides when analyzing ECCA score, physician and subject percentage improvement evaluation scores, and patient satisfaction scores [3].

> *Take Home Point:* Both NAFL monotherapy and alternating NAFL + MNRF significantly improved acne scarring ($P<.001$), and there was no significant difference in results between the 2 treatments.
>
> *Clinical Practice Point:* NAFL monotherapy may yield similar results to alternating therapy with NAFL and MNRF, therefore, monotherapy may be more cost-effective for patients.

Adverse Effects – Combination Therapy

Combination treatment is well-tolerated with a low risk profile that is safe for all skin types. Patients will experience transient erythema, edema, and burning or pruritic sensations with combined treatments [3,5,6]. There is risk of postinflammatory hyperpigmentation (PIH), acneiform eruptions, prolonged erythema, and scarring from NAFL and risk of folliculitis, PIH, prolonged erythema, crusting, and track marks from MNRF. There were no significant differences in pain score, no additional safety concerns, and no differences in the severity or duration of side effects with NAFL + MNRF combination treatment in comparison to NAFL monotherapy [3,5]. Importantly, no patients developed secondary infections or hypertrophic scarring when treated with combination therapy in these studies.

When a patient experiences a side effect from these energy-based treatments, there are treatment options. PIH is often treated with topical lightning agents such as topical hydroquinone, tranexamic acid, kojic acid, or vitamin C, as well as topical tretinoin or oral tranexamic acid. One study used topical 4% hydroquinone, 0.01% fluocinolone acetonide, and 0.05% tretinoin to improve PIH secondary to NAFL, while another used vitamin C, kojic acid, and arbutin after combination NAFL + MNRF therapy with good results [6,24]. Some providers also treat patients for several weeks to months prior to treatment with these lightning agents with the goal of preventing PIH [6]. Furthermore, decreased density and fluence are recommended in darker skin types when treating with NAFL. Prolonged erythema typically self-resolves within several months but can also be managed with the pulsed-dye laser. Acneiform eruptions and folliculitis are treated with medical therapy, such as topical clindamycin, topical benzoyl peroxide, oral doxycycline, and typically resolve with time. Secondary infection and scarring are unlikely with both treatments. Unlike AFL, prophylactic doxycycline, valacyclovir, or fluconazole are not needed for either of these treatments.

DISCUSSION

Combined NAFL + MNRF treatment demonstrates efficacy for the treatment of acne scarring with few side effects [6]. Sharad and colleagues evaluated alternating NAFL + MNRF treatments and demonstrated significant improvement in acne scarring [6]. Two studies, Kwon and colleagues and Hartmann and colleagues, explored the efficacy of a combined NAFL + MNRF versus NAFL monotherapy with contrasting results. Kwon and colleagues's same-day combined regimen showed significant improvement for patients compared to monotherapy, whereas the alternating approach by Hartmann and colleagues did not show a significant difference compared to monotherapy [3,5]. The alternating approach reduces the number of overall treatments the patients receive (ie, two if treated same-day vs one if alternating). Hartmann and colleagues [3] discussed limitations to perform both procedures on the same day, including patient cost and provider time. These limitations need to be weighed on an individual basis if there is greater benefit with same-day combined treatment, as Kwon and colleagues [5] suggested. Given these findings, further studies are warranted to determine best practice.

SUMMARY

The treatment of acne scarring, a common sequela of acne vulgaris, persists as a clinical challenge. As acne scarring can vary widely in type and severity, individualized treatment plans are essential for achieving optimal outcomes, and multimodal approaches are often recommended. This article has explored the role of combining NAFL + MNRF as complementary mechanisms for the treatment of acne scarring. Combined NAFL + MNRF demonstrate promise for the treatment of acne scarring, with tolerability in all skin types given the limited side effect profile. Further research is needed to determine the appropriate regimen that optimizes outcomes for patients and efficiency for both providers and patients.

FUTURE CONSIDERATIONS

Additional studies examining combination NAFL + MNRF versus NAFL monotherapy are needed to strengthen the evidence in the literature.

Given our review of the literature, a split-face study comparing combination NAFL + MNRF to alternating NAFL and MNRF would help clarify efficacy of same-day vs alternating combination treatment regimens.

No studies have compared combined NAFL + MNRF with MNRF monotherapy, and this could be evaluated in the future given that NAFL and MNRF monotherapies have similar effectiveness in the literature.

Further examination of combination treatments will allow providers to identify the most cost-effective options for patients.

CLINICS CARE POINTS

- Acne scarring can vary widely in type and severity, with most patients suffering from a combination of scar types. Individualized treatment plans are essential for achieving optimal outcomes, and multimodal approaches are often recommended.
- Both NAFL monotherapy and MNRF monotherapy demonstrate significant improvement in acne scarring, with similar efficacy in head-to-head studies.
- NAFL + MNRF combination therapy is efficacious in the treatment of acne scarring and is well-tolerated without additional side effects to monotherapy, making it a safe treatment option for all skin types.
- Further studies are needed to determine the difference in efficacy between NAFL monotherapy and NAFL + MNRF combination therapy, as well as the appropriate regimen of combination therapy to optimize patient outcomes in the treatment of acne scarring.

DISCLOSURE

The authors have no relevant disclosures.

REFERENCES

[1] Jacob CI, Dover JS, Kaminer MS. Acne scarring: a classification system and review of treatment options. J Am Acad Dermatol 2001;45:109–17.

[2] Salameh F, Shumaker PR, Goodman GJ, et al. Energy-based devices for the treatment of Acne Scars: 2022 International consensus recommendations. Lasers Surg Med 2022;54(1):10–26.

[3] Hartman N, Loyal J, Borsack S, et al. Alternating treatment with nonablative fractional laser and radiofrequency microneedling for the treatment of acne scars: a prospective, randomized, split-face study. Dermatol Surg 2024;50(1):81–5.

[4] Chae WS, Seong JY, Jung HN, et al. Comparative study on efficacy and safety of 1550 nm Er:Glass fractional laser and fractional radiofrequency microneedle device for facial atrophic acne scar. J Cosmet Dermatol 2015;14(2):100–6 [published correction appears in J Cosmet Dermatol 2016;15(3):303. doi:10.1111/jocd.12233].

[5] Kwon HH, Park HY, Choi SC, et al. Novel device-based acne treatments: comparison of a 1450-nm diode laser and microneedling radiofrequency on mild-to-moderate acne vulgaris and seborrhoea in Korean patients through a 20-week prospective, randomized, split-face study. J Eur Acad Dermatol Venereol 2018;32:639–44.

[6] Sharad J. Evaluation of the cumulative effect of radiofrequency microneedling and fractional Erbium: glass 1565 laser in moderate to severe acne scars in skin of color. J Cosmet Dermatol 2022;21(3):991–7.

[7] Boen M, Jacob C. A review and update of treatment options using the acne scar classification system. Dermatol Surg 2019;45:411–22.

[8] Mandavia R, Cariati M, Shahidi S, et al. Combination radiofrequency microneedling and carbon dioxide laser for acne scarring: a systematic review and retrospective case series across two centers. J Cosmet Dermatol 2022;21:5672–9.

[9] Tan MG, Jo CE, Chapas A, et al. Radiofrequency microneedling: a comprehensive and critical review. Dermatol Surg 2021;47:755–61.

[10] Sadick NS, Cardona A. Laser treatment for facial acne scars: a review. J Cosmet Laser Ther 2018;20:424–35.

[11] Kim J, Lee SG, Choi S, et al. Combination of fractional microneedling radiofrequency and ablative fractional laser versus ablative fractional laser alone for acne and acne scars. Yonsei Med J 2023;64:721–9.

[12] Tatlıparmak A, Aksoy B, Shishehgarkhaneh LR, et al. Use of combined fractional carbon dioxide laser and fractional microneedle radiofrequency for the treatment of acne scars: a retrospective analysis of 1-month treatment outcome on scar severity and patient satisfaction. J Cosmet Dermatol 2020;19:115–21.

[13] Narurkar VA. Nonablative fractional laser resurfacing. Dermatol Clin 2009;27:473–8, vi.

[14] Alster TS, Tanzi EL, Lazarus M. The use of fractional laser photothermolysis for the treatment of atrophic scars. Dermatol Surg 2007;33:295–9.

[15] Hedelund L, Moreau KE, Beyer DM, et al. Fractional nonablative 1,540-nm laser resurfacing of atrophic acne scars. A randomized controlled trial with blinded response evaluation. Lasers Med Sci 2010;25:749–54.

[16] Bencini PL, Tourlaki A, Galimberti M, et al. Nonablative fractional photothermolysis for acne scars: clinical and

in vivo microscopic documentation of treatment efficacy. Dermatol Ther 2012;25:463–7.

[17] Hu S, Chen MC, Lee MC, et al. Fractional resurfacing for the treatment of atrophic facial acne scars in asian skin. Dermatol Surg 2009;35:826–32.

[18] Al-Dhalimi M, Jaber A. Treatment of atrophic facial acne scars with fractional Er:Yag laser. J Cosmet Laser Ther 2015;17:184–8.

[19] Alexis AF, Coley MK, Nijhawan RI, et al. Nonablative fractional laser resurfacing for acne scarring in patients with Fitzpatrick skin phototypes IV-VI. Dermatol Surg 2016;42:392–402.

[20] Cho SI, Chung BY, Choi MG, et al. Evaluation of the clinical efficacy of fractional radiofrequency microneedle treatment in acne scars and large facial pores. Dermatol Surg 2012;38:1017–24.

[21] Chandrashekar BS, Sriram R, Mysore R, et al. Evaluation of microneedling fractional radiofrequency device for treatment of acne scars. J Cutan Aesthet Surg 2014;7:93–7.

[22] Vejjabhinanta V, Wanitphakdeedecha R, Limtanyakul P, et al. The efficacy in treatment of facial atrophic acne scars in Asians with a fractional radiofrequency microneedle system. J Eur Acad Dermatol Venereol 2014;28:1219–25.

[23] Kaminaka C, Uede M, Matsunaka H, et al. Clinical studies of the treatment of facial atrophic acne scars and acne with a bipolar fractional radiofrequency system. J Dermatol 2015;42:580–7.

[24] Rongsaard N, Rummaneethorn P. Comparison of a fractional bipolar radiofrequency device and a fractional erbium-doped glass 1,550-nm device for the treatment of atrophic acne scars: a randomized split-face clinical study. Dermatol Surg 2014;40(1):14–21.

[25] Wang JV, Friedman PM, Rodeberg D, et al. Enhancing skin uptake of topical antioxidants with 1,440-nm nonablative fractional diode laser pretreatment. Dermatol Surg 2022;48:927–31.

[26] Kwon HH, Park HY, Choi SC, et al. Combined fractional treatment of acne scars involving non-ablative 1,550-nm erbium-glass laser and micro-needling radiofrequency: a 16-week prospective, randomized split-face study. Acta Derm Venereol 2017;97(8):947–51.

Advances in Cosmetic Surgery 8 (2025) 97–106
ADVANCES IN COSMETIC SURGERY

Endpoints in Laser & Light-Based Devices

Morgan Murphrey, MD, MS[a,b,*], Molly Wanner, MD, MBA[a]
[a]Department of Dermatology, Massachusetts General Hospital, Harvard Medical School, Boston, MA, USA; [b]Wellman Center for Photomedicine, Massachusetts General Hospital, Boston, MA, USA

KEYWORDS
• Endpoints • Indicators • Laser-tissue interactions • Treatment settings

KEY POINTS

- Laser and energy based devices communicate device-tissue interactions via signs on the skin termed endpoints and indicators.
- Therapeutic endpoints are indicative of a successful treatment, and suggest that a treatment will be effective. Warning endpoints are signs that point toward skin damage or undesired outcomes.
- Rather than using a cookbook approach, treatment settings should be tailored until therapeutic endpoints are achieved, and warning endpoints are avoided.

INTRODUCTION

When treating patients with lasers and light-based devices, distinct signs on the skin relay important messages to the device operator. It is imperative to watch for and understand these signs, first and foremost for patient safety. Warning signs should prompt the practitioner to discontinue treatment until appropriate setting adjustments have been made. Similarly, subtherapeutic signs should result in setting adjustments until there is a therapeutic result, or *endpoint*. The term *endpoints* refers most specifically to devices that harness the theory of selective photothermolysis and reflect laser-chromophore-tissue interactions. The term *indicators* refers to the laser-tissue interactions of other light-based devices.

This article will briefly provide an overview of laser-tissue interactions, as well as a review of both therapeutic and warning endpoints. Understanding and application of these concepts is imperative for success when using laser and light-based devices. While it can be easy to follow templates or suggested settings, these should serve only as starting points, and treatment parameters should ultimately be adjusted until appropriate endpoints are obtained. As a result, patients will benefit from successful, selective treatments, and will be spared from deleterious side effects.

LASER-TISSUE INTERACTIONS

Understanding the principles of laser-tissue interactions is the first step to understanding endpoints. Laser light interacts with different components, called *chromophores,* in the skin (epidermis or dermis). The primary chromophores relevant to dermatology include water, hemoglobin, and pigment, including melanin. Chromophores absorb wavelengths of light in varying degrees, and the higher the selective absorption, the

*Corresponding author. Wellman Center for Photomedicine, Massachusetts General Hospital, 50 Blossom Street, Boston, MA 02114. *E-mail address:* mmurphrey@mgh.harvard.edu

https://doi.org/10.1016/j.yacs.2024.12.006 www.advancesincosmeticsurgery.com
2542-4327/25/

ABBREVIATIONS	
PWBs	port wine birthmarks
PWSs	port wine stains

better a wavelength is suited for a chromophore. When a highly absorbed wavelength is beamed at a chromophore in the skin, the result is heating and/or destruction of the chromophore. The principle of *selective photothermolysis,* or *The Anderson Principle,* describes something of a Goldilocks phenomenon: if the light energy absorbed is *just enough* to destroy the target chromophore, surrounding tissues will be spared and left intact. Therefore, 2 additional components are key to laser-tissue interactions: the *pulse duration,* or time the chromophore is exposed to the laser light, and the *fluence,* or energy delivered per unit area.

When considering the appropriate laser modality and treatment settings, the chromophore directs the wavelength, and the size of the chromophore directs the pulse duration. Smaller targets (ie melanosomes) require very short pulse durations to selectively absorb laser energy, while larger targets (ie blood vessels) require longer pulse durations for adequate destruction and therapeutic effect. In general, the fluence should be titrated based on tissue endpoints, within limits. If an endpoint is not achieved despite appropriate setting adjustments, the laser operator must ask if there is another explanation. For example, an anemic patient may never respond to a pulsed dye laser (595 nm), despite hemoglobin's selective absorption at this wavelength, as anemia results in low hemoglobin, and therefore inadequate chromophore.

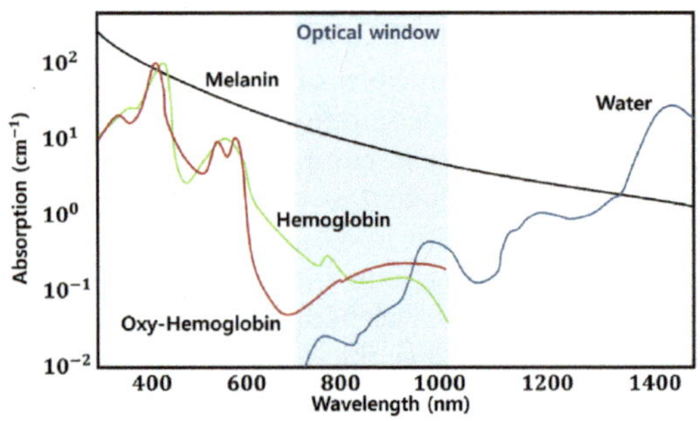

FIG. 1 Absorption spectrum of hemoglobin, deoxyhemoglobin, and melanin. *Data from* Lee J, Jeong I, Kim K, Cho J. Design and Implementation of Embedded-Based Vein Image Processing System with Enhanced Denoising Capabilities. Sensors (Basel). 2022;22(21)

THERAPEUTIC ENDPOINTS

When extrapolating laser-tissue interactions to clinical settings, these fundamental principles correlate to treatment settings. This section will describe specific clinical conditions and the appropriate skin endpoints for therapeutic efficacy. The following section will provide warning and catastrophic endpoints, which should be avoided by starting low and going slow.

Vascular Lesions

Vascular lesions are treated by targeting the chromophore hemoglobin. Based on the absorption spectrum of hemoglobin (Fig. 1) [1], this is best targeted with the commercially available 595 nm pulsed dye laser (PDL) or 532 nm potassium titanyl phosphate (KTP) laser. It is important to note that the absorption curve of oxyhemoglobin differs from that of deoxyhemoglobin, which has a unique absorption peak at around 755 nm. Consequently, venous lesions can be effectively and selectively treated at 755 nm, using an Alexandrite laser.

Port wine birthmarks

Port wine birthmarks (PWBs), also known as port wine stains (PWSs), are vascular birthmarks caused by endothelial cell proliferation resulting in ectatic, venous venule-like structures [2]. While they typically start as flat lesions, they often become larger and can develop vascular outpouchings, termed *blebs,* over time. PWBs typically result from sporadic genetic mutations but

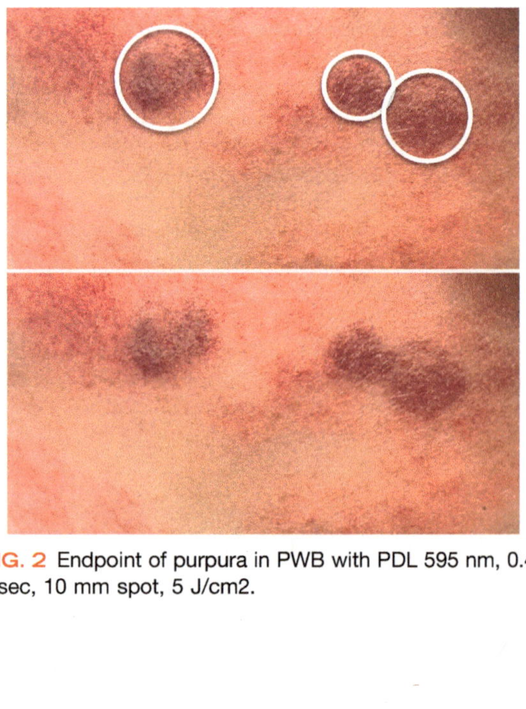

FIG. 2 Endpoint of purpura in PWB with PDL 595 nm, 0.45 msec, 10 mm spot, 5 J/cm2.

can present as part of Sturge-Weber Syndrome, or other genetic syndromes.

Treatment of PWBs should begin early, while the lesions are as flat as possible. They typically recur and require maintenance over time. When treating PWBs, the appropriate endpoint is purpura (Fig. 2). Notably, PWB in newborns may not have this endpoint. We typically use the 595 nm PDL (7–10 mm spot size) with short (0.45–3 msec) pulse durations at moderate to high fluences (4–9 J/cm2) to achieve this endpoint. As treatments progress and the chromophore becomes less dense, we often resultantly increase the fluence with treatments. The 532 nm KTP laser [3] is also an appropriate and effective choice.

Care should be taken when treating heterogenous lesions as areas saturated with more chromophore may result in bulk heating and skin injury. Settings may need to be titrated across a lesion based on clinical findings of deeper red or purple-blue hues within the lesion. Additionally, nonresponsive PWBs, or those more blue-purple in color, can be treated with the 755 nm Alexandrite laser. The long pulsed 755 nm laser has a narrow therapeutic window. It is good practice to pick the darkest area of the birthmark and treat at, but not above, the fluence that achieves purpura. Distinct blebs in PWBs should be treated with care due to chromophore density.

Infantile hemangiomas

In the past, infantile hemangioma treatment was limited, and lasers were especially useful. However, new treatment modalities, including topical timolol and oral propranolol [4], are highly safe and effective for treatment of infantile hemangiomas. As such, the use of lasers has declined over the years. Still, lasers are useful in combination with medical therapy or for treatment of hemangiomas resistant to medical therapy.

Infantile hemangiomas are dense in chromophore and can be susceptible to bulk overheating. Therefore, the desired immediate endpoint should be subtle, light, or even transient purpura. Frank purpura should prompt a decrease in fluence. Transient or very subtle purpura should be monitored as darkening of the lesion may occur post-treatment.

Telangiectasias

Telangiectasias are a common concern of patients and are typically responsive to PDL or KTP laser treatment. Perinasal telangiectasias can be refractory and typically require multiple treatments, with high recurrence rates. However, with appropriate counseling, treatment of telangiectasias can be very rewarding for clinician and patient. Immediate vessel darkening can be a therapeutic endpoint, but immediate vessel clearance is the preferred endpoint. We typically accomplish this using a 595 nm laser (3x10 or 7 mm spot size) with pulse durations ranging from 10 to 40 msec, depending on the size of the target vessel, with fluences ranging from 8 to 15 J/cm2. With increases in spot size, we typically decrease the fluence.

Cherry angiomas

Small, flat cherry angiomas respond best to 595 nm or 532 nm laser light. The ideal endpoint is immediate purpura, without petechiae (Fig. 3A–C). This typically indicates that the lesion will clear or lighten. We accomplish this with small spot sizes (3 mm) and short pulse durations (0.45–1.5 msec). Thick or large lesions may take multiple treatments. When using 595 nm or 532 nm light, if the ideal endpoint is not achieved with the first pulse, additional pulses may be fired after adequate skin cooling (typically 30 seconds–1 minute). Multiple lesions can be treated in one session, and any inadequately treated lesions can be retreated at the end of the session. When using 1064 nm laser light, pulse stacking should not be performed.

The technique of applying a glass slide to flatten the lesion, thereby increasing your chance of targeting a larger portion of the lesion, can be useful. However, care should be taken as the glass slide prevents epidermal cooling by cryogen cooling spray and cannot be used with ultrasound gel. Another technique we recommend is gentle outward stretching of the nearby skin, which can make the lesion flatter for the pulse.

Angiokeratomas can also be treated with the pulsed dye or KTP laser, including scrotal and labial angiokeratomas. A small spot size, short pulse duration, and moderately high fluence is generally required to achieve the therapeutic endpoint of purpura. Cooling should be high, and you can consider icing before and after treatment for comfort. The patient should be made aware that areas such as the scrotum and labia are prone to pigmentary changes.

Venous malformations

In addition to hemoglobin-rich vascular lesions, patients also present with deoxyhemoglobin-rich venous lesions. Large, soft, or disfiguring venous malformations should be treated surgically. However, some venous lesions, such as periorbital veins, spider veins, and venous lakes can be successfully treated with lasers. Typically, these vessels are larger, and therefore require longer pulse durations. Preferred wavelengths include 755 nm and 1064 nm. We treat periorbital veins using

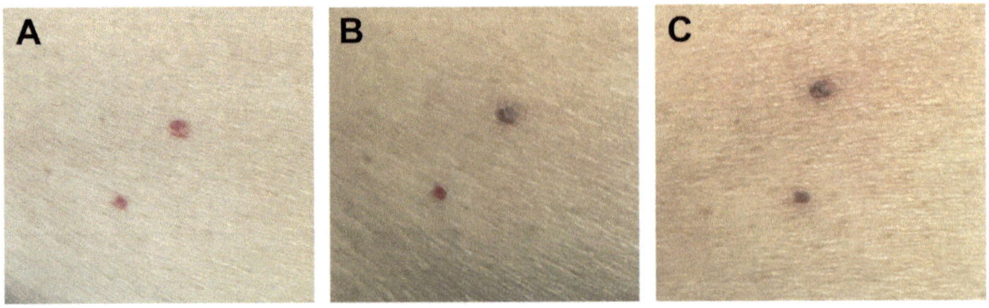

FIG. 3 (*A*) Before and immediately after treatment of the 1st (*B, superior lesion*) and 2nd (*C, inferior lesion*) cherry angioma with a pulsed dye laser at purpuric settings.

1064 nm light, with a therapeutic endpoint of visible darkening or immediate disappearance of the vessel. We use small spot sizes (3–5 mm), and march along the vessel with longer pulse durations (20–50 msec) and relatively high fluences.

Pulse stacking should not be performed when using this wavelength (1064 nm). Care should be taken to avoid overlap of pulses because of methemoglobin production from the laser pulse. The absorption of methemoglobin at 1064 nm is high, and overlap can result in ulcerations. When treating periorbital veins, caution should be used around the eye due to the depth of this wavelength.

Other venous lesions, such as cutaneous leg veins or *spider veins,* can also be treated with lasers. Patient selection is important as large or tortuous vessels may require sclerosing therapy or surgical interventions. Small (<3 mm) blue vessels can be targeted with 1064 nm laser light using moderately long pulse durations (10–40 msec). The ideal endpoint is immediate disappearance or graying of the vessel. Small red and purple vessels on the legs respond well to the pulsed dye laser or KTP laser, similar to telangiectasias on the face (Image 3). Delayed endpoints (2–5 minutes) include a cat scratch or wheal-like appearance, and slightly purpuric areas of hemorrhage can be seen (Fig. 4A–C).

Hyperpigmentation is more common on the lower extremity. Treating a tan patient should be avoided as this can cause undesired hypopigmentation or hyperpigmentation. Venous lakes, found on the vermillion lip, respond well to diode (810 nm) and Nd:Yag (1064 nm) laser light. Relatively long pulse durations should be used. Pulse stacking should be avoided and may cause bulk heating and necrosis. The ideal endpoint is purpura with darkening of the lesion to a dark blue-black color. Often, a tactile *pop* can be felt, like a kick back, when treating these growths.

Hair Removal and Pigmented Lesions

In addition to the hemoglobin in vascular lesions, pigment is also an effective chromophore for photothermolysis. Melanin has decreasing absorption over increasing wavelengths (see Fig. 1).

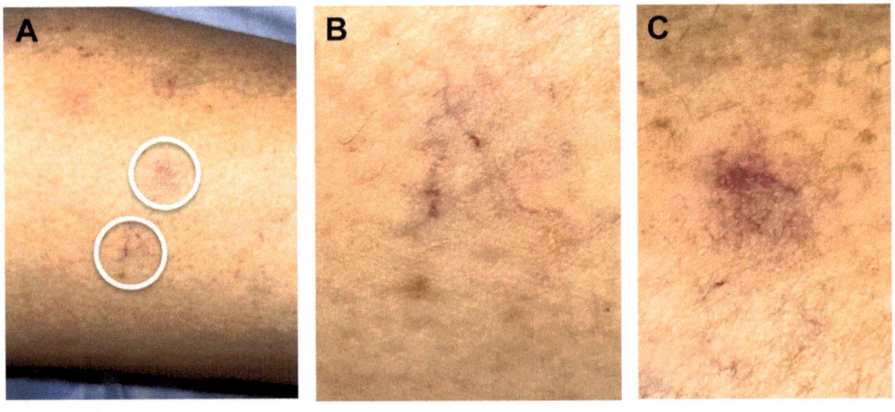

FIG. 4 (*A*) Comparison of untreated (*B*) and treated (*C*) cutaneous leg veins with 532 nm KTP laser.

When performing *laser hair removal*, the melanin pigment within the hair shaft is the primary chromophore, which is why red, blonde, and gray hair cannot be effectively treated. Because the hair shaft is the target, longer millisecond pulse durations are most effective.

When treating pigmented lesions such as lentigines, epidermal pigment is the primary target, most specifically the melanosomes found in the basal layer. While melanin has a high affinity at 595 and 532 nm wavelengths, intrinsic epidermal melanin is a notable competitive absorber. For deeper, dermal lesions, such as tattoos or Nevus of Ota, ultrashort pulses of deep penetrating light (755 nm or 1064 nm) can result in effective and selective treatment. At these ultrashort pulse durations, there are also mechanical effects, which help destroy the particles, in addition to the thermal effects described by the Anderson principle.

Hair removal

Hair removal is accomplished by targeting melanin in the hair shaft, which then transmits heat to the hair bulb, destroying the residing stem cells. Adequate destruction can result in permanent removal of the hair. This is termed the *extended theory of selective photothermolysis* [5], where a chromophore is not the primary target, but rather is used to generate and conduct heat to the desired target structure. In general, this requires longer pulse durations (ie, in the millisecond domain) at higher energies to be effective.

Melanin absorbs light well in the red and infrared range (600–1100 nm), and at these longer wavelengths deeper penetration allows for more selective targeting of dermal hair shaft melanin versus epidermal pigment. The ideal endpoint is perifollicular edema with or without erythema, with prominent follicles visible after a successful treatment. In skin of color, erythema can be subtle and should be monitored for carefully. It may take several minutes for the endpoint to develop. This is generally achieved at pulses in the millisecond duration (1–200 msec), with small hairs more effectively treated with shorter pulse durations, and thicker, coarser hairs best addressed with longer pulse durations.

Occasionally, an urticarial reaction can be seen, and is temporary. For patients who demonstrate this reaction, oral antihistamines can be used pre-treatment, and topical corticosteroids can be used post-treatment. In patients with darker skin types, a 1064 nm wavelength laser should be used. A thin layer of a high potency topical steroid immediately after treatment may decrease risk of post inflammatory pigment changes.

Lentigines

Lentigines and other brown macular lesions such as seborrheic keratoses can be treated with ultrashort pulsed 532 nm, 694 nm, and 755 nm lasers as well as long pulsed 532 and 595 nm lasers, or intense pulsed light. Other treatment modalities include liquid nitrogen cryotherapy and cautery; these can be especially useful for thicker lesions. When treating lentigines with nanosecond and picosecond pulses, the therapeutic endpoint is immediate whitening, resulting from gas bubble release by the targeted melanosomes [5] (Fig. 5). When treating with longer pulse durations, the appropriate endpoint is subtle darkening and associated mild erythema, which is also the appropriate endpoint when treating with liquid nitrogen or cautery. It takes several minutes for the endpoint to be visible.

Nevi

Treating nevi with lasers, especially papular nevi, is generally avoided. Treating nevi may result in histologic and dermatoscopic changes that raise concern, and lead to unnecessary biopsies. Nevi, and all pigmented lesions, should be carefully examined and evaluated under dermoscopy before treatment, ensuring that any concerning lesions are biopsied rather than addressed cosmetically.

Nevus of Ota

Oculodermal melanocytosis, also called *Nevus of Ota*, is a collection of dermal pigment and melanocytes around the eye, most commonly in the 1st and 2nd division of the trigeminal nerve. This condition, which disproportionately affects darker skin types, is most effectively treated by ultrashort pulsed lasers [5]. Picosecond duration pulses at 755 or 1064 nm are generally used, given their depth of penetration. The appropriate endpoint is dermal edema and immediate dermal whitening (Fig. 6). Edema and erythema will often develop and progress after the initial pulse. In darker skin types, post-treatment with a thin layer of clobetasol, or other potent topical steroid is recommended.

Tattoos

Tattoos similarly respond to ultrashort pulse durations, which cause both thermal and mechanical energy to break down tattoo pigment particles [5], releasing small gas bubbles. These small gas bubbles cause whitening of the tattoo, which is the appropriate therapeutic endpoint when treating tattoos (Fig. 7). The laser wavelength used correlates to the color of the tattoo ink and should be pulsed in the nanosecond or picosecond

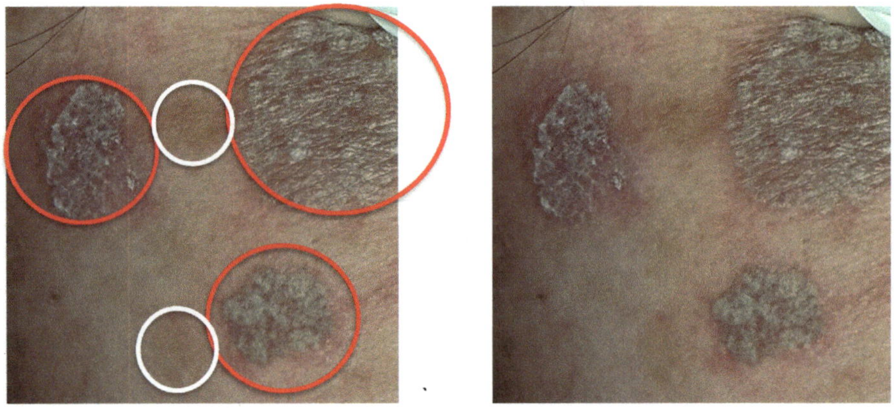

FIG. 5 Treated (red circle) and untreated (white circle) lentigines using a 755 nm Q-Switched laser.

pulse domain. Intense pulsed light (IPL) should never be used.

Lasers Without Specific Endpoints

Lasers with wavelengths in the near-infrared and infrared spectrum target the chromophore water. Commonly available wavelengths include 10,600 nm (CO_2), 2940 nm (erbium), 1927 nm (thulium), and 1550 nm. CO_2 and erbium lasers, which have a very high affinity for water, are termed *ablative* because they cause epidermal destruction through vaporization of water. Near-infrared and mid-infrared lasers (1927 nm, 1550 nm) are termed *nonablative* because they have a lower affinity for water, and therefore cause less epidermal ablation and can penetrate deeper into the skin. These wavelengths can be applied at full density or fractionally.

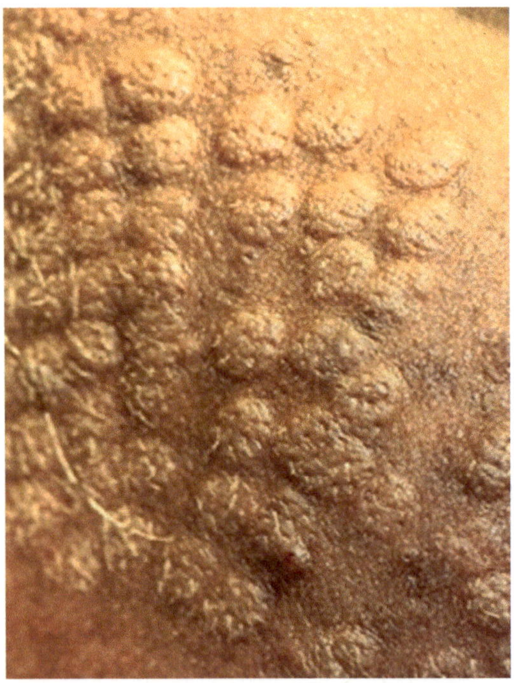

FIG. 6 Nevus of Ota status-post Q-Switched 1064 nm laser, with obvious dermal edema and faint whitening.

Full-field laser ablation causes erythema, edema, whitening, bleeding, and can cause contraction. Fractional ablative endpoints include erythema, pinpoint whitening or holes, and pinpoint bleeding. Fractional nonablative laser treatments result in mild edema and erythema, which may increase with time, before resolving. White dots can also be seen.

WARNING ENDPOINTS AND HOW TO AVOID THEM

When using lasers and energy-based devices, warning endpoints are important clues that too much energy has been delivered and skin damage is impending or

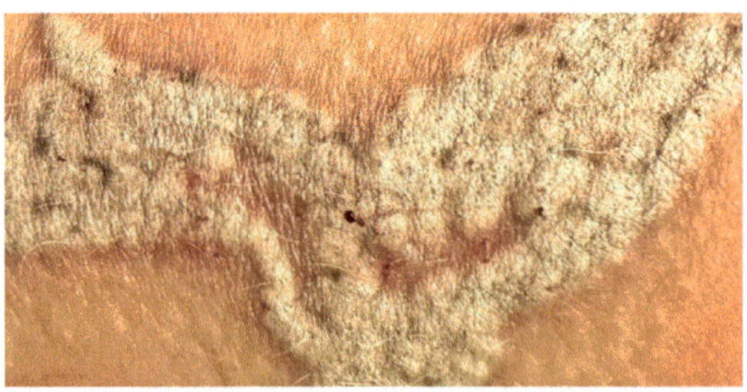

FIG. 7 Endpoint of whitening with mild dermal edema in a tattoo with black ink, using a 1064 nm picosecond laser, 4 mm spot, 1.8 J/cm2.

has occurred. When choosing a laser and selecting treatment settings, a keen understanding of laser tissue interactions will help guide treatment; it is always best to *start low* and *go slow*. In other words, start at low fluences, and take time to evaluate endpoints and think critically when adjusting parameters. Endpoints should be observed and monitored, as they can progress with time. In patients where there is a concern for adverse outcomes such as hyperpigmentation, test spots can be used, but there is no guarantee that the outcome of the test spot will be the same as the outcome of the procedure.

Cooling Related Injuries

Laser cooling is accomplished in 3 primary ways: contact cooling; cryogen spray cooling; and forced cold air. When cooling is accomplished by contact cooling, there is generally a cold sapphire tip, which is placed on the skin atop a layer of gel or other substance. With this method of cooling, it's important to ensure that the glass tip remains clean and free of *char* (as in with laser hair removal), and that the gel is intact. When cryogen spray cooling is in use, it's imperative to ensure the spray is not overly strong or long. The handpiece should be articulated at exactly 90°, or perpendicular, to the skin to avoid misalignment of the laser and cooling, which can result in *crescent-moon-like burns*. Finally, when using forced cold air, always ensure the device is plugged in and attached to the laser, and do not treat without cooling. Audible clues, such as the sound of the cooling device, can be useful cues to avoid errors.

Nikolsky Sign

Vesiculation of the skin or a dusky gray color change that results in a blister with gentle pressure is a sign of immediate skin damage and necrosis. Epidermal sloughing with gentle pressure is known as the *Nikolsky sign*. If this is seen, the treatment should be stopped. The Nikolsky sign arises when an area has been bulk overheated. Pulse stacking, inadequate cooling, or use of an inappropriate wavelength can result in this warning endpoint.

When using water-targeting lasers, avoiding high fluences or densities can help prevent skin necrosis and damage. Care should be taken not to repeat passes in small areas without adequate cooling between each pass. Observation of the skin after initial passes before laying down further energy is helpful.

Shrinkage, Contraction, Puckering, and Charring

Tissue shrinkage occurs when type 1 collagen is heated, causing the shape to morph from a helix to a coil. This coiled collagen is dense, and therefore the tissue shrinks, which can result in contraction and puckering (Fig. 8). Chemical bond change occurs in the setting of significant thermal damage to the dermis. If the thermal damage primarily involves the epidermis, char can be seen. Char can deposit on the skin if it accumulates

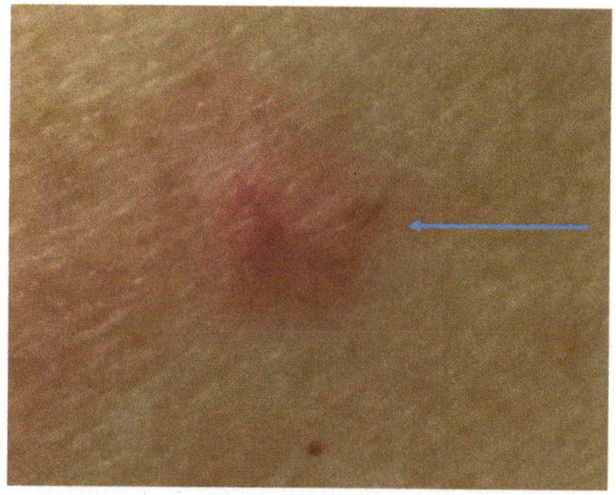

FIG. 8 Pucker sign as indicated by the blue arrow.

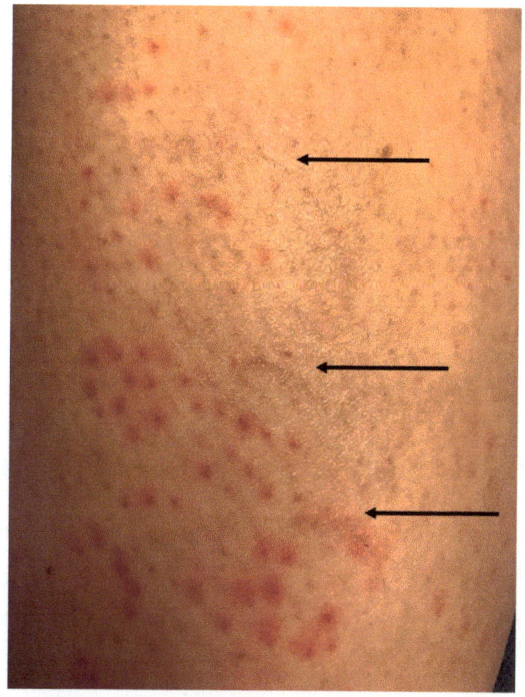

FIG. 9 Semi-circle shaped burn from charred hair via contact cooling that accumulated on the tip and deposited on the skin. The resulting shape is from char, which has absorbed the light.

on the laser tip. The handpiece should be cleaned throughout the treatment. While char accumulation is higher risk with contact cooling, it can happen with any type of handpiece (Fig. 9).

When using ablative lasers such CO2 or erbium, some degree of shrinkage and immediate contraction is desired. This indicates that ablation has occurred and represents water vaporization. When using fractionally ablative lasers, or targeting other chromophores such as pigment or hemoglobin, shrinkage and contraction are never desired endpoints and signal skin damage, with risk for adverse outcomes such as scarring.

Chrysiasis and Paradoxical Darkening

Chrysiasis results when an ultrashort laser pulse is used in a patient who has a history of systemic gold exposure. Gold was used as a treatment for immune conditions such as rheumatoid arthritis, Sjogren's syndrome, and lupus until the 1990s. In patients with a history of this treatment, exposure to nanosecond or picosecond energy can cause alterations of the gold particles, resulting in a blue-gray discoloration or darkening. This complication is difficult to remedy, and is minimally responsive to other laser treatments. The primary modality by which to avoid this undesired endpoint and complication is taking a thorough history of all patients treated with Q-switched or picosecond lasers. Those patients who have a history of systemic gold therapy should not be treated.

Paradoxical tattoo darkening occurs in patients with a history of white or pink tattoos. This was first described in 1993, when a white tattoo was treated inadvertently during a treatment for melasma [6], resulting in paradoxical tattoo darkening. Patients should be extensively counseled for this potential complication when treating white or pink tattoos. Improving this paradoxical discoloration is difficult and not always effective, but can be attempted with ultrashort pulsed 755 and 1064 nm light.

Metallic Gray, Impending Epidermal Necrosis, and Pain

Signs of epidermal death are the most concerning when wielding a laser. These signs should not be missed or overlooked, and warrant a marked decrease in laser strength before further treatment. Various devices, when used at inappropriate settings, can cause necrosis. When treating vascular lesions with the long pulsed 755 nm laser, metallic-gray blanching of skin is a sign of impending skin necrosis. This *dusky* appearance, which as dermatologists we typically associate with skin findings such as the overhanging border of pyoderma gangrenosum, represents acute separation of the dermis and epidermis and dermal overheating resulting in impending skin necrosis or death. Sometimes these findings take a moment to evolve, and pain or tenderness can be an important indicator; this should not be minimized or overlooked. If a pulse is overly painful, care should be taken to observe for endpoints before administering additional laser pulses.

Contact Dermatitis and Numbing Related Side Effects

A final concern and potential complication of laser or light-based procedures relates to the numbing and anesthesia used before administering any given device. There are a variety of commercially available topical numbing agents. Additionally, injectable lidocaine or other esther/amide anesthetics can be considered. It is important to assess for allergies before administering these anesthetics. It is also relevant to consider anesthesia limits (3.5 mg/kg without epinephrine, 7 mg/kg with epinephrine).

Topical anesthesia can cause irritant and allergic dermatitis, with tetracaine a frequent offender. This has resulted in many avoiding this topical anesthetic altogether. In addition to our anecdotal experience, this has been reported specifically in patients of Asian descent [7]. An immediate vesicular eruption in the setting of topical numbing agents should raise concern for allergic or irritant dermatitis. Topical numbing should be removed immediately with prompt application of a topical corticosteroid. Care should be taken to avoid offending ingredients in the future.

NEW FRONTIERS AND NEXT DIRECTIONS

As with all technologies, innovation in the field of laser and energy-based devices is constant. There has been significant work underway to better understand and identify endpoints and laser-tissue interactions. Additionally, there is persistent work to continue identifying chromophores to target in the epidermis and dermis for selective photothermolysis. This final portion of the article will focus on new frontiers, and the next directions in laser and energy-based devices and endpoints.

Targeting New Chromophores

The debilitating effects of acne vulgaris cannot be overstated, and this has led to a push to determine an appropriate chromophore for lasers in acne. Over the last 15 years, scientists and clinicians have worked together to use the problem and pathogenesis of acne as a jumping

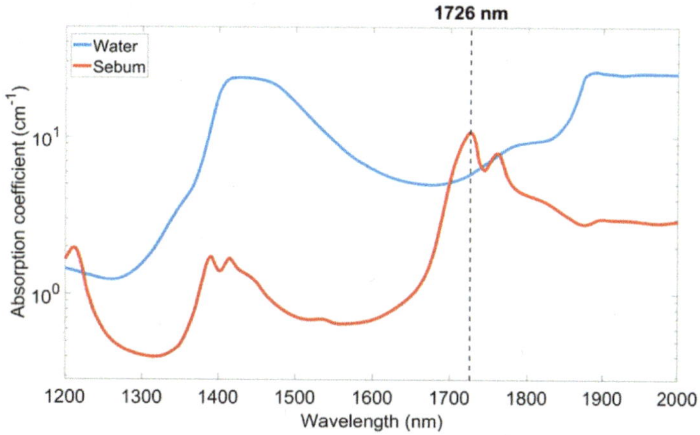

FIG. 10 Absorption spectrum of sebum. (*Adapted from* Sakamoto FH, Doukas AG, Farinelli WA, et al. Selective photothermolysis to target sebaceous glands: theoretical estimation of parameters and preliminary results using a free electron laser. Lasers Surg Med. 2012;44(2):175–183.)

point for future curative options facilitated by lasers and light-based devices. In 2012, the initial parameters for a sebum specific-laser were tested; from this early work comes the 1726 nm laser, selective for sebum and sebaceous glands (Fig. 10) [8].

In 2022, two 1726 nm laser devices were Food and Drug Administration (FDA) cleared for the treatment of acne. These lasers have the potential to revolutionize the treatment of acne and sebaceous lesions. In patients who are not candidates for medications such as isotretinoin, the 1726 nm laser offers a solution for targeting sebaceous glands, one of the primary contributors to acne, for resolution and improvement of skin lesions. These devices are successful for the treatment of acne, with durable treatment responses. In the future, this wavelength may prove to be beneficial for the treatment of other skin concerns related to sebaceous glands, such as sebaceous hyperplasia or sebaceomas.

Endpoints Versus Indicators

All energy-based devices are not created equal. While lasers and light-based devices function on similar principles, the specificity of lasers often makes them particularly useful when targeting conditions in a heterogenous organ like the skin. The term *endpoints* reflects laser-tissue interactions resulting from targeting of a specific chromophore, causing thermal destruction in a selective way. On the other hand, indicators refer to all skin reactions related to lasers and energy-based devices, and are more nonspecific. As technologies continue to emerge, this distinction is an important foundation in understanding the skin's response to energy.

Endpoints and Artificial Intelligence

As the world of artificial intelligence and augmented reality continues to develop, there will likely be implications for lasers, energy-based devices, and laser-tissue interactions. While new technologies such as confocal and optical coherence tomography are useful for determining real-time tissue interactions and responses, there are limitations in that these modalities are dependent on operators and their interpretations of study results. As we continue to better understand lasers and energy-based devices, there is a reasonable next step of creating machine learning models to help automate and interpret these advances. This technology is already being implemented in fields such as ophthalmology [9], and will likely become more prevalent in dermatology and aesthetic medicine.

SUMMARY

When treating patients with lasers and energy-based devices, each treatment should be individualized based on the patient and his or her response to the treatment. If a patient is demonstrating inadequate or warning endpoints, a thorough evaluation should ensue: is the laser firing appropriately? Is the cooling on and functional? Is there adequate chromophore in the skin?

The decision of which laser or energy-based device to use depends on the devices available, the chromophore at hand, and the patient's unique characteristics. Following a *cookbook* approach is, at best, ineffective, and at worst, harmful for patient care. While it may seem easy or simple to adhere to readily available or published *recipes*, a careful and keen eye is required to provide patients with safe and effective laser and light-based device treatments. Relying on the signs of endpoints and indicators allows for safe and effective treatments, resulting in satisfaction for patients and providers alike.

CLINICS CARE POINTS

- Laser and energy-based devices communicate device-tissue interactions via signs on the skin termed endpoints and indicators.
- When using devices that harness selective photothermolysis, resulting signs on the skin are termed *endpoints*. When using other energy-based devices, resulting signs on the skin are termed *indicators*.
- Therapeutic endpoints are indicative of a successful treatment, and suggest that a treatment will be effective. Warning endpoints are signs that point toward skin damage or undesired outcomes.
- Rather than using a cookbook approach, treatment settings should be tailored until therapeutic endpoints are achieved, and warning endpoints are avoided.

DISCLOSURE

M. Wanner receives grant funding from Bausch Health, Canada. Dr M. Wanner has equity and receives consulting fees from EllaOla, Sorette. She has equity with Akeyna, Clarity Cosmetics, MK2002.

REFERENCES

[1] Lee J, Jeong I, Kim K, et al. Design and implementation of embedded-based vein image processing System with enhanced denoising capabilities. Sensors (Basel) 2022; 22(21):8559.

[2] Nguyen V, Hochman M, Mihm MC Jr, et al. The pathogenesis of port wine stain and sturge weber syndrome: complex interactions between genetic alterations and aberrant MAPK and PI3K activation. Int J Mol Sci 2019; 20(9):2243.

[3] Nguyen L, Seeber N, Kautz G, et al. 532-nm potassium titanyl-phosphate laser versus 595-nm pulsed dye laser for port-wine birthmarks: a prospective, randomized, split-side study. J Eur Acad Dermatol Venereol 2024; 38(6):1140–6.

[4] Han K, Wei J, Zheng H, et al. Efficacy and safety of oral propranolol or topical timolol for the treatment of superficial infantile hemangiomas. J Craniofac Surg 2024.

[5] Ibrahimi OA, Avram MM, Hanke CW, et al. Laser hair removal. Dermatol Ther 2011;24(1):94–107.

[6] Anderson RR, Geronemus R, Kilmer SL, et al. Cosmetic tattoo ink darkening. A complication of Q-switched and pulsed-laser treatment. Arch Dermatol 1993;129(8): 1010–4.

[7] Vij A, Markus R. Immediate vesicular eruption caused by topical 23% lidocaine 7% tetracaine ointment in a patient scheduled for laser therapy: a new adverse drug reaction. J Cosmet Dermatol 2011;10(4):307–10.

[8] Sakamoto FH, Doukas AG, Farinelli WA, et al. Selective photothermolysis to target sebaceous glands: theoretical estimation of parameters and preliminary results using a free electron laser. Lasers Surg Med 2012;44(2):175–83.

[9] Khonina SN, Kazanskiy NL, Efimov AR, et al. A perspective on the artificial intelligence's transformative role in advancing diffractive optics. iScience 2024;27(7):110270.

Advances in Cosmetic Surgery 8 (2025) 107–119
ADVANCES IN COSMETIC SURGERY

Adjustments to the Maxillofacial Skeleton to Improve Facial Harmony

Kevin B. Coppelson, MD, DDS*
Private Practice, The Breathe Institute and Greater Ventura Oral and Facial Surgery, 10921 Wilshire Boulevard, Suite 912, Los Angeles, CA 90024, USA

KEYWORDS
• Maxillofacial surgery • Orthognathic surgery • Facial harmony • Skeletal adjustments • Virtual surgical planning • Custom implants • Facial esthetics

KEY POINTS

- Maxillofacial skeletal adjustments enhance facial harmony by refining proportions, improving symmetry, and achieving esthetically balanced outcomes.
- Virtual surgical planning for corrective jaw surgery and custom implants allow precise modifications tailored to each patient's unique esthetic needs.
- Techniques like LeFort I osteotomies, mandibular adjustments, and genioplasty optimize facial contours and incisor display for improved esthetic appeal.
- Addressing facial proportions, including thirds and fifths, and correcting asymmetry significantly impact overall attractiveness and patient satisfaction.

INTRODUCTION

Facial harmony and balance are foundational to esthetic appeal. Subtle variations in the proportions of facial structures can make a significant impact on perceived attractiveness. The maxillofacial skeleton—the maxilla, mandible, zygomatic arches, and surrounding structures—plays a central role in defining these proportions and supporting the overlying soft tissues. Adjustments to the maxillofacial skeleton can significantly enhance facial balance, improving esthetics and functionality.

This article explores surgical modifications aimed at optimizing facial harmony by adjusting the maxillofacial skeleton. These adjustments cater to a range of patient needs, from correcting congenital asymmetries to addressing age-related changes and enhancing natural features. Specialists across cosmetic surgery disciplines—including plastic surgeons, facial plastic surgeons, oculoplastic surgeons, and cosmetic dermatologists—will find these insights valuable for understanding how targeted skeletal changes can elevate surgical outcomes.

The article outlines key anatomic structures, principles of facial proportions, and surgical techniques used for skeletal adjustments. It will also cover advancements in custom orthognathic surgery, virtual surgical planning, custom facial implants, and minimally invasive midface expansion options that support facial enhancement. Practical case studies illustrate the application of these concepts, emphasizing the balance between esthetics and functional health. The aim is to provide a comprehensive overview that integrates current best practices and future directions in maxillofacial surgery.

*Corresponding author. *E-mail address:* kevin.coppelson@gmail.com

https://doi.org/10.1016/j.yacs.2025.01.001
www.advancesincosmeticsurgery.com
2542-4327/25/

ABBREVIATIONS

CPAP	continuous positive airway pressure
DOME	distraction osteogenesis maxillary expansion
EASE	endoscopically assisted surgical expansion
HA	hydroxyapatite
MARPE	miniscrew-assisted rapid palatal expansion
MIND	minimally invasive nasomaxillary distraction
MMA	maxillomandibular advancement y6
OSA	obstructive sleep apnea
SARPE	surgically assisted rapid palatal expansion
TMJ	temporomandibular joint
UARS	upper airway resistance syndrome
VSP	virtual surgical planning

ANATOMY OF THE MAXILLOFACIAL SKELETON

A thorough understanding of the maxillofacial skeleton is fundamental for making precise surgical adjustments that enhance facial harmony. This section outlines the key skeletal structures, their relationships with soft tissues, and the importance of their interactions in achieving aesthetic and functional outcomes.

Key Structures

The maxillofacial skeleton comprises several critical components that shape the face [1].

Maxilla

The upper jawbone forms much of the midface and supports the upper teeth. The maxilla plays a critical role in the projection and width of the midface, influencing incisor show, the smile arc, and the relationship between the nose and lips. Moreover, the nasal cavity volume and width of the nasal floor are determined by transverse maxillary development. Abnormal positioning or growth of the maxilla can lead to issues with occlusion, nasal obstruction, insufficient tongue space, and aesthetic imbalances in the midface.

Mandible

The lower jawbone defines most of the lower third of the face and contributes to jawline definition and facial symmetry. Variations in mandibular position, shape, and size can impact occlusion, pharyngeal airway size, chin projection, and overall facial harmony.

Zygomatic arch

The zygomatic bones form the cheekbones, creating lateral projection in the midface and contributing significantly to facial width and contour. The prominence of the zygomatic arches influences midface balance and can be a focal point in achieving facial harmony, in anterior and lateral projection.

Nasal and orbital bone

Nasal and orbital bone plays a central role in facial symmetry, nasal projection, periorbital esthetics, and overall facial balance. However, alterations to these structures are not discussed in this article.

Relationship of Soft Tissues to the Facial Skeleton

The overlying soft tissues of the face are significantly influenced by the underlying skeletal framework. The bone structure serves as the foundation for facial contours, determining the positioning of the skin, muscles, and fat [2].

Soft tissue support

The maxillofacial skeleton shapes soft tissue draping, affecting youthfulness and proportion. Inadequate skeletal support, such as insufficient maxillary projection, can reduce incisor show and prematurely age the face [3].

Response to skeletal changes

Adjusting bone structures affects soft tissue support. Maxillary advancements improve midface projection and the nasolabial angle, while mandibular changes can reduce jowls and marionette lines. A retruded jawline contributes to sagging skin and deepened lines, but surgical skeletal expansion enhances support and minimizes aging signs.

PRINCIPLES OF FACIAL PROPORTIONS AND INCISOR SHOW

Jaw deformities can impact the shape, size, position, orientation, and symmetry of the maxilla and mandible [4]. Facial harmony requires aligning skeletal and soft tissue elements based on established proportions. Although influenced by cultural and personal aesthetics, these ratios guide balance. This section explores key concepts, including the golden ratio, symmetry, skeletal positioning, and the role of incisor display and lip length in achieving esthetic outcomes.

Ideal Facial Proportions

Facial proportions are typically divided into distinct regions, providing a reference for surgical adjustments [5].

Facial thirds

The face is divided horizontally into 3 equal sections (Fig. 1): upper third (trichion to glabella), middle third (glabella to subnasale), and lower third (subnasale to menton). Within the lower third, the ideal ratio between the upper lip and lower lip-to-chin distance is approximately 1:2. Deviations in this ratio can disrupt harmony in the lower face, impacting aesthetic and functional outcomes.

Facial fifths

The face is divided vertically into 5 equal sections, establishing ideal spacing between the eyes, nose, and lateral facial edges. Proper alignment in these regions contributes to lateral symmetry and overall width (Fig. 2).

Golden ratio

The golden ratio (1.618:1) is a classic guide in facial aesthetics, applied to dimensions like face width to height, eye spacing, nose width, and mouth. Alignment with this ratio is often associated with perceived attractiveness [6].

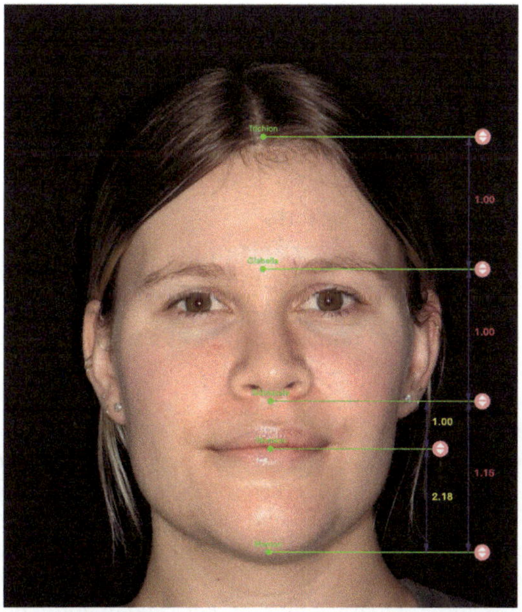

FIG. 1 Illustration of facial thirds, dividing the face into 3 proportional sections: the upper third (trichion to glabella), the middle third (glabella to subnasale), and the lower third (subnasale to menton). The lower facial third is further analyzed to evaluate the ratio of upper lip length to lower lip length, which plays a critical role in achieving balanced proportions and aesthetic harmony during orthognathic surgery planning.

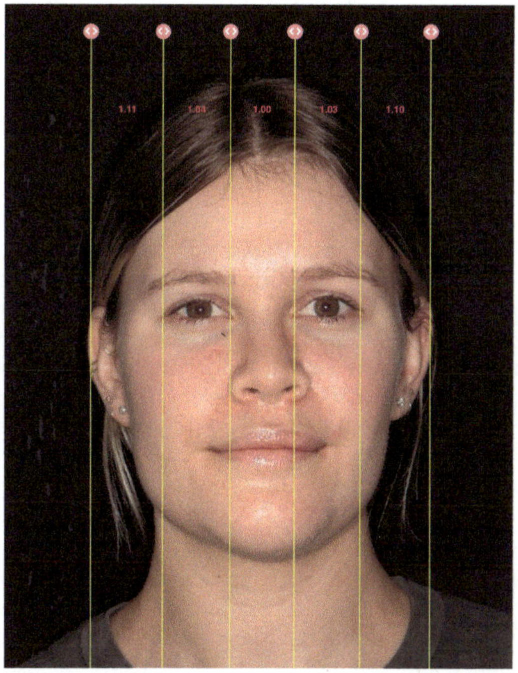

FIG. 2 Illustration of facial fifths, dividing the face vertically into 5 equal sections. This analysis measures the widths of the eyes, nose, and mouth relative to the facial width, emphasizing the importance of symmetry and proportionality in achieving aesthetic harmony during orthognathic surgery planning.

Facial Symmetry

Symmetry is a fundamental aspect of facial attractiveness, with balanced, mirror-like halves contributing to a harmonious appearance. Skeletal adjustments in maxillofacial surgery are often guided by the goal of enhancing symmetry, especially in the midface and jawline. Surgical plans frequently aim to correct asymmetries that may exist in bone structure, providing a more cohesive foundation for soft tissue draping and overall facial aesthetics [7].

Skeletal Proportions

Skeletal proportions play a critical role in defining forward maxillary position, chin positioning, and overall skeletal harmony. Certain reference lines and landmarks are used to assess these positions.

Andrews' six elements of orofacial harmony and the GALL line

This analysis outlines the ideal positioning of maxillary and mandibular structures for facial balance, with particular emphasis on maxillary projection relative to the forehead [8]. The ideal maxillary position is when the midpoint of the upper incisor aligns with goal anterior-limit line (GALL), which is parallel to the head's frontal plane and passes through a line connecting the foreheads anterior-limit line and the glabellar vertical line.

Chin positioning and holdaway analysis

Ideal chin prominence can be assessed through the holdaway analysis, which measures the relationship between the most forward point on the chin (pogonion) and the NB line (a line drawn from the nasion to the B point). In a balanced profile, the pogonion should be approximately 2 mm behind the NB line, matching the ideal distance of the lower incisor's most forward point (L1) from the NB line [9].

Control of Incisor Show

A key component in achieving an aesthetically pleasing smile is controlling the amount of maxillary incisor display. Proper incisor show contributes to facial vibrancy and youthfulness, while excessive or insufficient display may distort facial balance [10]. Surgical adjustments to the maxilla can control incisor display include

- Vertical maxillary impaction, which reduces maxillary height to correct excessive incisor show and a gummy smile, improving smile aesthetics and facial proportions
- Downgrafting, which increases incisor display in cases of inadequate visibility, enhancing balance and facial aesthetics
- Cant or roll correction, which addresses maxillary asymmetry to improve uneven incisor display, enhancing facial harmony and smile aesthetics

Lip Length Considerations

The relationship between lip length and incisor display is critical for balanced facial proportions [11]. When lip length is excessive, incisor show may be minimized, resulting in an aged or less vibrant appearance. Conversely, normal lip length allows for optimal control of incisor display through skeletal adjustments alone.

Excessive lip coverage

In cases where lip length conceals the maxillary incisors excessively, surgical interventions such as lip lifts may be considered to adjust the balance between lip and incisor display [12].

Normal lip length

For patients with standard lip length, precisely controlled maxillary adjustments, such as those listed previously, can optimize incisor display without altering the lips themselves [13].

Ethnic and Gender Variations

Perceptions of ideal facial proportions and incisor display vary across different ethnicities and genders [14,15]. These variations influence surgical planning, as patient expectations and anatomic baselines vary. Recognizing these factors allows practitioners to tailor adjustments to align with individual and cultural aesthetic preferences. The principles outlined here emphasize the role of facial proportions in achieving balanced, personalized outcomes, forming a foundation for maxillofacial surgery that enhances aesthetics and function.

SURGICAL ADJUSTMENTS TO THE MAXILLOFACIAL SKELETON

Surgical adjustments to the maxillofacial skeleton are essential for enhancing facial harmony, correcting translation discrepancies, addressing orientation issues, and achieving symmetry. By modifying key structures such as the maxilla, mandible, chin, and zygomas, surgeons can significantly impact facial proportions and balance. This section outlines the primary surgical techniques used to adjust these structures.

Maxillary Adjustments

Maxillary adjustments are performed to correct vertical, horizontal, transverse, or orientational discrepancies, impacting everything from incisor display to midface projection. The primary surgery performed on the maxilla is the LeFort 1 osteotomy.

LeFort I osteotomy

This transoral procedure involves horizontal sectioning of the maxilla at the LeFort I level (just above the roots of the teeth and a few millimeters above the floor of the nose) [16]. This osteotomy separates the maxilla from the surrounding facial bones, allowing it to be mobilized. Using virtual surgical planning (VSP) and titanium hardware for fixation, this technique provides nearly full 3-dimensional control over the positioning of the maxilla.

High LeFort I osteotomy

A variation of the standard LeFort I osteotomy, this approach raises the osteotomy level to sometimes include the lower part of the zygoma [17]. This modification enables enhanced midface projection, which can be beneficial for patients with midface hypoplasia.

Transverse Maxillary Expansion Techniques

All methods of transverse maxillary expansion widen the dental arch, reducing negative spaces and enhancing the patient's smile. Additionally, these techniques broaden the palate, increasing tongue space to improve airway function and expanding the volume of alveolar bone, which facilitates better orthodontic alignment.

Segmental LeFort expansion

Performed during orthognathic surgery, this technique broadens the maxilla and nasal floor to increase transverse width. It primarily addresses occlusal issues and increases tongue space with minimal impact on nasal breathing. A key advantage is the completion of expansion during surgery, although it is limited to approximately 6 mm [18].

Traditional two-piece LeFort I osteotomy

Also called surgically assisted rapid palatal expansion (SARPE) [19] or distraction osteogenesis maxillary expansion (DOME) [20], this technique combines a midline maxillary split with a LeFort I osteotomy to achieve significant transverse expansion. It addresses occlusal issues, increases tongue space, and moderately improves nasal breathing, with expansion limited by the palatal distractor.

Minimally invasive midface expansion techniques

Recent minimally invasive methods, such as MARPE (miniscrew-assisted rapid palatal expansion), allow expansion not only at the LeFort I level but across the entire midface [21,22]. Additionally, techniques like MIND (minimally invasive nasomaxillary distraction) [23]and EASE (endoscopically-assisted surgical expansion) [24] enable controlled midface expansion in complex cases. The benefits of midface expansion include 3-dimensional widening of the entire nasal cavity, significantly reducing nasal obstruction and airway resistance, and enhancing zygomatic (cheekbone) projection, which can also be cosmetically beneficial.

Mandibular Adjustments

Mandibular surgeries correct chin prominence, jaw asymmetry, and occlusion, enhancing the lower facial third and jawline definition. These procedures often improve oropharyngeal airway size, benefiting patients with sleep-breathing disorders.

Bilateral sagittal split osteotomy

This commonly performed intraoral procedure enables forward, backward, and orientational adjustments of the distal mandible to correct prognathism or retrognathism, enhancing jaw alignment and facial balance. However, it is less suitable for patients with reduced mandibular ramus height [25].

Inverted-L osteotomy

This is used for vertical elongation, large advancements, and orientational adjustments of the mandible. Traditionally performed extraorally, it can now be completed intraorally with VSP and custom hardware. Bone grafting is required to fill the gap created by the osteotomy [26].

Additional Mandibular Procedures

Genioplasty

Genioplasty reshapes the chin to enhance lower facial balance, allowing precise control over chin position, height, width, and projection. By advancing or setting back the chin, surgeons can influence profile harmony [27]. Additionally, a wedge resection can be used to narrow or widen the chin, while vertical modifications allow for control over lower facial height [28].

Mandibular contouring and angle reduction

Cosmetic contouring of the mandibular body and angles can soften overly prominent structures, refining the jawline for a more harmonious and aesthetically pleasing appearance [29].

Mandibular angle and chin implants

These are available in stock or custom-made designs, and they improve jawline definition and chin prominence. Custom implants precisely match the patient's anatomy for optimal symmetry and contour, while stock implants provide a cost-effective option. These implants enhance lower facial width, projection, and overall aesthetic harmony [30,31].

Zygomatic (Malar) Adjustments

Zygomatic, or malar, adjustments impact midface width, cheekbone prominence, and facial symmetry. Techniques include augmentation and reduction to achieve balanced contours.

Zygomatic (malar) augmentation

Stock implants, custom implants, and hydroxyapatite (HA) are used to enhance cheekbone projection [32]. Custom implants are tailored to the patient's anatomy for precise control over symmetry, projection, and contour, while HA and stock implants offer more economical options. This approach is ideal for adding volume and definition to flat or underprojected cheekbones.

Zygomatic reduction

For overly prominent or wide cheekbones, zygomatic reduction narrows midface width, softening lateral projection to create a balanced appearance. This procedure is particularly popular in Asia [33].

The combination of these surgical techniques allows practitioners to customize facial adjustments based on each patient's unique anatomy and aesthetic goals. Each intervention is planned to address a patient's specific needs, creating a harmonious, individualized result.

VIRTUAL SURGICAL PLANNING AND PATIENT-SPECIFIC HARDWARE

Advancements in VSP and custom 3-dimensional printed titanium (patient-specific) hardware have revolutionized maxillofacial surgery by enabling unparalleled facial skeletal analysis, surgical planning, precision, and customization. These technologies allow surgeons to preoperatively simulate procedures, predict outcomes, and develop tailored solutions that enhance functional and aesthetic results [34,35].The integration of custom facial implants further expands the potential for achieving optimal outcomes, especially in complex cases.

Virtual Surgical Planning

VSP involves the use of advanced 3-dimensional imaging and modeling software to map the patient's anatomy and design a surgical plan with pinpoint accuracy. Key benefits of VSP include diagnosis, mapping, and preoperative simulation.

Diagnosis and mapping

VSP employs 3-dimensional cephalometry and skeletal measurements to diagnose dentofacial issues. By analyzing proportions in 3 dimensions, it identifies discrepancies that may not be apparent in traditional imaging or clinical examinations, improving diagnosis and treatment planning.

Preoperative simulation

VSP enables simulation of osteotomies, adjustments, and hardware placement, minimizing intraoperative guesswork and enhancing accuracy. Visualizing outcomes allows surgeons to refine approaches, achieving functional and aesthetic goals with greater predictability.

Traditional corrective jaw surgery uses VSP in conjunction with prefabricated occlusal splints that aid in jaw positioning before fixation.

Patient-Specific Hardware

Patient-specific hardware refers to custom-designed plates and surgical guides created using the patient's unique anatomy. These components, designed in conjunction with VSP, improve the accuracy and efficiency of maxillofacial procedures [36,37]. Key features include surgical guides and custom plates.

Prefabricated surgical guides allow for accurate osteotomies, bone reduction, and predrilling of screw holes, ensuring precise execution of the surgical plan.

Designed to match the patient's bone contours, custom plates minimize intraoperative adjustments, reducing surgical time. When paired with surgical guides, they ensure precise plan execution. Their 3-dimensional printed rigidity also enhances postoperative stability compared with traditional hardware.

Integration of Custom Facial Implants

Custom facial implants designed through the VSP process expand the possibilities for achieving optimal aesthetic and functional outcomes. These implants address deficiencies in midface projection, jawline definition, and areas not fully correctable with skeletal osteotomies. They can also be precisely designed to integrate with 3-dimensional printed titanium plates, ensuring accurate placement during surgery.

FUNCTIONAL CONSIDERATIONS

Functional considerations are paramount in maxillofacial surgery, as skeletal adjustments traditionally address both aesthetic goals with improvements in critical functions such as breathing, chewing, swallowing, and speaking [38]. Functional improvements often align with aesthetic goals, as proper skeletal alignment enhances appearance and mechanical performance. Addressing these issues not only enhances the patient's quality of life, but also ensures long-term health and stability.

Airway Obstruction and Sleep Apnea

Skeletal adjustments can significantly impact airway size and function, making breathing optimization a primary focus of maxillofacial surgery. Documented cases of obstructive sleep apnea (OSA) unresponsive to conservative measures, such as continuous positive airway pressure (CPAP) or oral appliances, often require surgical intervention.

- Maxillomandibular advancement (MMA): Bimaxillary advancement surgery is one of the most effective treatments for sleep-disordered breathing, such as OSA. This procedure expands the oropharyngeal airway, reducing airway resistance and improving breathing [39].
- Maxillary/midface expansion: Techniques that expand the maxilla or midface help reduce nasal obstructions and airway resistance, leading to improved breathing.

Chewing and Swallowing Difficulties

Impairments in chewing and swallowing caused by skeletal discrepancies can significantly affect a patient's ability to process food effectively. Surgical interventions aim to align the jaws and teeth properly, enabling efficient mastication.

Speech Disorders

Speech articulation problems can arise because of jaw misalignment. These issues often require surgical correction to improve the positioning of the jaws.

Temporomandibular Joint Disorders

Temporomandibular joint (TMJ) disorders are frequently linked to jaw misalignment. Maxillofacial surgery can relieve TMJ stress by achieving proper jaw alignment and dental occlusion.

By addressing airway management, chewing, swallowing, speech, and TMJ health, maxillofacial surgery not only enhances facial esthetics but also significantly improves functional outcomes and quality of life.

CASE STUDIES AND EXAMPLES

Case Study 1: Comprehensive Orthognathic Surgery for Functional and Aesthetic Improvement

Patient overview

A 23-year-old woman presented with jaw tension, difficulty chewing, and speech articulation.

Clinical and radiographic findings included class III skeletal underbite, macrogenia with a wide chin, broad mandibular bodies, and insufficient incisor display despite normal lip length.

Surgical intervention included

1. LeFort I osteotomy, 3-pieces: the maxilla was advanced, downgrafted, and expanded horizontally to improve incisor display and enhance midface projection
2. Bilateral sagittal split osteotomies (BSSOs)
3. T-genioplasty, which narrowed the chin with a wedge resection
4. Mandibular contouring, which reduced the width of the mandibular body to create a more harmonious jawline

The surgical outcomes demonstrated significant functional and aesthetic improvements. Functional outcomes included jaw alignment relieved tension that allowed for proper chewing, improved articulation, and improved sleep quality. Aesthetic outcomes included more

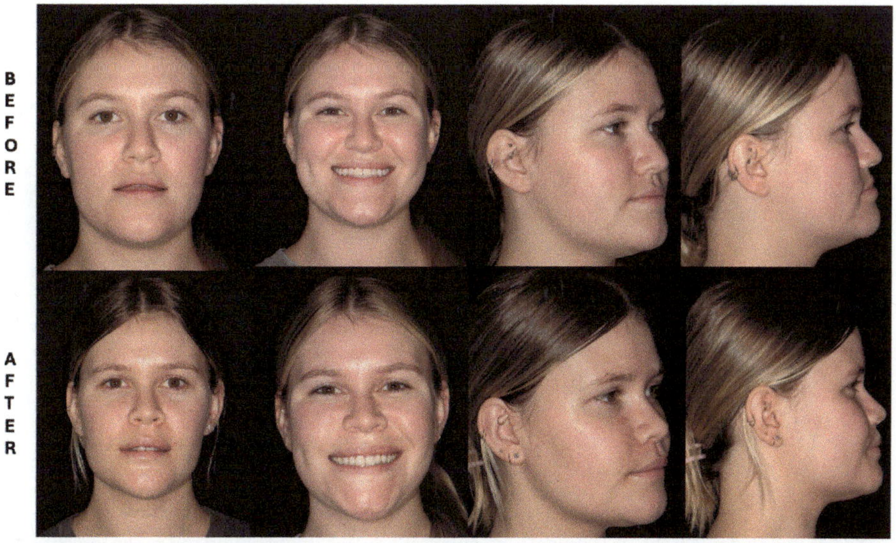

FIG. 3 Preoperative and postoperative facial photographs. The images highlight improved maxillary incisor show in relaxed and smiling positions, enhanced facial harmony, and reduced width of the mandibular body and chin.

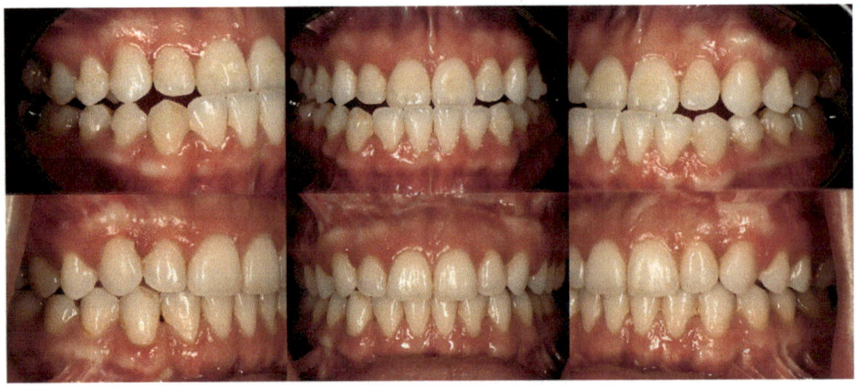

FIG. 4 Preoperative and postoperative occlusion photographs. The images illustrate corrected overbite and overjet of the incisors, along with improved overall occlusion, contributing to enhanced chewing efficiency and speech function.

proportional facial appearance with enhanced balance in frontal and lateral views, narrower chin and softened jawline created a more refined lower face, and appropriate incisor display enhanced the patient's natural beauty.

Discussion

The coordinated approach using maxillary and mandibular adjustments, combined with chin narrowing and mandibular contouring, addressed skeletal discrepancies and soft tissue harmony. The result was a comprehensive improvement in the patient's quality of life and facial appearance (Figs. 3–5).

Case Study 2: Comprehensive Orthognathic Surgery and Custom for Post-Trauma Jaw Asymmetry and Sleep Apnea

Patient overview

A 40-year-old man presented with functional impairments and severe mandibular asymmetry caused by prior jaw trauma. Symptoms include nasal obstruction, chewing, mild OSA, and jaw pain. Despite multiple reconstructive surgeries, he continued to experience poor function and asymmetry.

Clinical and radiographic findings included severe mandibular asymmetry with significant loss of height and width of the left angle and ramus of the mandible, severe malocclusion, and significant nasal deviation.

Surgical intervention included

1. LeFort I osteotomy (3-piece), which realigned the maxilla and allowed for transverse and vertical adjustments to improve occlusion and midface symmetry
2. BSSO, which corrected the mandibular asymmetry and repositioned the jaw to restore alignment
3. Custom PEEK implant for the left mandibular angle, which addressed severe asymmetry in the height and width of the left mandibular angle

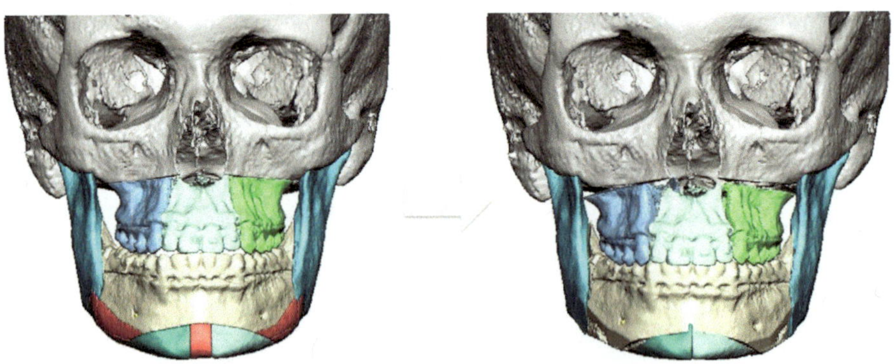

FIG. 5 The left image depicts the VSP model with segmented jaws, highlighting red areas indicating planned bone reduction on the mandibular bodies and the wedge resection used to narrow the chin. The right image shows the final jaw positions after surgery.

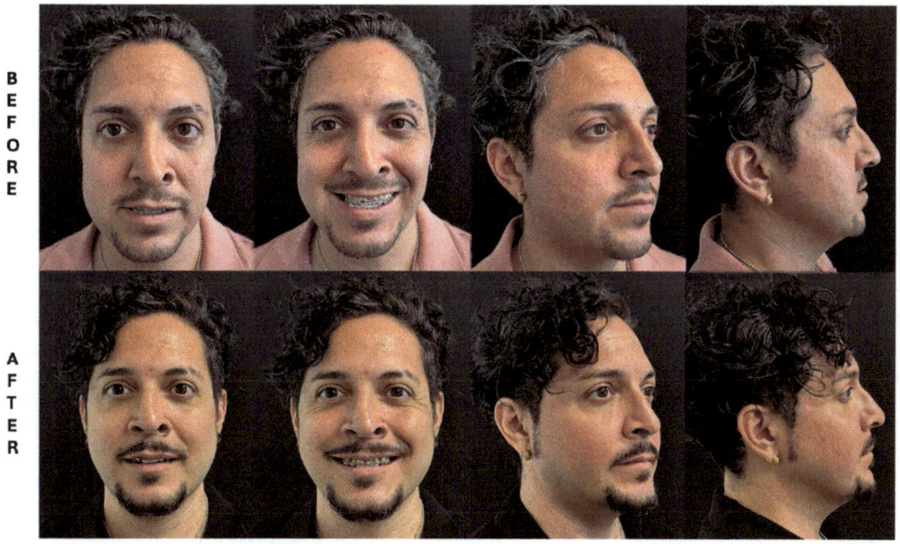

FIG. 6 Preoperative and postoperative facial photographs. The preoperative images highlight the severe mandibular asymmetry and overall facial distortion, including deviation of the nose and septum to the left. The postoperative images demonstrate significantly improved facial symmetry and balance, with even the nose appearing straighter despite no formal open septal rhinoplasty.

Results

Functional outcomes included significant improvement in chewing, nasal obstruction, and sleep quality, as well as reduction in jaw joint pain, locking, and shifting during opening.

Aesthetic outcomes included marked improvement in facial symmetry and balance, with alignment of the jawline and correction of mandibular asymmetry. Additionally, nasal deviation and midline alignment improved significantly, despite not performing a formal open septal rhinoplasty.

Discussion

Comprehensive orthognathic surgery, combined with custom implant technology, offers effective solutions for complex deformities. This case underscores the

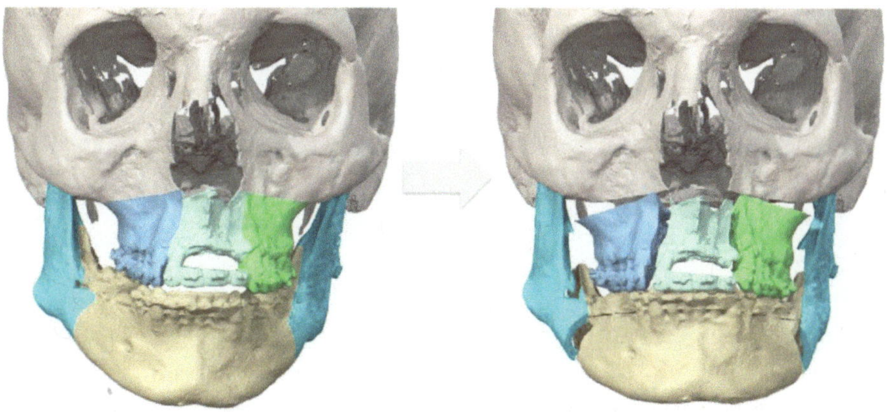

FIG. 7 VSP images demonstrate the alignment achieved through a three-piece LeFort I osteotomy and BSSO. Despite maximizing alignment using the patient's own bones, a significant asymmetry remains between the left and right sides of the mandible, necessitating additional intervention.

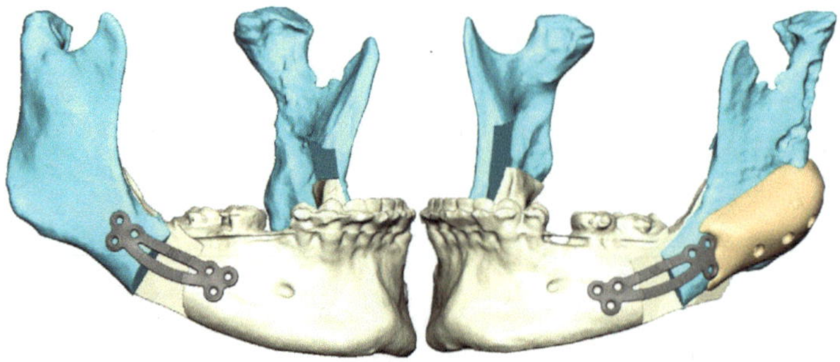

FIG. 8 VSP images of the custom PEEK left angle implant. The implant was designed to mirror the anatomy of the contralateral side, correcting asymmetry. Note how the implant was precisely fabricated to fit seamlessly against the custom BSSO hardware for optimal placement and stability.

transformative potential of modern maxillofacial surgical techniques to restore function and aesthetics in challenging cases (Figs. 6–8).

Case study 3: Orthognathic Reconstruction for Severe Mandibular Hypoplasia and Upper Airway Resistance Syndrome

Patient overview

A 38-year-old woman reported lifelong fatigue, jaw pain, and ear problems starting at age 7, coinciding with mandibular retrusion.

Clinical and radiographic findings included severe mandibular hypoplasia with significant loss of height and length bilaterally, as well as malocclusion contributing to functional impairments, including difficulty chewing, articulating certain sounds, and upper airway resistance syndrome (UARS).

Surgical interventions included

1. LeFort I osteotomy, performed to improve orientation and enhancing midface projection
2. Bilateral inverted-L osteotomies of the mandible, which allowed for vertical elongation and lengthening of the mandible, addressing the severe loss of height and length bilaterally
3. Genioplasty, which augmented chin projection and balanced the lower facial third to improve overall aesthetics and profile harmony

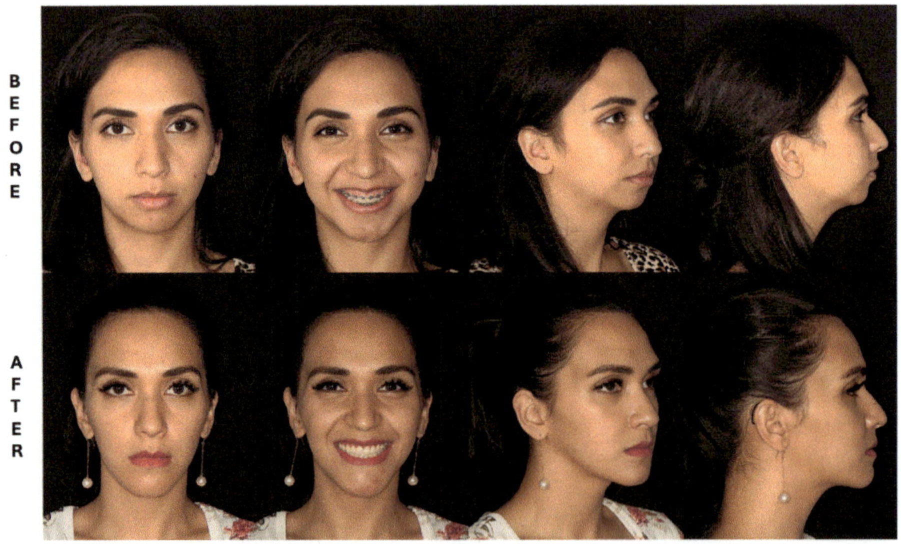

FIG. 9 Preoperative and postoperative facial photographs. The preoperative images highlight the severe mandibular hypoplasia, significant loss of mandibular height and length, and associated facial disproportions. Postoperative images demonstrate restored mandibular contour and profile symmetry, improved chin projection, and harmonized facial proportions.

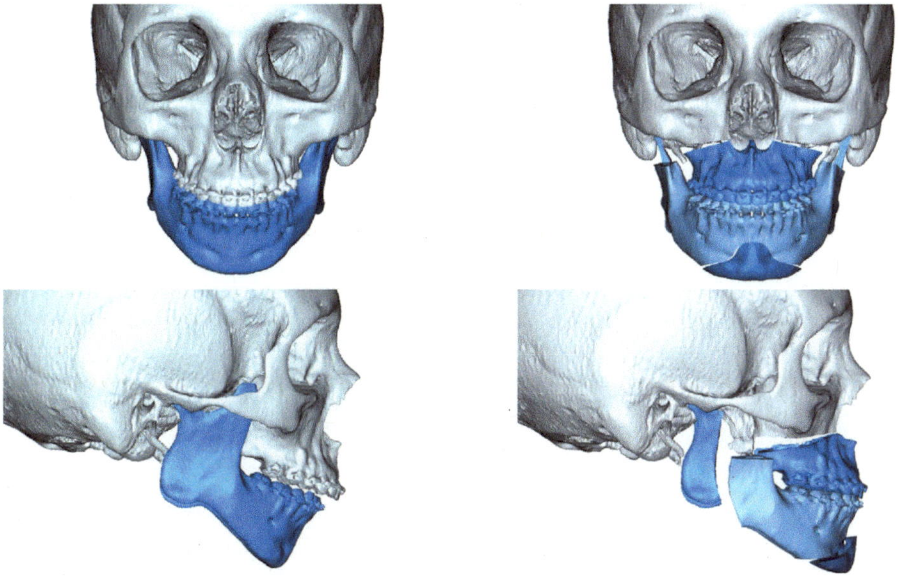

FIG. 10 VSP images illustrating the planned movements for the LeFort I osteotomy, bilateral inverted-L osteotomies, and genioplasty. The VSP highlights the precise adjustments required to restore mandibular height, length, and symmetry, and the enhanced chin projection and maxillary repositioning.

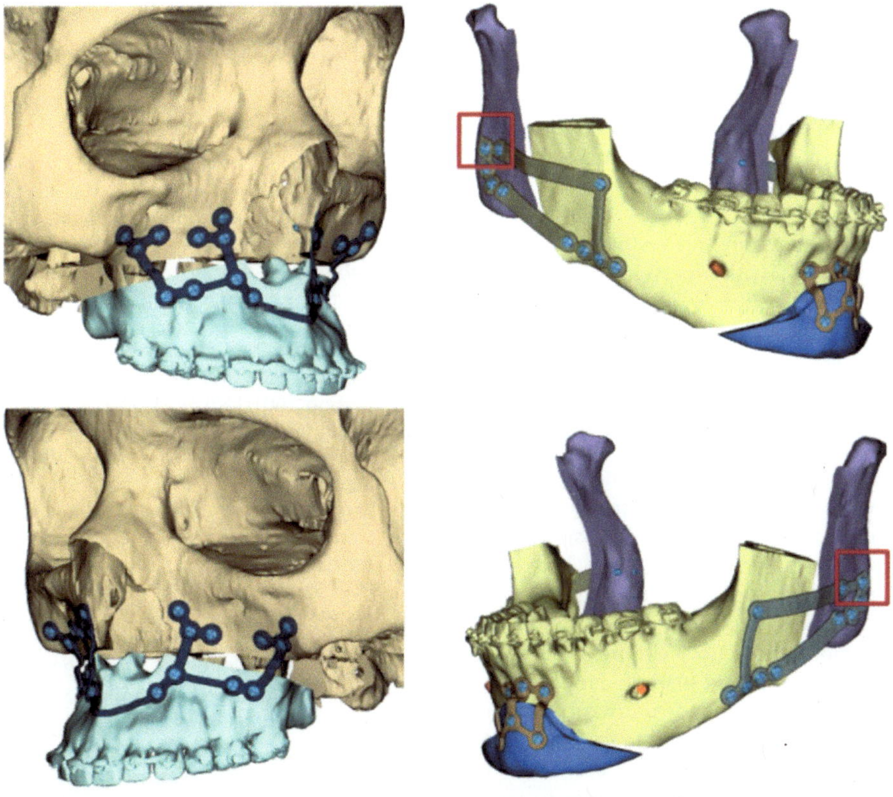

FIG. 11 Custom patient-specific hardware designed to execute the VSP and facilitate the bilateral inverted-L osteotomies through intraoral incisions. The hardware ensures precise bone movements and accurate alignment, minimizing surgical invasiveness and optimizing outcomes.

Results

Functional outcomes included improved chewing, articulation, and airway function leading to better sleep quality and reduced daytime fatigue.

Aesthetic outcomes included improved mandibular contour with restoration of mandibular height and length andharmonized facial proportions, including a more balanced lower third.

Discussion

This case underscores the critical role of mandibular reconstruction in addressing functional impairments and facial harmony. The combination of LeFort I osteotomy and bilateral inverted-L osteotomies allowed for comprehensive correction of severe mandibular hypoplasia and the associated loss of height and length. The addition of genioplasty refined the lower facial third, enhancing aesthetics and functional balance (Figs. 9–11).

SUMMARY AND FUTURE DIRECTIONS

Orthognathic surgery is one of the most effective tools for enhancing facial aesthetics. By leveraging advancements in surgical techniques, VSP, and patient-specific hardware, the field continues to evolve, offering increasingly precise and individualized care. Each case underscores the transformative potential of these interventions to improve quality of life while achieving aesthetic balance and functional harmony.

The integration of function and aesthetics is central to orthognathic surgery, with interventions designed to simultaneously improve airway dynamics, occlusion, and jaw function while enhancing facial appearance. Advances in technology, such as VSP, custom implants, and patient-specific hardware, have revolutionized surgical precision, reducing variability and improving esthetic outcomes.

Looking to the future, ongoing innovation will continue to shape the field. The incorporation of bioresorbable materials may enhance postoperative healing and reduce the need for long-term hardware. Artificial intelligence and predictive modeling are anticipated to play a growing role in surgical planning, enabling more accurate predictions of outcomes based on patient-specific anatomy and historic data.

Orthognathic surgery is driven by a commitment to enhancing functional and aesthetic outcomes. As technology and surgical techniques continue to advance, the potential to address even the most complex cases will grow. Through a patient-centered approach and ongoing research, the field is poised to achieve new milestones in precision, efficiency, and patient satisfaction [40].

CLINICS CARE POINTS

- Accurate analysis of facial proportions and symmetry is crucial for planning aesthetic maxillofacial surgery.
- Incorporating VSP ensures precise aesthetic outcomes by simulating surgical adjustments before the procedure.
- Custom implants provide personalized solutions for enhancing midface projection, jawline definition, and other aesthetic concerns.
- Skeletal adjustments, such as maxillary impaction or cant correction, are effective for refining incisor display and smile esthetics.
- Balancing soft tissue response with skeletal changes is essential to achieving a harmonious and natural appearance.

DISCLOSURE

The author has nothing to disclose.

REFERENCES

[1] Standring S, Borley NR, Gray H. Gray's Anatomy: The Anatomical Basis of Clinical Practice (41tsted., anniversary edition). Edinburgh: Churchill Livingstone/Elsevier; 2008.

[2] Kahn DM, Shaw RB. Overview of current thoughts on facial volume and aging. Facial Plast Surg 2010;26(5): 350–5.

[3] Sarver DM. The importance of incisor positioning in the esthetic smile: the smile arc. Am J Orthod Dentofacial Orthop 2001;120(2):98–111.

[4] Gateno J, Alfi D, Xia JJ, et al. A geometric classification of jaw deformities. J Oral Maxillofac Surg 2015;73(12 Suppl):26–31.

[5] Farkas LG, Hreczko TA, Kolar JC, et al. Vertical and horizontal proportions of the face in young adult North American Caucasians: revision of neoclassical canons. Plast Reconstr Surg 1985;75(3):328–38.

[6] Marquardt SR. Dr. Stephen R. Marquardt on the golden decagon and human facial beauty. Interview by Dr. Gottlieb. J Clin Orthod 2002;36(6):339–47.

[7] Little AC, Jones BC, DeBruine LM. Facial attractiveness: evolutionary based research. Philos Trans R Soc Lond B Biol Sci 2011;366(1571):1638–59.

[8] Andrews LF. The 6-elements orthodontic philosophy: treatment goals, classification, and rules for treating. Am J Orthod Dentofacial Orthop 2015;148(6):883–7.

[9] Holdaway RA. A soft-tissue cephalometric analysis and its use in orthodontic treatment planning. Part I. Am J Orthod 1983;84(1):1–28.

[10] Sarver DM, Ackerman MB. Dynamic smile visualization and quantification: Part 2. Smile analysis and treatment strategies. Am J Orthod Dentofacial Orthop 2003;124: 116–27.

[11] Sarver DM, Ackerman MB. Dynamic smile visualization and quantification: part 1. Evolution of the concept and dynamic records for smile capture. Am J Orthod Dentofacial Orthop 2003;124(1):4–12.

[12] Benjamin T. The modified upper lip lift: advanced approach with deep-plane release and secure suspension: 823-patient series. Facial Plast Surg Clin North Am 2019; 27(3):385–98.

[13] Panossian AJ, Block MS. Evaluation of the smile: facial and dental considerations. Oral Maxillofac Surg 2010; 68(3):547–54.

[14] Vig RG, Brundo GC. The kinetics of anterior tooth display. J Prosthet Dent 1978;39(5):502–4.

[15] Hyeon-Shik H, Wang-Sik K, McNamara JA Jr. Ethnic differences in the soft tissue profile of Korean and European-American adults with normal occlusions and well-balanced faces. Angle Orthod 2002;72(1):72–80.

[16] Bell WH, Proffitt WB, White RP. Surgical correction of dentofacial deformities. Philadelphia (PA): W.B. Saunders Co.; 1980.

[17] Sugahara K, Koyachi M, Odaka K, et al. A safe, stable, and convenient three-dimensional device for high Le Fort I osteotomy. Maxillofac Plast Reconstr Surg 2020;42:32.

[18] Bailey LJ, White RP Jr, Proffit WR, et al. Segmental LeFort I osteotomy for management of transverse maxillary deficiency. J Oral Maxillofac Surg 1997;55(7):728–31.

[19] Strömberg C, Holm J. Surgically assisted, rapid maxillary expansion in adults. A retrospective long-term follow-up study. J Cranio-Maxillo-Fac Surg 1995;23(4):222–7.

[20] Liu SY, Guilleminault C, Huon LK, et al. Distraction osteogenesis maxillary expansion (DOME) for adult obstructive sleep apnea patients with high arched palate. Otolaryngol Head Neck Surg 2017;157(2):345–8.

[21] Suzuki H, Moon W, Previdente LH, et al. Miniscrew-assisted rapid palatal expander (MARPE): the quest for pure orthopedic movement. Dental Press J Orthod 2016;21(4): 17–23.

[22] Cantarella D, Dominguez-Mompell R, Moschik C, et al. Midfacial changes in the coronal plane induced by microimplant-supported skeletal expander, studied with cone-beam computed tomography images. Am J Orthod Dentofacial Orthop 2018;154(3):337–45.

[23] Coppelson K. Multidisciplinary approach to tongue space surgery. Int J Orofacial Myology 2022;48(1):5.

[24] Li K, Quo S, Guilleminault C. Endoscopically-assisted surgical expansion (EASE) for the treatment of obstructive sleep apnea. Sleep Med 2019;60:53–9.

[25] Epker BN. Modifications in the sagittal osteotomy of the mandible. J Oral Surg 1977;35(2):157–9.

[26] McMillan B, Jones R, Ward-Booth P, et al. Technique for intraoral inverted 'L' osteotomy. Br J Oral Maxillofac Surg 1999;37(4):324–6.

[27] Strauss RA, Abubaker AO. Genioplasty: a case for advancement osteotomy. J Oral Maxillofac Surg 2000; 58(7):783–7.

[28] Grime PD, Blenkinsopp PT. Horizontal-T genioplasty–(a modified technique for the broad or asymmetrical chin). Br J Oral Maxillofac Surg 1990;28(4):215–21.

[29] Han K, Kim J. Reduction mandibuloplasty: ostectomy of the lateral cortex around the mandibular angle. J Craniofac Surg 2001;12(4):314–25.

[30] Yaremchuk MJ. Facial skeletal reconstruction using porous polyethylene implants. Plast Reconstr Surg 2003;111(6): 1818–27.

[31] Saponaro G, Doneddu P, Gasparini G, et al. Custom made onlay implants in peek in maxillofacial surgery: a volumetric study. Childs Nerv Syst 2020;36(2): 385–91.

[32] Agostino AD, Trevisiol L, Favero V, et al. Hydroxyapatite/collagen composite is a reliable material for malar augmentation. J Oral Maxillofac Surg 2016;74(6):1238.

[33] Kim Y-H, Cho B-C, Lo L-J. Facial contouring surgery for Asians. Semin Plast Surg 2009;23(1):22–31.

[34] Xia JJ, McGrory JK, Gateno J, et al. A new method to orient 3-dimensional computed tomography models to the natural head position: a clinical feasibility study. J Oral Maxillofac Surg 2011;69(3):584–91.

[35] Sheng-Pin Hsu S, Gateno J, Bell RB, et al. Accuracy of a computer-aided surgical simulation protocol for orthognathic surgery: a prospective multicenter study. J Oral Maxillofac Surg 2013;71(1):128–42.

[36] Suojanen J, Leikola J, Stoor P. The use of patient-specific implants in orthognathic surgery: a series of 32 maxillary osteotomy patients. J Cranio-Maxillo-Fac Surg 2016; 44(12):1913–6.

[37] Rückschloß T, Ristow O, Müller M, et al. Accuracy of patient-specific implants and additive-manufactured surgical splints in orthognathic surgery - a three-dimensional retrospective study. J Cranio-Maxillo-Fac Surg 2019; 47(6):847–53.

[38] Schneider SA, Gateno J, Coppelson KB, et al. Validity of medical insurance guidelines for orthognathic surgery. J Oral Maxillofac Surg 2021;79(3):672–84.

[39] Zaghi S, Holty JE, Certal V, et al. Maxillomandibular advancement for treatment of obstructive sleep apnea: a meta-analysis. JAMA Otolaryngol Head Neck Surg 2016;142(1):58–66.

[40] Rhodes G. The evolutionary psychology of facial beauty. Annu Rev Psychol 2006;57:199–226.

Advances in Cosmetic Surgery 8 (2025) 121–131
ADVANCES IN COSMETIC SURGERY

Facial Rejuvenation and Orthodontics; Is There a Connection?

Dimitrios Mavreas, DDS, MS, PhD*
Private Practice, 238 Kifissias Avenue, Chalandri 15231, Greece

KEYWORDS
• Adult orthodontics • Facial rejuvenation • Guidelines

KEY POINTS

- Age-related changes to facial bones, fat, muscles, ligaments, skin, teeth, and smile.
- Orthodontics promotes the rejuvenation of faces affecting directly the dentoalveolar bone and the teeth, and indirectly the rest of the facial tissues.
- Orthodontic treatment planning guidelines for rejuvenation.
- Self-esteem and confidence increase.
- Synergistic effect of orthodontics and other medical cosmetic interventions.

INTRODUCTION

Facial aging is a process that is influenced by numerous environmental factors [1], as well as intrinsic (genetic) factors [2] affecting the different components of the facial anatomy such as the skin, fat, muscles, ligaments, skeleton, and the teeth with the surrounding dentoalveolar bone. Seminal orthodontic research has contributed to the understanding of the alterations occurring at the craniofacial complex associated with postmaturation and aging [3], and newer evidence on dental [4] and lip changes is continuously emerging [5]. Despite the broad belief that the craniofacial skeleton is expanding throughout life in general, it has been well documented that specific areas of it undergo resorption impacting the aging pattern [6], emphasizing the stigmata of the aging face.

Aging and the reversal or amelioration of its consequences had led to an increase in the number of minimally invasive cosmetic procedures to more than 25 million in the year 2023 in the United States alone. It is the elder Generation X and Younger Boomers who dominate the facial enhancement procedures category [7]. Adult patients seeking orthodontic treatment have increased from 15% to 35% of new case starts in orthodontic practices, with a rising tendency [8]. Orthodontic treatment has anecdotally been perceived to service the demand for addressing problems relating to dental esthetics but adults have often complex treatment needs. Since the skeleton of the face has a significant effect on an individual's appearance, it should be expected that elderly patient satisfaction and treatment uptake could be enhanced if facial rejuvenation can be among the anticipated outcomes of treatment. To rejuvenate the aging face effectively, it is necessary to understand the dynamic aging processes and the imbalances between these components that lead to the characteristics of the aged face [9]. The under-projection of the elderly facial bones if overlooked and managed incorrectly with conventional facelift soft-tissue techniques may lead to unpleasant esthetic results [10]. It would be beneficial thus for the elderly individuals if the aging process could be managed from both the bone and

*Corresponding author. *E-mail address:* mavreas@otenet.gr

https://doi.org/10.1016/j.yacs.2025.01.002 www.advancesincosmeticsurgery.com
2542-4327/25/

ABBREVIATIONS

VDO	vertical dimension of occlusion
W/H	width-to-height

soft-tissue aspects with the minimum invasive techniques, providing the maximum in esthetics.

The aims of this article are (a) to briefly describe the skeletal changes to the maxilla, mandible, soft tissues, and smile/teeth induced by aging, and (b) present the effect orthodontics may have on elderly faces, rejuvenating them at the dentoalveolar/skeletal and the "facial mask" level, altering the initial perception of a patient's cosmetic needs and possibly augment the result of any cosmetic procedure(s) that may follow. If these aging aspects as well as those associated with the smile are addressed prior to any cosmetic treatment, the final approach may need to be significantly modified [11].

BONE CHANGES OF THE MIDFACE AND THE MANDIBLE

There is change in the relative dynamics between bone resorption and expansion in the aging craniofacial skeleton and the process is not purely the atrophy of the bone. Computed tomography images of the face have shown that aging reduces the height of the maxilla relatively to the orbit which had increased from infancy to youth and that further actual decrease in vertical maxillary height in the medial plane occurs secondary to the normal skeletal remodeling in the dentate individuals [12]. Clockwise rotation and recession of the maxilla has been repeatedly observed in various studies [13–16] which appear to undermine midfacial support and projection, and the findings seem to be more profound in women than they are in men [17,18]. Also, the rate of facial aging tends to increase after the age of 50 with a higher pace for women [19]. In general, the maxillary skeleton exhibits primarily signs of retrusion and deterioration [20,21].

The mandible can be considered the pillar supporting the lower part of the face. The shape of the mandible changes, becoming less convex with age, as some areas continue to grow faster than others according to the principle of differential growth [22]. Ramus height, mandibular body height, and mandibular body length decrease significantly with age for both genders, whereas the mandibular angle increases significantly for both genders with increasing age, the processes being mainly those of contraction [23]. The aging process of the mandible often involves resorption of bone in the chin region [24]. The presence of the dentition is of predominant importance in mandibular morphology [25,26], and the vertical dimension [27] which plays a significant role in facial esthetics. In general, there is an appreciable reduction in facial height, which is mainly due to changes in the maxilla and mandible, and a modest increase in facial width and depth [28]. Even with bony changes of small magnitude, the effects can be dramatic through amplification via the overlying structures [29].

SOFT TISSUE CHANGES

The skeletal changes described earlier when combined with the changes in soft tissues lead to the characteristic appearance of the aged face. The main external factors responsible for skin aging are ultraviolet radiation, pollution, and smoking while intrinsic aging also contributes to the appearance of fine rhytids and skin laxity [30]. With intrinsic aging, the skin thins and weakens as the dermis atrophies from changes related to deterioration of these components. The rate of collagen breakdown increases, whereas the rate of collagen synthesis decreases [31]. Volumetric changes and gravitational descent of the facial fat are considered responsible for some of the changes observed during aging [32]. It is the redistribution and demarcation of fat that gives the senile face an unbalanced appearance [28]. Permanent muscle contractures, loss of mass volume, and changes in physiology are also accountable for facial wrinkles and volume loss that signify aging [33]. Although muscles may weaken with age, their relative pull is greater on the less resistant tissues and dermis and can result in hyperdynamic expressions [31]. The zygomatic, the orbital retaining, and the mandibular retaining ligaments are the most affected by aging and are weakened, which in combination with the bony changes affecting the point of origin of all the facial ligaments promote the appearance of the facial sagging [33].

SMILE/TEETH CHANGES

The maxillary anterior teeth are key elements for smile esthetics, and the display of the maxillary incisors at rest and on smile is a characteristic of youthful appearance [34]. The upper lip elongation is a continuous process and in the third and fourth decades of life, after growth of the craniofacial skeleton is minimal, elongation of the upper lip exceeds vertical growth of the face in different populations [35,36]. As age advances, the loss of resting muscle tone and increased flaccidity and redundancy contribute more in lowering of the smile height than the decreased muscle's ability to create a smile [36,37]. Dynamic smile analysis showed that as a person ages, the smile gets narrower vertically and wider transversely. The result is a significant decrease in incisor display at rest, speech, and smile, along with a greater display of mandibular incisors [36,38,39]. It should be noted that crowding in the lower anterior area increases, especially in females, with age [40] making the image less esthetically pleasing. Natsumeda and colleagues [41] followed a group of subjects with normal occlusions for 5 decades and noticed significant changes in proportions (due to shortening of crown height), color, angulation, and gingival step between central and lateral incisor which are all factors impairing dental and smile esthetics, and attractiveness. Faces with more white dentition are perceived to be younger across all age groups and gender of judges [42]. Elderly adults may have fewer teeth, edentulous spaces, failing restorations, teeth with uncertain prognosis, more wear and abrasion, more artificial crowns, advanced periodontal tissue destruction, pronounced gingival recessions, higher frequency of uneven gingival margins due to combinations of supraeruption and wear, and a greater need for implants, preprosthetic orthodontic treatment, and orthodontic molar uprighting [43] all of which make the restoring of the dentition more challenging.

There is a close link between physical appearance and self-esteem, family life, social attractiveness, and professional life. Attractiveness would therefore seem to make an essential contribution to an individual's self-fulfillment and Quality of Life [44,45]. Facial tissues change over time, and the orthodontist's training is to understand the principles of dental and skeletal development, maturation, and aging in addition to the many other facets of dental practice. Given the substantial variations in the substrate, the treatment planning for adults may well deviate from that for younger individuals, for whom conventional orthodontic protocols are more readily applicable. Orthodontic treatment has been shown that it cannot only correct an existing or acquired malocclusion and provide a beautiful smile but it can also contribute to the rejuvenation of an elderly face when properly planned [46]. Guidelines for orthodontic management of the aged face have been developed and cases treated according to these guidelines are presented.

REJUVENATION AND ORTHODONTICS—GUIDELINES

- When facial rejuvenation is a treatment objective, comprehensive facial evaluation should be prioritized, and a sound diagnosis of macro-esthetic needs (esthetics of the face), should be made [46].
- Posterior displacement of the skeletal elements inferior to the orbit, accompanied by bone loss at the pyriform process, is associated with a deepening of the nasolabial fold. This suggests that maintaining the maxilla-mandibular skeleton in a forward position can be esthetically advantageous.
- As the height of the upper part of the lower face increases with aging, the lower part should also be increased to maintain harmony and balance.
- A decrease in the maxillary and mandibular body heights combined with loss of tooth structure also supports methods to increase lower face height. In a periodontally healthy environment, creating a posterior open bite at the start of treatment and promoting eruption of the posterior teeth into the space created could prove advantageous for the elderly patient.
- A decrease in maxillary anterior teeth exposure may be managed by combining the above with clockwise rotation of the occlusal plane; any deep bite correction required should be carried to the lower teeth. Disarticulating the occlusion at the most posterior teeth in the arch and combining extrusion of upper and lower teeth anterior to it can promote rotation around this artificially created fulcrum point. Once the desired rotation and vertical height are established and the overjet has been improved (clockwise rotation of the occlusal plane may also benefit the decrease of the overjet), the disarticulation point can be transferred anteriorly, behind the central incisors where it may act as a stable determinant of the final anterior lower face height.
- An increase in the mandibular width with age that overthrows the width-to-height [W/H] facial ratio can be masked, and youthful looking W/H proportions could be restored by increasing lower face height, which is in agreement with the previous. If mesial movement of molars and lingual movement of first premolars and canines is present in elderly patients [4], uprighting and expansion of the lingually tipped teeth should be performed preferably.
- The square appearance of older faces due to facial fat descent and increase in submalar fullness may be also harmonized by increasing the lower face height.
- Individuals who present cephalometric characteristics of "long-face" could still require elongation of the lower face height in later adulthood.
- Dentoalveolar transverse development is strongly recommended—when it can be safely accomplished—since it may enhance the support of the

overlying loose and shrunk soft tissues, and may also compensate for lost fat, thus restoring "youthful" contours.

- Dentoalveolar posteroanterior development could also improve the skin appearance by stretching the perioral wrinkles.

CASE 1

A 54-year-old female who needed restoring of her worn upper anterior teeth (Fig. 1D) was referred by her dentist to assess the possible benefits from an orthodontic intervention. However, a comprehensive macro-esthetics evaluation revealed several facial abnormalities: severely short lower face height (Fig. 1A, right), distorted facial W/H ratio (W/H ≅ 1.13), thin and collapsed lips, deep nasolabial folds, prominent jowls (Fig. 1A, left), concave profile with an upward rotated chin (Fig. 1B), a blunt cervico-mandibular angle, and no teeth exposure upon smiling (Fig. 1C). The treatment deviated from the simple rearrangement of the teeth (which were relatively straight) and encompassed the normalization of as many of the impaired facial characteristics as possible. A new vertical dimension was immediately established by applying composite on the posterior teeth (as described above) resulting in a more harmonious facial appearance and allowing the unfolding of the depressed lips (Fig. 1E), and created space anteriorly for the temporary reconstruction of the anterior teeth with composite resin (Fig. 1F).

The posttreatment photographs demonstrate increased lower face height and improved facial W/H ratio (W/H ≅ 1.0) (Fig. 2A, right), increased upper lip length and nicely unfolded lips with normalized volume, softer nasolabial folds (Fig. 2A, left), straightened profile (Fig. 2C), adequate tooth exposure when smiling (Fig. 2B), and corrected occlusal relationships with temporary restorations on the anterior teeth (Fig. 2D). Any additional cosmetic medical intervention could have a synergistic effect, resulting in a multiplicative enhancement of the esthetic benefits for the patient.

CASE 2

A 68-year-old female was referred for evaluation following an accident, and trauma on her maxillary anterior teeth which combined with the existing deep bite (Fig. 3D) worsened the prognosis for these teeth. The initial request was to decrease the deep bite, and relieve the teeth from the heavy occlusal contacts present, in order to improve their long-term prognosis. Notice that as in the previous case there are no significant teeth irregularities. The systematic facial examination disclosed several typical aging signs like a retrusive midface, thin lips, marionette-like cheeks, prominent jowls, drooping corners of the mouth (Fig. 3A, left), short-lower face height and unfavorable facial W/H ratio (≅ 1.0) (Fig. 3A, right), and dished-in lower face (Fig. 3C). The smile was esthetically acceptable (Fig. 3B). The treatment was performed following the previously described guidelines. The final photographs show a balanced face with increased lower face height and better H/W ratio (≅ 0.9) (Fig. 4A, right), fuller lips, better midfacial support, more subtle nasolabial folds, and enhanced

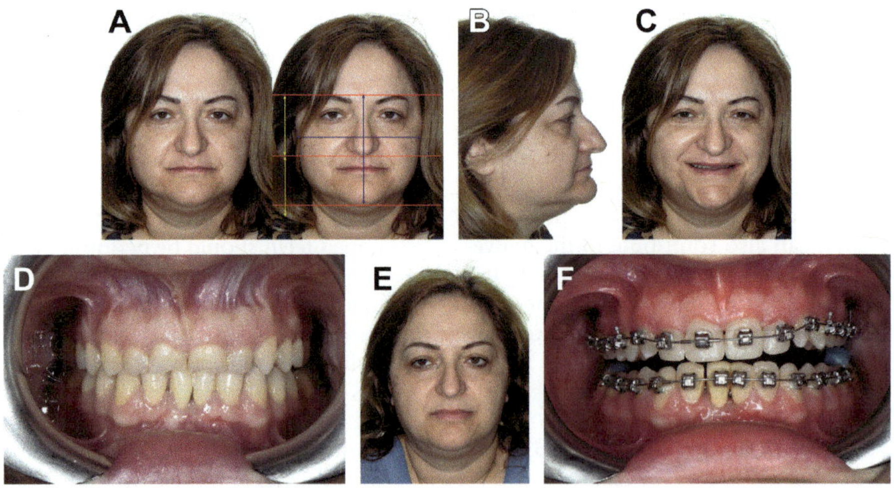

FIG. 1 **(A–F)** An adult patient displaying signs of an aged facial appearance prior to, and during orthodontic treatment.

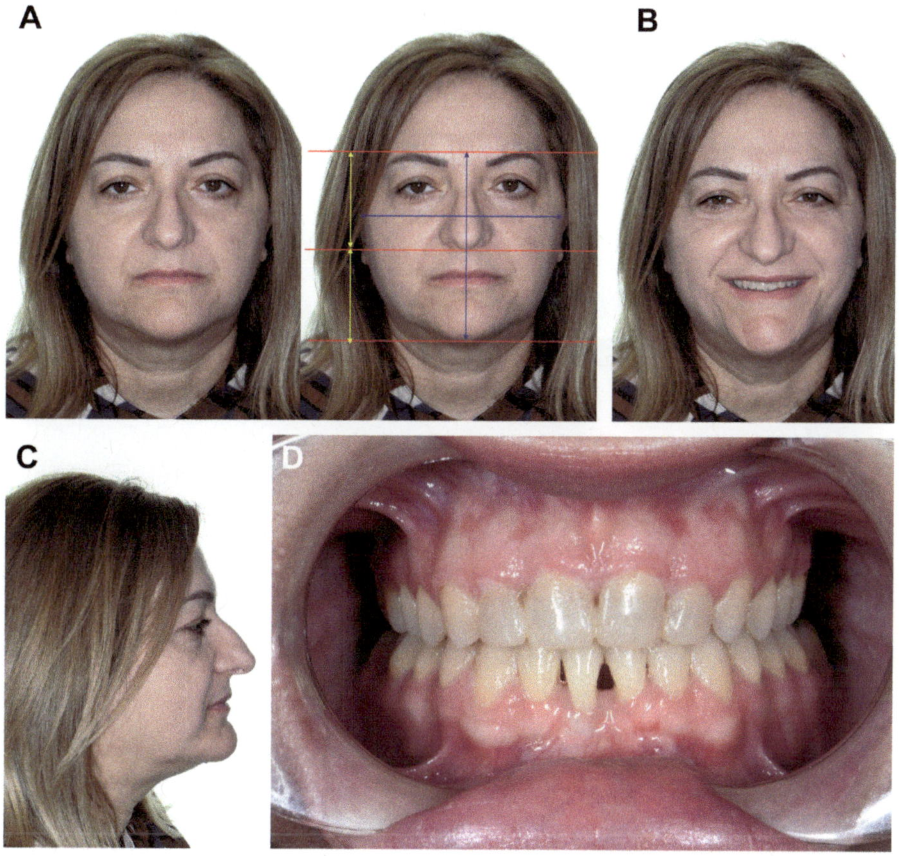

FIG. 2 (**A–D**) Changes in facial and smile esthetics, as well as occlusal changes after treatment.

cheek projection (Fig. 4A, left). The smile arc has been improved, the smile is fuller and more harmonious (Fig. 4B) following transverse and postero-anterior dentoalveolar development (Fig. 4C), and the deep bite which was the initial concern has been corrected (Fig. 4D).

DISCUSSION

Facial aging is a multifaceted process influenced by various interconnected factors but volume loss plays an essential role in this process which is dynamic, not uniform, and differs from one individual to another although the main pattern involves changes in all anatomic layers of the face: skeleton, muscles, adipose tissue, ligaments, skin, and teeth.

As the skin ages, collagen loss diminishes the mechanical tension that stimulates fibroblasts, resulting in their collapse and reduced collagen production. Consequently, treatments that stimulate fibroblasts indirectly through a stretching effect may induce collagen production, thereby slowing and replacing collagen loss [33]. As individuals age, the proportions of the face are disrupted and a ptotic tendency appears due to the vertical descent of fat compartments and fat volume loss from the middle third of the face, with the lower part gaining volume. Also, the deep fat deflates and this results to additional loss of the overlaying fat support [32]. The masseter and medial pterygoid muscles show a significant reduction in their cross-sectional area and density with age; women exhibiting more reduction than men [47]. Orbicularis oris muscle displays signs of decrease in thickness and flattening of cross-sectional conformation, which contributes to a flattening of the upper lip complex with age [48]. The facial ligaments fatigue and weaken and as their points of insertion either into the soft tissues (skin and muscles) or into the bone alter along with the aging alterations of these elements, they permit a change in position of the structures that they suspend [33,49].

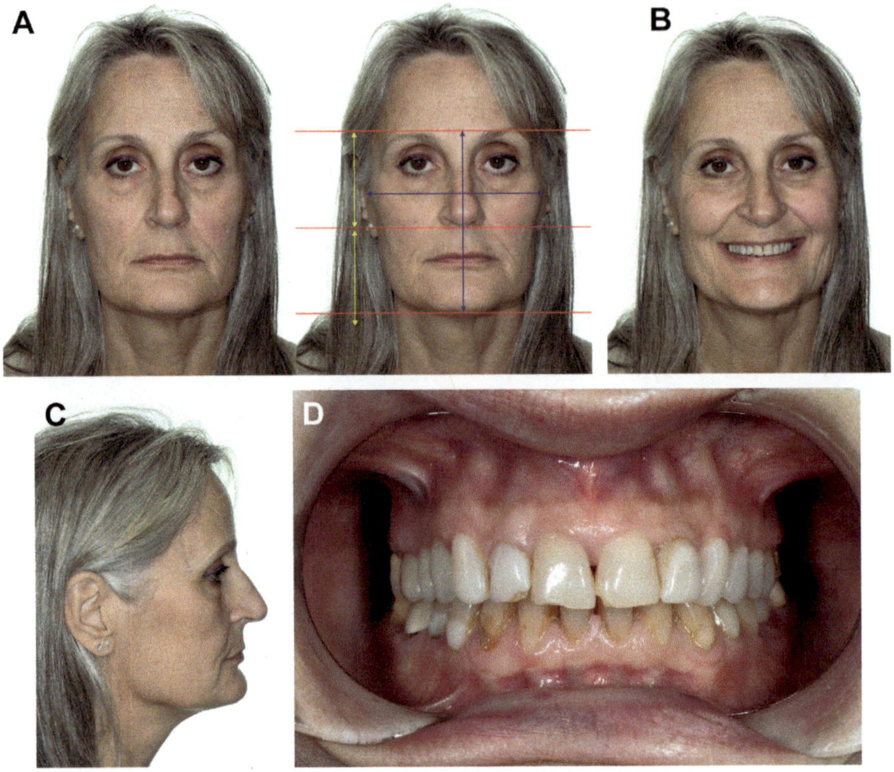

FIG. 3 **(A–D)** An elderly adult patient exhibiting typical facial characteristics associated with aging before orthodontic treatment.

The osseous components are essential for the contour of the face since they provide the framework to the soft tissues. The increased loss of soft tissue volume over the entire facial area may lead to decreased mechanical strain on the facial skeleton and could be one of the main factors contributing to bone loss, since craniofacial osseous remodeling is a major contributor to the facial aging process with recession being a predominant phenomenon. A mechanism leading to a vicious "tissue recessing" cycle, and the subsequent "folding in" of the overlying soft tissues may be argued [46]. Over a 40-year period females have shown maxillary and mandibular retrusion, nose and soft chin thickness increase, augmenting the perception of bi-retruded lips with aging [50]. From the age of 31 to 62, the upper and lower jaws showed minor retrognathism, the upper and lower incisors exhibited retroclination, with concomitant straightening of the soft tissue profile and thinning of the lips, and the distance from the lips to the esthetic line increased [51].

Loss of the Vertical Dimension of Occlusion (VDO) and subsequent forward rotation of the mandible, dentofacial bone remodeling after tooth wear, an edge-to-edge anterior tooth relationship after loss of vertical tooth height, and anterior positioning of the mandible due to the loss of anterior tooth guidance have all been associated with mandibular pseudo-prognathism which enhances the perception of the retruded lower middle face, alters the facial contours from the frontal view, narrows the vermillion borders, and over-closes the commissure [52]. It has been suggested that whenever indicated, permanent increase of the vertical dimension of occlusion (VDO) of up to 5 mm is a safe and predictable procedure without detrimental consequences [53,54]. Thus, the herein proposed and orthodontically induced increase of the VDO in these elderly patients can be performed safely without expecting any undesired sequelae [55]. In addition, transverse and postero-anterior developments of the dentoalveolar part further augment the bony part of the face. The esthetic improvements exhibited are not confined to the immediate perioral areas but they radiate to a larger part of the face (see Figs. 2 and 4). The mechanisms explaining these changes could be attributed to the fact

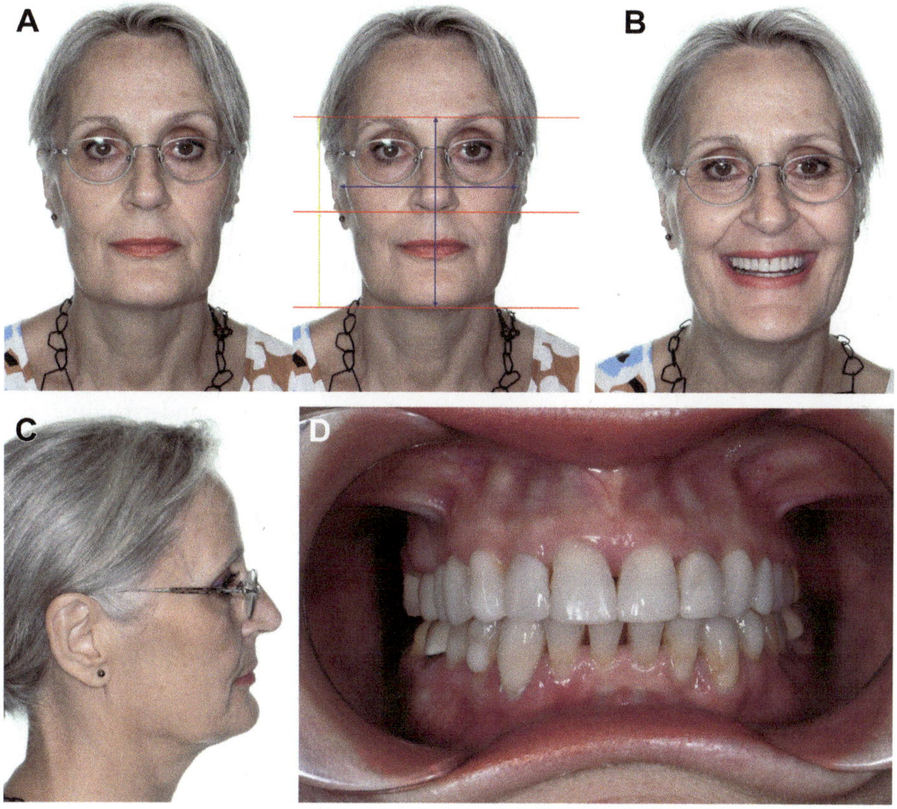

FIG. 4 (**A–D**) Esthetic and occlusal changes following orthodontic treatment.

that both muscles and bone respond to mechanical stimuli [56]. Stretching of the muscles, ligaments, and skin triggered by the above volumization of the dentoalveolar area may lead to increased protein activity causing hypertrophy, and change in muscle fiber composition, which in turn causes increased strain on the bones. This may cause an epigenetic regulation of the stretched bone cell genome, including its phenotypic expression [56]. Both muscle and bone tissue respond to mechanical signals for which bone depends on muscles, and for muscles stretch has been shown to be important as it induces protein synthesis and an increase in width as well as length of the muscle fibers. The latter involves the production of more sarcomeres in series so that the jaw muscles adapt to a new functional length following changes in vertical dimension of occlusion [57] which in turn causes increased strain on the bones. This leads to an increase in the bone density due to the activity of the osteocytes, a change in the architecture of the bone, and an increase in periosteal thickening. Stretch of the muscle fibers also induces release of mechano-growth-factor and insulin growth factor. This increased cellular activity seems to lead to an increased vascularity in the tissues and also prevents apoptosis [58]. Improvement in the chin, and tightening of the skin is apparent on the faces of these patients and this could be due to a possible redistribution of the fat to muscle ratio. The facial skin improves because of the stretching of the facial mask but there seems to be an improvement in the thickness of the skin itself. This may be due to increased collagen production, improved elasticity, and improved blood flow to the skin. The alterations in dentoalveolar height, width, and posteroanterior development influence the height/width of the smile window ratio. By increasing the height, these alterations favor the improvement of the vermillion show, as the disproportion between the transverse and vertical dimensions during maturation can cause the perceived imbalance.

Individuals who have growth deficiencies within their maxillofacial pattern by birth reveal them more intensely after the loss of soft tissue and contour occurring with aging, and this may reinforce the characteristic changes that we associate with aging [59]. This under-projection of facial bones which is coupled with lack of support at the facial mask can in certain cases be treated by a combination of orthodontics and orthognathic surgery which can be perceived as a "reverse face-lift." However, many complex malocclusions often can be resolved without the need of osteotomies by using temporary anchorage devices (TADs) which have become a common place in today's orthodontics, providing enhanced esthetic results (Fig. 5A–E and 6A–D). This practice normalizes the facial features at a younger age (early rejuvenation), potentially preventing premature aging. Individuals who exhibit a primary dentofacial deviation can be considered to be positioned at an advanced stage on an imaginary aging scale.

People with a corrected malocclusion tend to smile more with the eyes [60], and this might explain that the eyes in these patients appear much brighter, bigger, and more youthful. Psychosocial well-being is associated with the act of smiling [60]. The younger appearance of the smile might negate or ameliorate the impression given by the wrinkled skin around the eyes; it might act synergistically with skin products and botulinum toxin injections [61]. Also, a more beautiful smile would make people seem more intelligent, amiable, and popular [62].

A middle-aged face that has been subjected to "face lift" often presents the surgical stigma of mechanically tightened soft tissues, which is not only unnatural but also does not seem youthful or rejuvenated. Restoring the facial shape may be more preferable and this requires an accurate understanding of the anatomic changes that have occurred with aging and appreciating the importance of underlying skeletal support in formulating the treatment plan for each individual patient

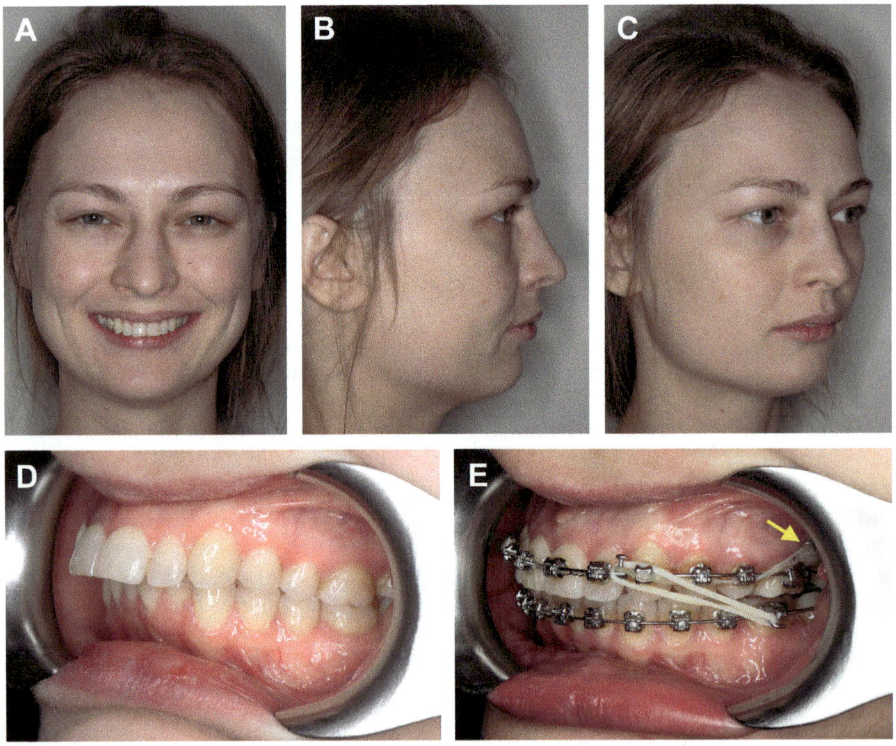

FIG. 5 (**A–E**) A young woman who had previously undergone unsuccessful orthodontic treatment presented with a severe mandibular retrognathism (**B, C**), a tendency for small lower face height (**B**), mild maxillary dentoalveolar protrusion (**A, B**), excessive overjet, and a deep bite (**D**).These findings place her on an advanced stage on the aging scale despite her young age. A standard approach would require surgical orthodontics and a sagittal split osteotomy to advance the mandible. However, this plan was declined by the patient and a pure orthodontic approach involving the bilateral use of temporary anchorage devices (TADs) (**E**) (*yellow arrow*) was implemented.

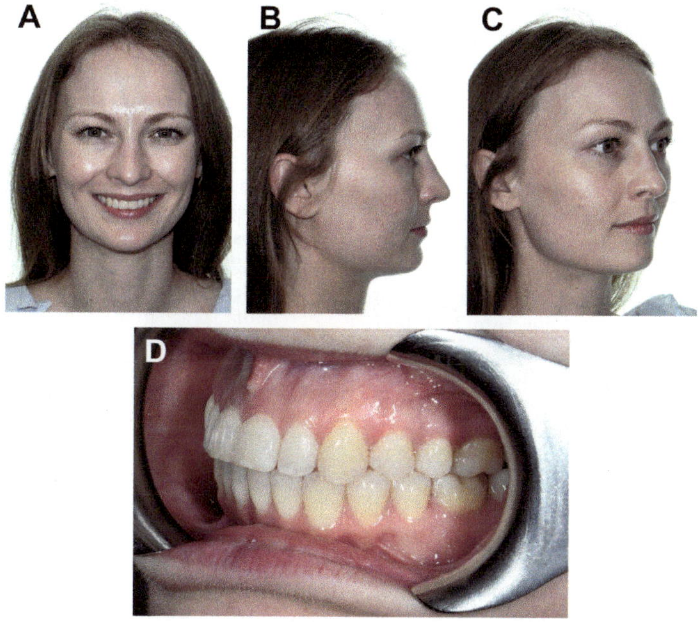

FIG. 6 (**A–D**) The result not only normalized her occlusion (**D**) but also harmonized the face by increasing the lower face height (**C**) camouflazing the persisting retrognathia, resolving the maxillary protrusion, providing a beautiful smile, and reversing the early "skeletal aging." A common observation in all these patients is that once they are treated and gained self-confidence, they start experimenting with their new look changing hairstyle or using make-up.

[46]. Indeed, treatment planning to restore facial shape can only be patient specific, and the volumetric requirements are influenced by the underlying skeletal support which is a key element to increasing consistency in face lifting [63]. Perioral soft-tissue rejuvenation techniques [64], specifically selected to enhance the orthodontic (and in some cases the adjunctive restorative) outcome can significantly reinforce the esthetic benefits for these patients.

SUMMARY

Orthodontics aims to improve the quality of life for the elderly by achieving esthetic and functional dental occlusion, facilitating social interaction [43,65]. Medical specialties involved with the treating of facial aging signs have similar goals [66,67]. Understanding the changes that can be induced by a successful orthodontic treatment on the skeletal framework of the face as well as the accompanying transformations occurring on the overlying tissues could greatly benefit those patients seeking assistance to restore a youthful appearance. Combining orthodontics with other medical disciplines dedicated to cosmetic alterations may yield synergistic and exponential effects. As individuals become increasingly concerned about the effects of aging on their faces, and as surgical corrective procedures gain popularity, it may be prudent to consider orthodontic intervention as an alternative before opting for direct cosmetic surgery.

CLINICS CARE POINTS

- Orthodontic treatment can be a significant aid in facial rejuvenation in a "from the-inside-out" approach.
- Skeletal and dentoalveolar optimization through orthodontics, and consequent soft tissue(s) reaction are the keys to successful rejuvenation.
- Establishing a new vertical dimension is usually the principal factor of success.

DISCLOSURE

The author has nothing to disclose.

REFERENCES

[1] Albert AM, Ricanek K, Patterson E. A review of the literature on the aging adult skull and face: implications for forensic science research and applications. Forensic Sci Int 2007;172(1):1–9.

[2] Rohrich RJ, Avashia YJ, Savetsky IL. Prediction of facial aging using the facial fat compartments. Plast Reconstr Surg 2021;147(1 2):38S–42S.

[3] Behrents RG. Craniofacial Growth Series, 17. Ann Arbor (MI): Center of Human Growth and Development, University of Michigan; 1985.

[4] Garib D, Miranda F, Massaro C, et al. Three-dimensional mandibular dental changes with aging. Am J Orthod Dentofacial Orthop 2021;159(2):184–92.

[5] Nam J-H, Choi Y, Lee KJ, et al. Differences in the 3-dimensional aging changes of the lips among female adults with skeletal Class I, II, and III malocclusion. Am J Orthod Dentofacial Orthop 2023;164(4):516–29.

[6] Mendelson B, Wong CH. Changes in the facial skeleton with aging: implications and clinical applications in facial rejuvenation. Aesthetic Plast Surg 2012;36(4):753–60.

[7] 2023 ASPS procedural statistics release Available at: 2023. https://www.plasticsurgery.org/news/plastic-surgery-statistics (Accessed 20 October 2024).

[8] Kravitz ND, Vogels D, Vogels P. 2023 JCO orthodontic practice study part 1: trends. J Clin Orthod 2023;57(10):567–84.

[9] Kahn DM, Shaw RB. Overview of current thoughts on facial volume and aging. Facial Plast Surg 2010;26(5):350–5.

[10] Lorente C, Hernández-Alfaro F, Perez-Vela M, et al. Surgical-orthodontic approach for facial rejuvenation based on a reverse facelift. Prog Orthod 2019;20(1). https://doi.org/10.1186/s40510-019-0287-8.

[11] Roberts J, Roberts W. Incorporating facial rejuvenation into the dental practice. Dent Today 2010;29(2).

[12] Pessa JE, Zadoo VP, Yuan C, et al. Concertina effect and facial aging: nonlinear aspects of youthfulness and skeletal remodeling, and why, perhaps, infants have jowls. Plast Reconstr Surg 1999;103(2):635–44.

[13] Fourgeot E, Graillon N, Savoldelli C, et al. Intra-individual aging of the facial skeleton. Aesthetic Surg J 2021. https://doi.org/10.1093/asj/sjab228.

[14] Pessa JE, Zadoo VP, Mutimer KL, et al. Relative maxillary retrusion as a natural consequence of aging: combining skeletal and soft-tissue changes into an integrated model of midfacial aging. Plast Reconstr Surg 1998;102(1):205–12.

[15] Pessa JE. An algorithm of facial aging: verification of lambros's theory by three-dimensional stereolithography, with reference to the pathogenesis of midfacial aging, scleral show, and the lateral suborbital trough deformity. Plast Reconstr Surg 2000;106(2):479–88.

[16] Shaw RB, Kahn DM. Aging of the midface bony elements: a three-dimensional computed tomographic study. Plast Reconstr Surg 2007;119(2):675–81.

[17] Richard MJ, Morris C, Deen BF, et al. Analysis of the anatomic changes of the aging facial skeleton using computer-assisted tomography. Ophthalmic Plast Reconstr Surg 2009;25(5):382–6.

[18] Bondevik O. Dentofacial changes in adults A longitudinal cephalometric study in 22–33 and 33–43 year olds. J Orofac Orthop 2012;73(4):277–88.

[19] Windhager S, Mitteroecker P, Rupić I, et al. Facial aging trajectories: a common shape pattern in male and female faces is disrupted after menopause. Am J Phys Anthropol 2019;169(4):678–88.

[20] Wulc AE, Sharma P, Czyz CNCC. The anatomic basis of midfacial aging. In: Hartstein M, Wulc A, Holck D, editors. Midfacial rejuvenation. New York: Springer; 2012. p. 15–28.

[21] Emre IE, Cakmak O. Ageing face, an overview - aetiology, assessment and management. Otorhinolaryngologist 2013;6(3):160–6.

[22] Pessa JE, Slice DE, Hanz KR, et al. Aging and the shape of the mandible. Plast Reconstr Surg 2008;121(1):196–200.

[23] Shaw RB, Katzel EB, Koltz PF, et al. Aging of the mandible and its aesthetic implications. Plast Reconstr Surg 2010;125(1):332–42.

[24] Romo T, Yalamanchili H, Sclafani AP. Chin and prejowl augmentation in the management of the aging jawline. Facial Plast Surg 2005;21(1):38–46.

[25] Ozturk CN, Ozturk C, Bozkurt M, et al. Dentition, bone loss, and the aging of the mandible. Aesthetic Surg J 2013;33(7):967–74.

[26] Chrcanovic BR, Abreu MHNG, Custódio ALN. Morphological variation in dentate and edentulous human mandibles. Surg Radiol Anat 2011;33(3):203–13.

[27] Rosa WG, Navarro Rde L, Conti AC, et al. Assessment of cephalometric characteristics in the elderly. Braz Oral Res 2015;29(1):1–9.

[28] Coleman SR, Grover R. The anatomy of the aging face: volume loss and changes in 3-dimensional topography. Aesthetic Surg J 2006;26(1 SUPPL). https://doi.org/10.1016/j.asj.2005.09.012.

[29] Shaw RB, Katzel EB, Koltz PF, et al. Aging of the facial skeleton: aesthetic implications and rejuvenation strategies. Plast Reconstr Surg 2011;127(1):374–83.

[30] Ko AC, Korn BS, Kikkawa DO. The aging face. Surv Ophthalmol 2017;62(2):190–202.

[31] Swift A, Liew S, Weinkle S, et al. The facial aging process from the "inside out.". Aesthetic Surg J 2021;41(10):1107–19.

[32] Wan D, Amirlak B, Rohrich R, et al. The clinical importance of the fat compartments in midfacial aging. Plast Reconstr Surg 2013;1(9):1–8.

[33] Guisantes E. Beauty and aging. In: Pinto H, Fontdevila J, editors. Regenerative medicine procedures for aesthetic physicians. Cham, Switzerland: Springer Nature Switzerland AG; 2019. p. 33–43. https://doi.org/10.1007/978-3-030-15458-5.

[34] Dickens ST, Sarver DM, Proffit WR. Changes in frontal soft tissue dimensions of the lower face by age and gender. World J Orthod 2002;3:313–20.

[35] Fudalej P. Long-term changes of the upper lip position relative to the incisal edge. Am J Orthod Dentofacial Orthop 2008;133(2):204–9.

[36] Singh B, Ahluwalia R, Verma D, et al. Perioral age-related changes in smile dynamics along the vertical plane A videographic cross-sectional study. Angle Orthod 2013; 83(3):468–75.

[37] Chetan P, Tandon P, Singh GK, et al. Dynamics of a smile in different age groups. Angle Orthod 2013;83(1):90–6.

[38] Drummond S, Capelli J. Incisor display during speech and smile: age and gender correlations. Angle Orthod 2016;86(4):631–7.

[39] Van Der Geld P, Oosterveld P, Kuijpers-Jagtman AM. Age-related changes of the dental aesthetic zone at rest and during spontaneous smiling and speech. Eur J Orthod 2008;30(4):366–73.

[40] Rajbhoj AA, Parchake P, Begnoni G, et al. Dental changes in humans with untreated normal occlusion throughout lifetime: a systematic scoping review. Am J Orthod Dentofacial Orthop 2021;160(3):340–62.e3.

[41] Natsumeda G, Miranda F, Massaro C, et al. Aging changes in maxillary anterior teeth in untreated individuals: an observational longitudinal study. Prog Orthod 2023; 24(1). https://doi.org/10.1186/s40510-023-00478-z.

[42] Newton JT, Subramanian SS, Westland S, et al. The impact of tooth colour on the perceptions of age and social judgements. J Dent 2021;112:103771.

[43] Zachrisson BU. JCO interviews. Bjorn U. Zachrisson, DDS, MSD, PhD, on current trends in adult treatment, part 1. J Clin Orthod 2005;39(4):231–44.

[44] Lecocq G, Truong Tan Trung L. Smile esthetics: calculated beauty? Int Orthod 2014;12(2):149–70.

[45] De Couto Nascimento V, De Castro Ferreira Conti AC, De Almeida Cardoso M, et al. Impact of orthodontic treatment on self-esteem and quality of life of adult patients requiring oral rehabilitation. Angle Orthod 2016; 86(5):839–45.

[46] Mavreas D, Athanasiou AE. Rejuvenation of the ageing face and the role of orthodontics: guidelines for management. J Orthod 2022;49(4):463–71.

[47] Newton JP, Yemm R, Abel RW, et al. Changes in human jaw muscles with age and dental state. Gerodontology 1993;10(1):16–22.

[48] Gerth DJ. Structural and volumetric changes in the aging face. Facial Plast Surg 2015;31(1):3–9.

[49] Ilankovan V. Anatomy of ageing face. Br J Oral Maxillofac Surg 2014;52(3):195–202.

[50] Garib D, Natsumeda GM, Massaro C, et al. Cephalometric changes during aging in subjects with normal occlusion. J Appl Oral Sci 2021;29:e20210199.

[51] Al-Taai N, Persson M, Ransjö M, et al. Craniofacial changes from 13 to 62 years of age. Eur J Orthod 2022;44(5): 556–65.

[52] Abduo J, Lyons K. Clinical considerations for increasing occlusal vertical dimension: a review. Aust Dent J 2012; 57(1):2–10.

[53] Abduo J. Safety of increasing vertical dimension of occlusion : a systematic review Safety of increasing vertical dimension of occlusion : a systematic review. Quintessence 2014;43(5):369–80.

[54] Muts EJ, Van Pelt H, Edelhoff D, et al. Tooth wear: a systematic review of treatment options. J Prosthet Dent 2014;112(4):752–9.

[55] Yadfout A, El Aoud J, Merzouk N, et al. Increasing vertical dimension of occlusion (VDO): review. Clin Cosmet Invest Dent 2024;16(April):135–42.

[56] Moss ML. The functional matrix hypothesis revisited. 1. The role of mechanotransduction. Am J Orthod Dentofacial Orthop 1997;112(1):8–11.

[57] Goldspink G. Cellular and molecular aspects of muscle growth, adaptation and ageing. Gerodontology 1998; 15(1):35–43.

[58] Mohindra NK, Bulman JS. The effect of increasing vertical dimension of occlusion on facial aesthetics. Br Dent J 2002;192(3):164–8.

[59] Levine RA, Garza JR, Wang PTH, et al. Adult facial growth: applications to aesthetic surgery. Aesthetic Plast Surg 2003;27(4):265–8.

[60] Mohammed H, Kumar R, Bennani H, et al. Malocclusion severity and smile features: is there an association? Am J Orthod Dentofacial Orthop 2023;164(1):14–23.

[61] Ganel T, Goodale MA. The effect of smiling on the perceived age of male and female faces across the lifespan. Sci Rep 2021;11(1):1–10.

[62] Pithon MM, Nascimento CC, Barbosa GCG, et al. Do dental esthetics have any influence on finding a job? Am J Orthod Dentofacial Orthop 2014;146(4):423–9.

[63] Stuzin JM. Restoring facial shape in face lifting: the role of skeletal support in facial analysis and midface soft-tissue repositioning. Plast Reconstr Surg 2007;119(1): 362–77.

[64] Niamtu J. Perioral soft-tissue rejuvenation techniques to enhance esthetic restorative dentistry. Compend Contin Educ Dent 2003;24(11):811–7.

[65] Zachrisson BU. Bjorn U. Zachrisson, DDS, MSD, PhD, on current trends in adult treatment, part 2. Interview by Robert G. Keim. J Clin Orthod 2005;39(5):285–96.

[66] Reilly MJ, Tomsic JA, Fernandez SJ, et al. Effect of facial rejuvenation surgery on perceived attractiveness, femininity, and personality. JAMA Facial Plast Surg 2015;17(3):202–7.

[67] Gupta MA, Gilchrest BA. Psychosocial aspects of aging skin. Dermatol Clin 2005;23(4):643–8.

Advances in Cosmetic Surgery 8 (2025) 133–140

ADVANCES IN COSMETIC SURGERY

Whitnall's Ligament Suspension Repair of Involutional Ptosis—The Old Is New

Jeffrey Schiller, MD[a,b,*], Andrea Cacciarelli, MD[a,c]

[a]JFK University Medical Center, Hackensack Meridian Health, Edison, NJ, USA; [b]Department of Ophthalmology, Rutgers-NJ Medical School, Newark, NJ, USA; [c]Clara Maass Medical Center, Montclair, NJ, USA

KEYWORDS

• Involutional ptosis • Whitnall's • Sling • Suspension • Repair

KEY POINTS

- Involutional ptosis is rather common in patients requesting cosmetic blepharoplasty and contributes to the appearance of fatigue.
- Ptosis repair is sometimes unpredictable and can be challenging to the casual ptosis surgeon.
- Whitnall's ligament suspension allows maximal reliable levator aponerurotic repair of involutional ptosis with minimal complications.

Ptosis often must be addressed in order to maximize the aesthetic result of upper blepharoplasty. Ptosis repair is one of the most common procedures performed in an oculofacial surgeon's practice.

Older patients frequently present with ptosis severe enough to interfere with activities of daily life, manifesting margin-to-reflex distance of 2 mm or less. Aesthetically, ptosis creates a tired, inattentive appearance, especially when combined with orbitomalar sulcus deflation and midface descent, and/or frank steatoblepharon. Patients are thought to be sleepy, under the influence of alcohol or drugs, or unintelligent, based on the appearance of upper eyelid drooping [1] Correction of ptosis when combined with upper and/or lower cosmetic blepharoplasty results in a refreshed younger more alert appearance and hence a more comprehensive facial rejuvenation than would be accomplished without ptosis repair. A series from the Mayo Clinic reported that "up to 21% of patients undergoing upper blepharoplasty required ptosis correction in addition to upper blepharoplasty" [2] (Fig. 1A, B, Fig. 2A, B).

Ptosis repair can be challenging to occasional and even frequent blepharoplasty surgeons. Approaches that are simple and reliable and that do not require secondary surgeries are highly desirable. One of these techniques is the Muller's muscle conjunctival resection (MMCR), which may be useful in patients with ptosis responsive to Neosynephrine. One disadvantage of the technique is that it requires an internal incision in addition to an external upper blepharoplasty incision (if needed if involutional aesthetic issues are to be addressed) which can result in increased swelling, and discomfort related to corneal irritation and chemosis.

For the past 8 years, I have been utilizing a technique of plication of the levator aponeurosis to Whitnall's ligament, which fulfills the above criteria with great success and a minimal reoperation rate. It is a valuable addition to the cosmetic surgeon's armamentarium.

*Corresponding author. 1550 Richmond Avenue, Suite 208, Staten Island, NY 10314. *E-mail address:* jeffschillermd@gmail.com

https://doi.org/10.1016/j.yacs.2025.01.009

www.advancesincosmeticsurgery.com

2542-4327/25/

ABBREVIATIONS	
LAA	levator aponeurotic advancement
MMCR	Muller's muscle conjunctival resection
UTZ	upper transitional zone

Herein, I will describe the anatomy necessary to an understanding of the procedure, the technique itself, and show some typical results.

CAUSES OF INVOLUTIONAL PTOSIS

Multiple causes of ptosis are well-described and include congenital ptosis, mechanical ptosis, myogenic ptosis, neurogenic ptosis, and neuromuscular junction-related. Involutional ptosis is the most common cause of aesthetic ptosis. Levator function is normal, and the upper lid crease is usually elevated with hollowing of the upper sulcus.

Changes in the aponeurosis or its relationships to adjacent eyelid tissues are generally thought to be the root cause of ptosis, with combinations of dehiscence, attenuation, or elongation described. A decline in levator palpebrae superioris function with age has also been recognized, and the severity of involutional ptosis has been shown to be associated with diminished levator function in many cases [3]. The variety of procedures espoused to correct involutional ptosis may, in part, be related to the variety of underlying pathoanatomic elements.

ANATOMY OF WHITNALL'S LIGAMENT

Whitnall's ligament was first described in 1910 by Dr Samuel Ernest Whitnall as a superior transverse ligament at the junction of the levator muscle and its aponeurosis [4]. Anderson and Dixon's seminal article in 1979 further elaborated the anatomy and function [5]. Further investigation was done by by Codère and colleagues [6]. The ligament originates medially at the superior border of the trochlea and the adjacent orbital bone and traverses horizontally to the lateral orbital wall between the palpebral and orbital lobes of the lacrimal gland, merging with the anterior fascia of the levator muscle. The ligament has variably been referred to as the anterior transverse ligament or check ligament [7]. It is composed of collagen and a variable amount of elastin. There is a less robust inferior transverse component beneath the levator muscle and aponeurosis, which also spans the orbit and is described as forming a sleeve around the levator muscle. This structure has been called the intermuscular transverse ligament [8], and it is said to contribute to the suspensory ligament of the superior

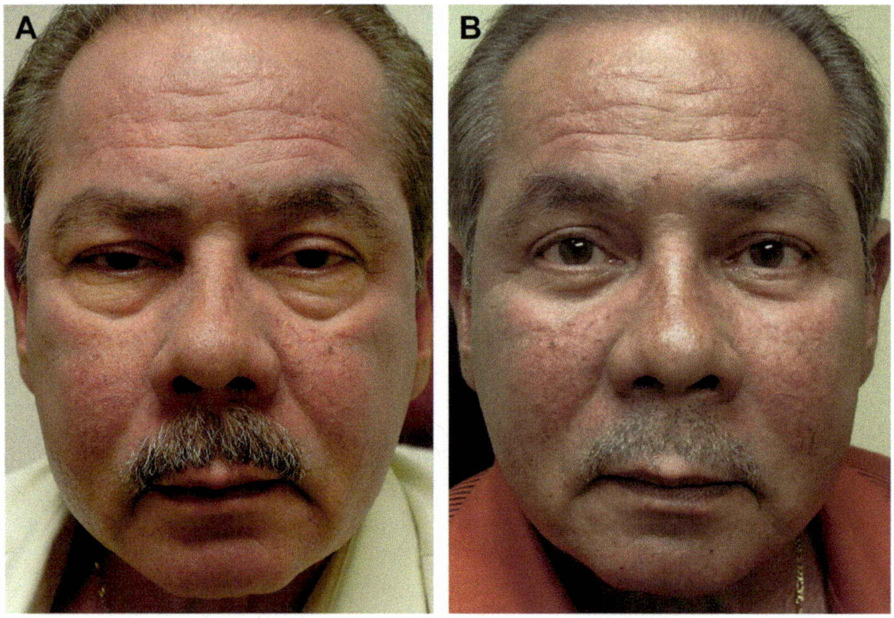

FIG. 1 (*A*, *B*) A 75 year old man 5 months after levator advancement to Whitnall's ligament, lower blepharoplasty with midface lift.

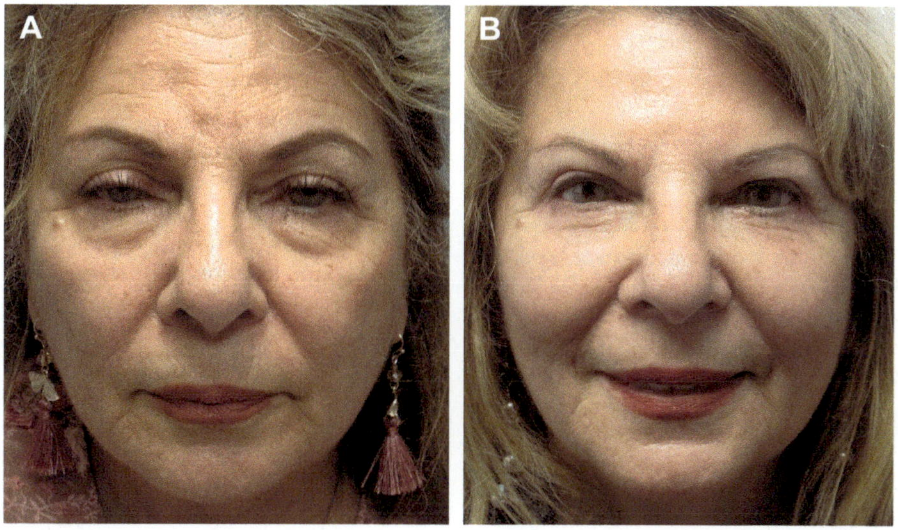

FIG. 2 (*A*, *B*) A 78 year old woman 6 months after levator advancement to Whitnall's ligament, upper and lower blepharoplasty with midface lift.

fornix together with the superior transverse ligament or Whitnall's.

The anatomy of Whitnall's varies widely in thickness, continuity, and branching as illustrated in Anderson and Dixon's original article in 1979 [5], which included photographs of a "poorly developed" and a "hypertrophic" Whitnall's ligament (their Figs. 5 and 6).

There has been some dispute regarding Anderson's suggestion that Whitnall's ligament provides a fulcrum directing the pull of the levator not only posteriorly but also superiorly. Goldberg and colleagues [9] presented MR images of the levator muscle action and Whitnall's motion during opening and closing of the upper eyelid.

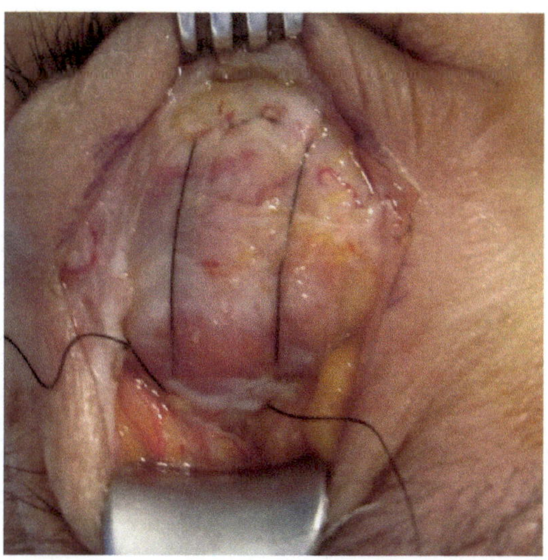

FIG. 3 Placement of 6-0 silk suture with 3 bites of tarsus above and mattress suture of Whitnall's below.

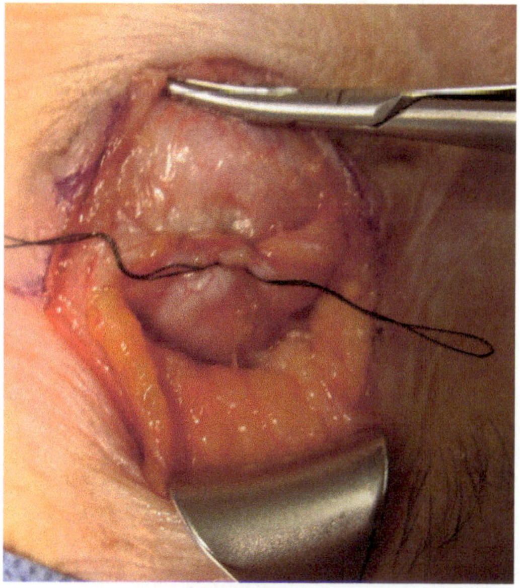

FIG. 4 Another case with the suture placed and tightened.

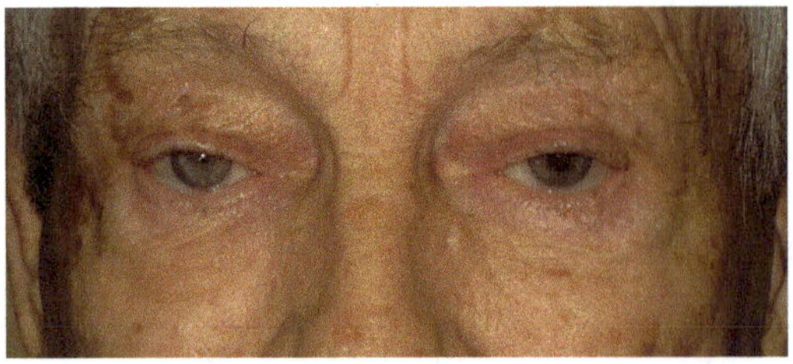

FIG. 5 An 85 year old man shows marked involutional ptosis with MRD 1 of 0 mm OU.

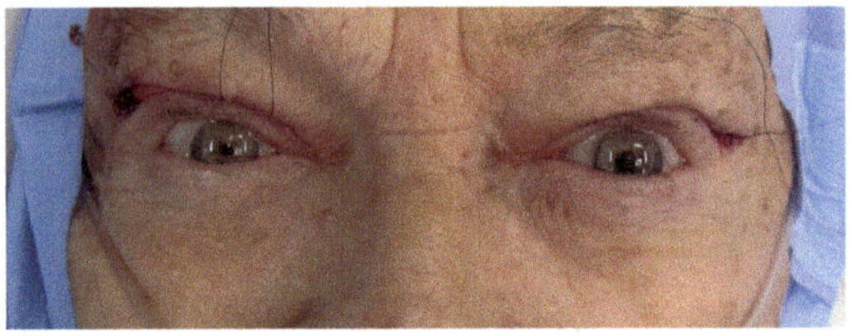

FIG. 6 Intraoperative adjustment done.

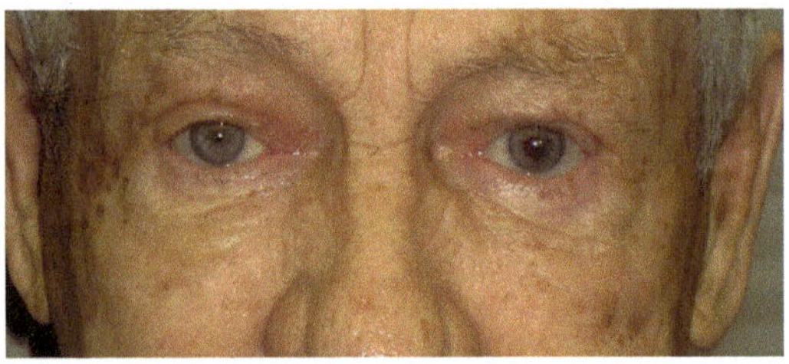

FIG. 7 Same patient 5 month postoperative with excellent symmetry and contours.

They concluded, "Whitnall's ligament …travels anteriorly and posteriorly with the excursion of the levator muscle." The elastic nature and vector of Whitnall's motion can easily be observed intraoperatively when the patient is asked to open the eyes, and the ligament follows the levator into and out of the orbit. One may observe a mild pulley action redirecting the vector, but primarily the ligament directly follows the levator muscle's movement.

In Anderson's article, his anatomic dissections demonstrate the inferior movement of Whitnall's with closure of the eye, which may allow closure even when it is sutured to the tarsus, and hence the absence of lagophthalmos noted after their "Whitnall's sling" procedure (Anderson and Dixon [5]; see Figs. 1A, B and 2A, B).

My experience performing this procedure has shown me that Whitnall's ligament is quite variable in structure and robustness, from dense to fibrillar and branching, and rarely can barely be discerned, and it occurs only very rarely as low as the superior margin of the aponeurosis.

Whitnall's Ligament and Ptosis Repair

The technique of Whitnall's suspension to correct ptosis has been described in the literature almost exclusively for the treatment of congenital ptosis with poor levator function. Its use has been advocated by Anderson as a "Whitnall's sling" [10] and others as a substitute for levator resection in severe congenital ptosis. Daoudi and colleagues [11] evaluated Whitnall's suspension alone in severe congenital ptosis with good results.

A 2020 report by Pfeiffer and colleagues [12] from Europe compared involutional ptosis repair by "simple reinsertion" of dehisced aponeurosis to tarsus, compared to "double reinsertion" suturing aponeurosis to tarsus and also suturing Whitnall's to tarsus. Anatomically, they describe an upper transitional zone (UTZ) of 1 to 5 mm or more between the upper edge of the aponeurosis and Whitnall's ligament in 70.5% of cases, which is consistent with my observations. They noted improved correction of ptosis using the Whitnall's suspension particularly in cases of a larger gap (UTZ) between the superior border of the aponeurosis and Whitnall's, supporting the Whitnall's technique in a majority of cases.

TECHNIQUES FOR CORRECTION OF INVOLUTIONAL PTOSIS

Two procedures are commonly used to correct involutional or aponeurotic ptosis. MMCR described by Alan Putterman [13] has the advantage of avoiding a skin incision and may be considered "minimally invasive." Several protocols have been advocated for determining the degree of resection to be performed, but none are definitive [14,15]. Multiple reports have compared levator aponeurotic advancement technique with MMCR, but the results appear similar [16–23].

It is reported that the incidence of reoperation is lower with MMCR. BenSimon and colleagues [24] compared MMCR to levator advancement and reported a slightly higher reoperation rate following aponeurotic advancement, but insofar as MMCR is often performed on patients with less severe ptosis, it is unclear whether the variable results are due to patient selection or the technique used. Chang and colleagues [17] concluded in a review that there is no level 1 evidence to compare the techniques.

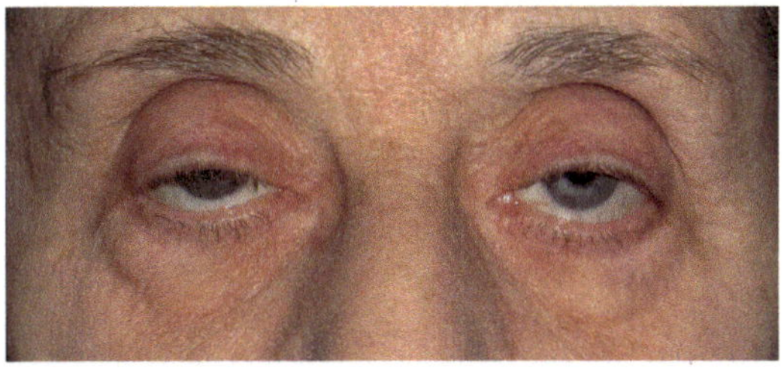

FIG. 8 A 72 year old woman with MRD 1 of −1 mm OD and −0.5 mm OS.

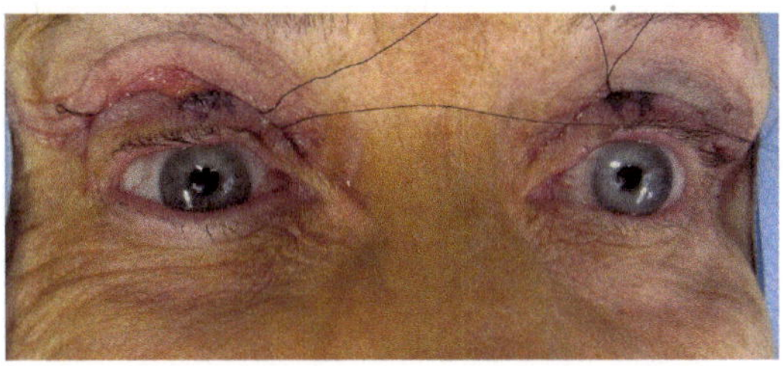

FIG. 9 Intraoperative adjustment done.

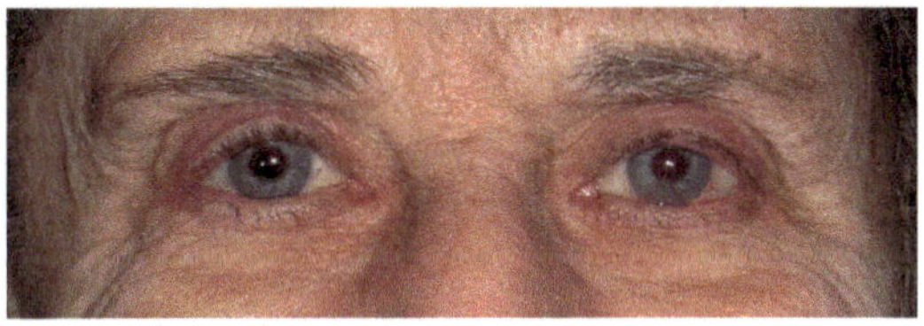

FIG. 10 Three months postop shows good symmetry and contours.

Levator aponeurotic repair or advancement (LAA) is usually performed under local anesthesia with mild intravenous sedation to allow patient cooperation opening and closing the eyes intraoperatively. In the case of frank dehiscence, the aponeurosis may be reapproximated to the tarsus. A common variation in technique is dissection posterior to the levator aponeurosis to allow full thickness advancement of the aponeurosis as a free flap. The commonest maximal use of the LAA involves plication from the tarsus to the superior margin of the aponeurosis. More lift can be achieved with partial tarsal resection.

One to three plicating sutures have been described. The patient is awakened and asked to open their eyes. The lids are then adjusted with attention to height, contour, and symmetry. The lid margin is placed 1 to 2 mm above the desired height to compensate for the loss of tone of the orbicularis due to local anesthesic infiltration. The elevation is limited to the superior edge of the aponeurosis as the sutures are generally not placed into the levator muscle itself in this procedure.

In my fellowship training with Stephen Bosniak and Serge Morax, a simplified approach to levator advancement was used, plicating the anterior surface of the aponeurosis to the anterior surface of the tarsus with no posterior dissection or resection.

For the past 8 years, I have been performing levator advancement plicating the anterior surface of the tarsus to Whitnall's ligament with one horizontal mattress suture of 6-0 silk in most cases of involutional ptosis with margin-reflex distance (MRD) of 2 mm or less and levator excursions of 8 mm or more with excellent results in several hundred cases. Because Whitnall's moves in concert with the levator muscle, I have had one case of mild lagophthalmos. If there is undercorrection, I can be certain that the maximal correction has been achieved without a more complex procedure such as levator resection, or aponeurotic advancement combined with tarsal and/or Muller's resection. If more lift is required, sometimes, revision by MMCR is helpful. The Whitnall's procedure is my default procedure for involutional ptosis repair.

SURGICAL TECHNIQUE

I have used CO_2 laser as a cutting tool since the early 1990s for almost all eyelid procedures. The laser causes less burning and charring than monopolar cautery, with the Bovie cautery operating at 1204 degrees C and the CO2 laser at 100 degree C (James Zins MD, 2019, personal communication), and hence I believe less stimulation of scarring and cicatricial issues of induration and contraction. The 0.2 mm laser spot is used in continuous mode at 5 to 6 W using stainless steel corneal protectors.

The upper eyelid creases are marked in the desired location, usually asking the patient to open and close and verifying symmetry with calipers centrally, medially, and laterally. If skin or skin and muscle resection is elected to correct excess skin weighing down the eyelids or to improve cosmesis, a pinch technique is used. With the eyes open, the apex of the eyelid contour is marked to locate the center of the plicating suture.

The skin and orbicularis are incised in a single layer and the skin muscle flaps excised exposing the orbital septum. The septum is tented and the preaponeurotic fat is exposed. The fat is peeled off the aponeurosis from inferior to superior with light passes of the laser

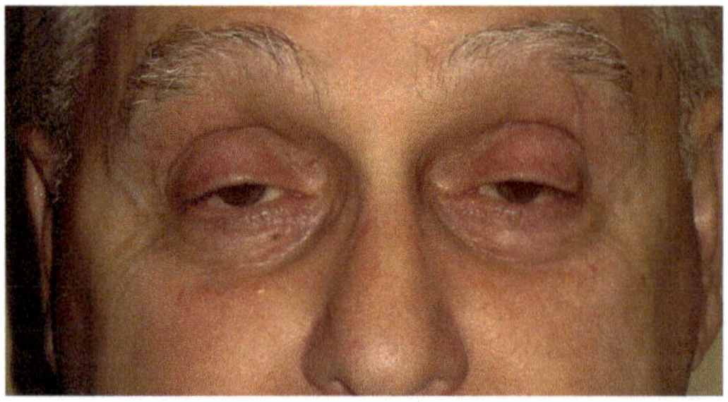

FIG. 11 A 79 year old man with MRD 1 of −1 mm OU.

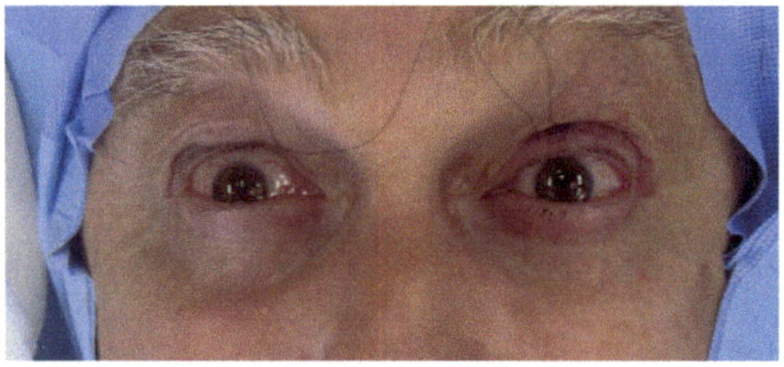

FIG. 12 Intraoperative adjustment.

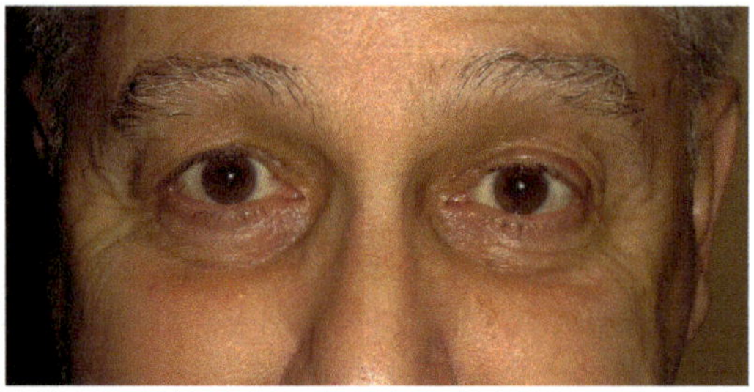

FIG. 13 Postop 5 months with excellent height and contours.

dividing the fine attachments until Whitnall's ligament is exposed. The anterior surface of the tarsus is exposed. There is generally minimal to no bleeding with the use of the CO_2 laser.

A double-armed 6-0 silk suture with a small spatula needle (Ethicon 769 - Rariton, NJ) is passed horizontally with three or four. half-depth bites of the tarsus centered on the apex of the contour 2 mm inferior to the superior border, taking care to avoid Mullers muscle. The small spatula needle facilitates the half -depth bite of the tarsus. The eyelid is everted to verify that the suture bites are not full thickness. The suture is then passed through Whitnall's ligament in a horizontal mattress manner as wide as the lateral and medial points of entry into and out of the tarsus and tied temporarily with a slip knot. Whitnall's has significant variation from very robust and thick to fibrillar and attenuated, occasionally with a diagonal orientation (Figs. 3 and 4). The patient is awakened and the corneal shields are removed and the lights moved off the field, and the patient is asked to open their eyes. The height, contour, and symmetry are observed (Figs. 5–13). Often the heights and contours are perfectly symmetric. This is one of the surprising advantages of this technique. Occasionally, there is some mild overcorrection or asymmetry, which a small hang-back can correct. The three or four bite tarsal stitch technique affords excellent contours in the vast majority of cases. The target height is between 1 mm below and 1 mm above the superior limbus with a higher level favored in patients with preoperative lesser levator excursions.

A small rake retracts the upper flap to expose the knot and the loop is cut and the free end of the suture is pulled out without disturbing the knot or lid height. Five throws are added. The orbicularis is closed with buried 7-0 vicryl incorporating bites of the inferior aponeurosis fusion with the septum medial and lateral again asking the patient to open their eyes to verify height, depth, and symmetry of the creases. The skin is closed with a running subcuticular 6-0 prolene suture.

In my experience progressing from initially using three mattress sutures to a single broad plicating suture, this technique has proven to reliably provide aesthetically pleasing and symmetric contours. Reoperations with this procedure are rare and are almost never required for contour abnormalities, overcorrection, or lagophthalmos. Undercorrection can occur occasionally in severe involutional cases, but if symmetric, I feel that I have maximized the levator advancement, and further surgery may require secondary approaches such as MMCR perhaps with tarsectomy. Overcorrection and lagophthalmos have been seen extremely rarely, perhaps because of the intraoperative adjustment. Using the CO_2 affords a relatively bloodless field and the operating time is under 30 minutes if other maneuvers such as fat sculpting are not added.

This surgery has become my standard procedure for correction of common involutional ptosis cases with MRD $\leq$ 2 mm for many years, and I perform it generally at least a few times each week. I have performed a handful of revisions over the years. Undercorrection can occur occasionally but usually there is marked improvement and a more aggressive procedure would have been necessary for a more dramatic outcome. A couple of patients had evidence of a broken plicating suture in the early postop period repaired in the office setting under local anesthesia.

Ointment is applied on the sutures in the operating room and often not thereafter. Sutures are removed later than non-laser procedures because the wounds tend to require a few additional days, generally at 8 to 10 days postoperatively.

SUMMARY

This procedure has mostly supplanted MMCR and levator aponeurotic advancement in my practice, which is a mixed cosmetic and functional practice. In my hands, it is more reliable and stable over time than aponeurotic surgery, does not require the second internal incision as with MMCR with its attendant concerns regarding direct contact with the ocular surface. It is a valuable adjunct to the cosmetic blepharoplasty surgeon's armamentarium with a low complication rate and a high rate of patient and surgeon satisfaction.

CLINICS CARE POINTS

- An alternative approach to ptosis repair.
- A viable alternative in patients where aponeurotic advancement or mullerectomy fail.
- A reliable procedure for repair of primary or reoperation ptosis.
- Can accompany cosmetic blepharoplasty in cosmetic patients.
- Adds to the oculoplastic cosmetic surgeons' armamentarium.

DISCLOSURE

The authors have nothing to disclose.

REFERENCES

[1] Richards HS, Jenkinson E, White P, Harrad RA. Patient reported psychosocial functioning following successful ptosis surgery. Eye 2022;36(8):1651–5.

[2] Falcon Rodriguez L, Kuruoglu D, Salinas CA, et al. Eyelid and Brow rejuvenation: Technical Pearls and outcomes of upper blepharoplasty with or without ptosis correction and Brow lift. Plast Reconstr Surg 2024;154(6): 1199–207.

[3] Lai HT, Weng SF, Chang CH, et al. Analysis of levator function and ptosis severity in involutional Blepharoptosis. Ann Plast Surg 2017;78(3):S58–60.

[4] Whitnall SE. Anatomy of the human orbit and accessory organs of vision. 2nd edition. NewYork: Oxford University Press inc; 1932. p. 148–63.

[5] Anderson R, Dixon R. Role of Whitnall's ligament in ptosis surgery. Arch Ophthalmol 1979;97(4):705–7.

[6] Codère F, Tucker NA, Renaldi B. The anatomy of Whitnall ligament. Ophthalmology 1995;102(12):2016–9, PMID: 9098310.

[7] Kakizaki H, Malhotra R, Selva D. Upper eyelid anatomy: an update. Ann Plas Surg 2009;63:336–43.

[8] Kakizaki H, Takahashi Y, Nakano T, et al. Whitnall ligament anatomy revisited. Clin Exp Ophthalmol 2011; 39(2):152–5, Epub 2010 Dec 16.PMID: 21040310.

[9] Goldberg RA, Wu JC, Jesmanowicz A, et al. Eyelid anatomy revisited. Dynamic high-resolution magnetic resonance images of Whitnall's ligament and upper eyelid structures with the use of a surface coil. Arch Ophthalmmol 1992; 110:1598–600.

[10] Anderson RL, Jordan DR, Dutton JJ. Whitnall's sling for poor function ptosis. Arch Ophthalmol 1990;108(11): 1628–32.

[11] Daoudi C, Chahdi KO, Lezrek O, et al. Technique de suspension au ligament de Whitnall dans le traitement chirurgical du ptosis. (Whitnall's ligament suspension technique in ptosis surgery). J Fr Ophtalmol 2017;40:763–9.

[12] Pfeiffer N, Pfeiffer M, Sainz AR, et al. Double reinsertion including Whitnall's ligament in aponeurotic ptosis surgery. Graefes Arch Clin Exp Ophthalmol 2021;259:1309–13.

[13] Putterman AM, Urist MJ. Mueller muscle-conjunctiva resection. Arch Ophthalmol 1975;93:619–23.

[14] Rootman DB, Sinha KR, Goldberg RA. Change in eyelid position following muller's muscle conjunctival resection with a standard versus variable resection length. Ophthalmic Plast Reconstr Surg 2018;34(4):355–60, PMID: 28914711.

[15] Saffari PS, Dallazadeh O, et al. The Utility of Preoperative Phenylephrine Testing in Muller Muscle Conjunctival Resection Surgery for Involutional Ptosis. Ophthal Plast Reconstr Surg 2025;41(1):90–3. https://doi.org/10.1097/IOP.0000000000002746.

[16] Cohen LS, Rootman DB. Blepharoptosis repair:external versus posterior approach surgery: Why I Select one over the other. Facial Plast Surg Clin N Am 2021;29: 195–208.

[17] Chang S, Lehrman C, Itani K, et al. A systematic review of comparison of upper eyelid involutional ptosis repair techniques: efficacy and complication rates. Plast Reconstr Surg 2012;129(1):149–57, PMID: 22186506.

[18] Matsuda H, Sakai T, Takahashi Y, et al. J Surgical outcomes of the anterior versus posterior approach for advancement of the levator aponeurosis in Japanese patients. Plast ReconstrAesthet Surg 2020;73(11):2001–9, Epub 2020 Aug 25.PMID: 32912723.

[19] PreamjitSaonanon, SupapanSithanon external levator advancement versus Müller muscle-conjunctival resection for aponeurotic blepharoptosis: a randomized clinical trial. Plast Reconstr Surg 2018;141(2):213e–9e.

[20] Allen RC, Saylor MA, Nerad JA. The current state of ptosis repair: a comparison of internal and external approaches. Curr Opin Ophthalmol 2011;22(5):394–9.

[21] Thomas GN, Chan J, Sundar G. S Amrith Outcomes of levator advancement and Müller muscle-conjunctiva resection for the repair of upper eyelid ptosis. Orbit 2017;36(1):39–42.

[22] Arslan N, Bahar A, Acar M, et al. GurdalC.Rom J the results of muller muscle conjunctival resection versus levator advancement for mild to moderate ptosis. Ophthalmol Times 2023;67(2):128–33, PMID: 3752 2026.

[23] Sweeney AR, Dermarkarian CR, Williams KJ, et al. Outcomes after Müller muscle conjunctival resection versus external levator advancement in severe involutional blepharoptosis. Am J Ophthalmol 2020;217:182–8, Epub 2020 May 6.PMID: 32387434.

[24] Ben Simon GJ, Lee S, Schwarcz RM, et al. External levator advancement vs Muller's muscle-conjunctival resection for correction of upper eyelid involutional ptosis. Am J Ophthalmol 2005;140(3):426–32.

Advances in Cosmetic Surgery 8 (2025) 141–151
ADVANCES IN COSMETIC SURGERY

Filler Rhinoplasty

Beatrice Ching-Chen Go, MD[a], Anne Sun Lowery, MD[a], Kirkland N. Lozada, MD[b,*]
[a]Department of Otorhinolaryngology–Head & Neck Surgery, University of Pennsylvania, 3400 Spruce Street, Ravdin 5, Philadelphia, PA 19103, USA; [b]Division of Facial Plastic & Reconstructive Surgery, Department of Otorhinolaryngology–Head & Neck Surgery, University of Pennsylvania, 503 Ramblewood Drive, Bryn Mawr, PA 19010, USA

KEYWORDS
• Filler • Rhinoplasty • Liquid rhinoplasty • Nonsurgical rhinoplasty • Facial plastics

KEY POINTS

- Nonsurgical rhinoplasty (NSR) utilizes filler injection to augment and improve aesthetic concerns of the nose.
- Hyaluronic acid is the most commonly used material.
- Advantages include low cost, quick recovery times, convenience, and low risk profile without the added risk of general anesthesia.
- Injection techniques closely mirror graft placement in traditional rhinoplasty.
- Vascular compromise leading to blindness is a major complication and requires immediate attention.

INTRODUCTION

Traditional rhinoplasty involves the surgical correction of nasal deformities to improve cosmetic appearance and/or functional status of the nose. Continuous innovation in the field has resulted in refinement of surgical techniques and approaches with the goal of producing natural results with minimal scarring and complications. Nonsurgical rhinoplasty (NSR) is a novel, popular approach that involves the injection of filler, most commonly hyaluronic acid (HA), into various areas to augment the nose and correct cosmetic concerns. Several advantages of this technique include natural results, lower associated costs, rapid recovery, ability to perform in the clinic, and temporary nature of the procedure, all without the added risks of general anesthesia and surgery. While there are a variety of injection techniques, an in-depth understanding of nasal anatomy is critical to achieve optimal results and reduce risks of significant adverse effects, namely vascular compromise.

RELEVANT ANATOMY

The nose can be best described in thirds comprising the bony upper third, the cartilaginous middle third, and the tip (Fig. 1A, B). The upper third consists of paired nasal bones extending from the frontal bone toward the rhinion, or the junction of the nasal bone and the upper lateral cartilages (ULCs). The nasofrontal angle consists of 2 lines tangent to the glabella and to the nasal dorsum intersecting at the nasion, with the ideal angle dependent on gender and ethnicity [1]. Nasal bones articulate with the lacrimal bone superolaterally, the nasomaxillary processes inferolaterally.

The middle third of the nose consists of paired ULCs, which articulate with the nasal bones and septum to form the keystone area. One critical area in the middle third is the internal nasal valve (INV), which is formed by the ULCs, septum, and head of the inferior turbinate. As the narrowest area in the nasal cavity, collapse in this area can lead to complaints of obstruction while exacerbating sinus and middle ear pathology [2].

*Corresponding author. *E-mail address:* drkirklozada@gmail.com

https://doi.org/10.1016/j.yacs.2025.01.007 www.advancesincosmeticsurgery.com
2542-4327/25/

ABBREVIATIONS	
CaHa	calcium hydroxyapatite
HA	hyaluronic acid
INV	internal nasal valve
LLCs	lower lateral cartilages
NSR	nonsurgical rhinoplasty
SMAS	superficial musculoaponeurotic system
ULCs	upper lateral cartilages

The tip consists of paired lower lateral cartilages (LLCs) formed from lateral, intermediate, and medial crura, which define tip shape, structure, and support. The medial crura join to form the columella with the caudal septal cartilage sitting just behind, extending from upper lip to the tip. The caudal border of the ULCs articulates with cephalic margins of the LLCs in the scroll area. The scroll; the shape, size, and strength of LLCs; and the attachment of medial crura to the caudal septum represent the 3 major tip support mechanisms of the nose. In addition, the minor support mechanisms include the anterior nasal spine, membranous septum, dorsal septum, lateral sesamoid cartilages, interdomal ligaments, and skin and soft tissue envelope [3]. Understanding the intricate nuances of each unique nasal tip is essential to improving esthetic appearance while preserving function.

Layers of the nose include skin, superficial fat, fibromuscular layer (superficial musculoaponeurotic system [SMAS]), deep fatty layer (loose areolar tissue), and perichondrium [4]. Skin is thickest at the radix and tip, while thinnest at the rhinion. Crucial blood vessels supplying the nose typically lie in the deep fatty layer along the lateral sidewalls of the nose. An understanding of the complex vascular supply to the nose is essential to avoiding filler-related complications with the acknowledgment that there are variations in individual anatomy (Fig. 2). The ophthalmic artery branches into anterior ethmoid artery, posterior ethmoid artery, and dorsal nasal artery that supply the lateral nasal wall/septum, superior turbinate/septum, and dorsal aspect of external nose, respectively [5]. The floor of the nose and internal structures receive blood supply from the greater palatine artery and sphenopalatine artery via the maxillary artery. The facial artery has multiple prevalent branches that supply the external nose. The alar and septal branches of the superior labial artery are responsible for alar and septal perfusion while the angular artery, which runs along the nasal sidewall, is responsible for tip, dorsum, and lateral wall supply [6].

FILLER SELECTION

Many types of filler including silicone, HA, and calcium hydroxyapatite (CaHa) have been used over the years in NSR, with HA as the most common [7]. When selecting

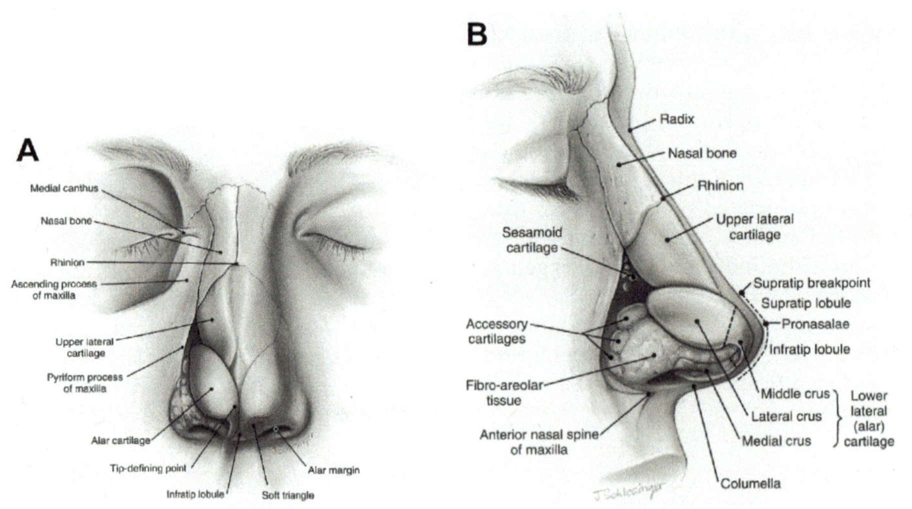

FIG. 1 (**A**) Frontal view of external nose. (**B**) Lateral view of external nose. (Used with permission from Oneal RM, Beil RJ. Surgical anatomy of the nose. Clin Plast Surg 2010;37(2):191–211. https://doi.org/10.1016/j.cps.2009.12.011.)

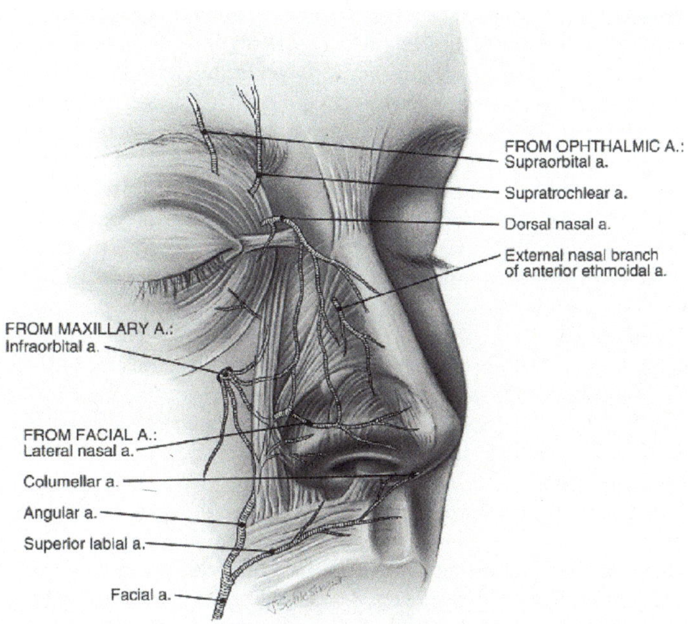

FIG. 2 Vascular supply of external nose. (Used with permission from Oneal RM, Beil RJ. Surgical anatomy of the nose. Clin Plast Surg 2010;37(2):191–211. https://doi.org/10.1016/j.cps.2009.12.011.)

an appropriate filler for NSR, ideal characteristics should include reversibility, long duration, and stiffness. Storage or elastic modulus (G′) is a rheological characteristic that represents the elastic behavior of the material and how likely it is to retain its shape [8]. Higher G′ has an elevated resistance to deformation and increased stiffness as a result, making this feature an ideal option for NSR.

HA is a naturally occurring compound that is composed of polymeric disaccharides with the ability to form stable structures in aqueous solutions. Due to its low immunogenicity and relative ease of use, HA has been used in various areas of the face to enhance facial features [9–12]. HA is a good choice for the precision required for NSR due to its low immunogenicity and high G′ options resulting in strong structural support, reversibility in event of adverse effects or patient preference, and low potential for tissue distortion. While CaHa has a significantly higher G′ than any HA product on the market, the ease of reversal makes HA a more common choice in practice today. In cases of complication, vascular injury, or patient dissatisfaction, reversibility offers an advantage to the patient and peace of mind to the injector. Compared to CaHa and other long-lasting semipermanent fillers, HA fillers can typically last between 6 and 12 months, depending on concentration, cross-linking, and density [13]. Permanent fillers such as silicone, poly-L-lactic acid (Sculptra, Galderma, La Tour-de-Peilz, Switzerland), polymethylmethacrylate (Bellafill, Suneva Medical, CA, USA) should be avoided in the nose due to the potential for permanent complications including vascular injury and granulomas. Advantages and disadvantages of filler options should be thoroughly discussed with the patient, and optimal filler selection may depend on independent patient characteristics and preferences.

PATIENT SELECTION

As with all cosmetic procedures, patient selection is one of the most critical aspects in achieving a positive outcome. In-depth knowledge of the strengths and limitations of NSR is absolutely critical in choosing patients who are optimal candidates for injection. At its most fundamental, NSR adds volume to the nose to help camouflage, blend, and/or balance the nose. It cannot make the nose smaller. Relationships such as raising dorsal height can give the *illusion* of smaller tip projection, but the fundamental length of the tip cannot be made smaller with NSR. This principle seems obvious to the reader but is worth emphasizing. Patients who desire a smaller overall nose (including smaller bridge height, smaller tip position, or shape) should be counseled that a surgical rhinoplasty may be the best option and referred for surgical consultation.

INJECTION TECHNIQUE

The procedure begins with a detailed conversation on ideal nose shape with the patient and obtaining informed consent. Local anesthetic ointment and ice to the nose may be applied for anesthesia and vasoconstriction, respectively. The nose should be cleansed thoroughly with antiseptic. The dorsal midline and ideal radix position should be marked to prevent asymmetry. A discussion of injection principles is warranted as they can help achieve an ideal outcome and minimize risk at the same time. The ideal layer for filler injection is just above the perichondrium or periosteum in the deep fatty layer as the superficial fatty layer and SMAS are rich in blood vessels (Fig. 3). Deep injection, use of small needles, small boluses, and low injection pressure are all strategies to reduce the risk of vascular infiltration and will be discussed further.

A linear threading technique with either a blunt or sharp needle tip with small boluses (<0.03 cc) is one option. Injection via cannula is another technique that is commonly used in the nose. The author's preferred technique involves small bolus injections using back-filled insulin syringes. It is important to avoid larger gauge needles provided in the filler packaging for higher G′ fillers. These 27 G needles are ideal for deep injections in large areas of the face such as the cheeks but are much too large for NSR. Using smaller needles in theory helps achieve a higher level of safety and patient comfort. A 27 G needle increases the risk of vascular injury, allows for a higher extrusion force of the product, and places a larger bolus than smaller needles. The author backfills 0.5 cc 31 G insulin syringes with 0.1 to 0.2 cc of product in each syringe by removing the plunger and placing product into the syringe and replacing the plunger pushing the product to the front of the syringe (Fig. 4). This technique allows smaller aliquots of filler to be used per injection with a much smaller extrusion force.

Product should be placed deep: either on the periosteum of the bone or perichondrium of the cartilage. In reality, perfect placement in these 2 planes may not always be realistic but the emphasis on deep injections is the key principle. Avoiding injections in the subdermal tissue will at least *attempt* to lower the risk of intravascular injury. Needle aspiration prior to injection may not be clinically useful in NSR as the small gauge of the needle may prevent backflow into the syringe and prevent the "flash" seen with larger needles. A 2 hand injection technique should be employed, using the nondominant hand to guide and stabilize the needle tip and then shape/smooth the tissue to the desired effect. Gentle massage of the site after injection can smoothen lumps, and touch ups should be offered after 2 weeks to allow for edema to decrease [14]. Capillary refill (<2 seconds) should be tested on completion to insure no blanching.

There are numerous approaches to NSR depending on the overall desired esthetic outcome and deformity

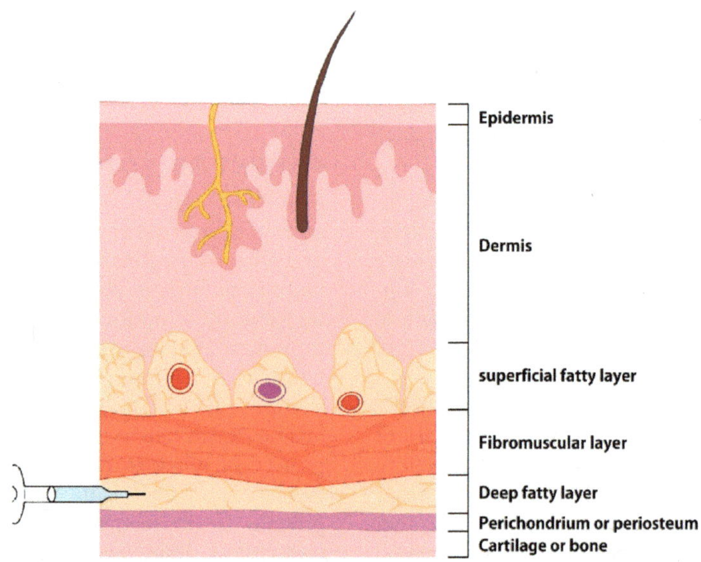

FIG. 3 Layers of the nose. Ideal layer of filler injection is into deep fatty layer to avoid vasculature. (Used with permission from Moon HJ. Injection rhinoplasty using filler. Facial Plast Surg Clin North Am 2018;26(3):323–30. https://doi.org/10.1016/j.fsc.2018.03.006.)

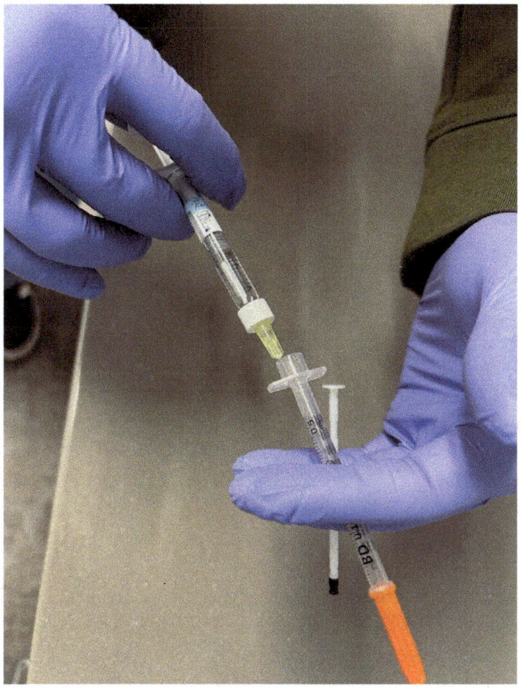

FIG. 4 Backfilling an insulin syringe is accomplished by removing the plunger, placing filler into the syringe, and replacing the plunger.

type/location. One proposed strategy to improve overall contour is to inject in the order of radix, rhinion, tip, and then supratip area [15]. Another useful concept is replicating a known graft that exists in surgical rhinoplasty with filler instead to achieve similar results of augmentation and camouflage. A detailed discussion of injection technique by area is included later.

Radix

The radix, or root of the nose, refers to the upper bony portion of the nasal bones. Injection along the radix allows for treatment of a dorsal hump by moving the radix breakpoint superiorly and creating the effect of a straight bridge, similar to a radix graft in surgical rhinoplasty (Fig. 5) [16]. An important anatomic concept in this region is the relationship of the dorsal height to tip projection. When one raises the dorsal height with filler, it will provide the illusion of a shorter or less projected tip. This is ideal for most patients as creating a smaller appearing nose is a common esthetic goal. Prior to injection, lifting or manipulating of the skin of the radix can help simulate a straight dorsum to approximate the end goal. For extremely large dorsal humps, filling the radix to create a straight dorsum may raise the height past the point of esthetic balance. If this occurs, the nose tends to "blend" into the forehead without any distinct break point. This is unnatural and should be avoided. When this is anticipated, it is advised to discuss using NSR to "soften" the dorsal hump but not eliminate it entirely. If the patient's desire is a completely straight dorsum, referral for a surgical rhinoplasty consultation is warranted.

One technique initially described by Segreto and colleagues [17] utilizes the "pinch, push, and pull" method by the nondominant hand to reduce risk of intravascular injection. Using the index and thumb fingers of the nondominant hand, the dorsal skin is pinched medially then pushed laterally onto the nasal bone to

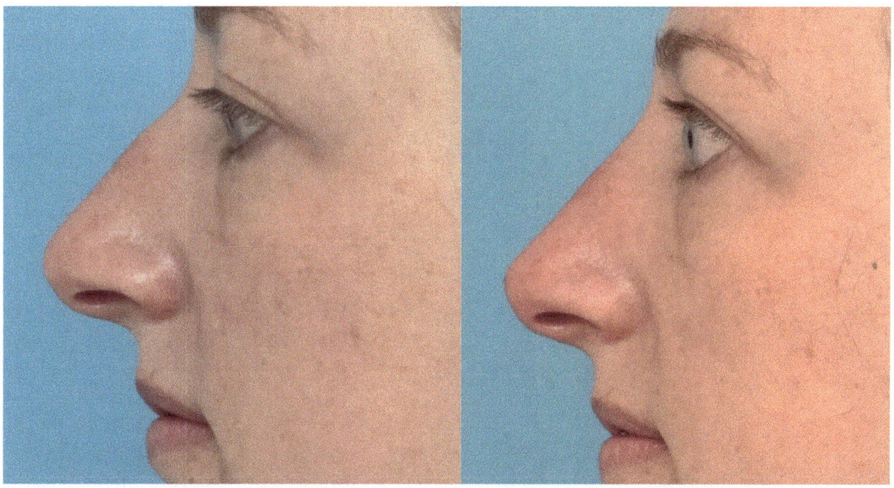

FIG. 5 Lateral view of before (*left*) and after (*right*) nonsurgical rhinoplasty for dorsal hump augmentation.

compress vessels. The needle is then inserted at the midline to the depth of the periosteum or perichondrium, and the skin slowly pulled up prior to slow injection of HA. The author prefers vertical injections deep onto the periosteum or perichondrium, utilizing small boluses of filler and blending with a finger to achieve a smooth outcome (Fig. 6). Sometimes, a straight object such as a cotton tip application can be useful to achieve a straight dorsum similar to a level. While Segreto and colleagues suggests not injecting below the hump to avoid blunting the supratip, the technique described by Moon [15] recommends augmenting superior and inferior to the bump for better camouflage. Injection below the bump is frequently useful, but it is important not to inject the supratip excessively. Raising the supratip above the tip creates a situation similar to a surgical pollybeak deformity, creating an excessively round tip and losing any tip definition that previously existed.

Midvault

Common esthetic and functional concerns in the midvault include deviation, depressions, concavity, and INV collapse. Achieving a straighter nose in the frontal view is a common reason for performing NSR. The structural cause of the twisted nose stems from the position and shape of the nasal septum. While NSR cannot change the position of the septum or improve breathing, it can improve symmetry and straightness. Another common indication for midvault injections includes fixing issues after a surgical rhinoplasty. Rhinoplasty can produce depressions, shadows, and asymmetries that may be too small to warrant a revision. In these cases, NSR is the perfect option. As mentioned before, mirroring known rhinoplasty cartilage grafts help the injector create a successful injection plan. Popular surgical rhinoplasty techniques in this region include dorsal onlay grafts, lateral nasal wall grafts, and camouflage grafts. The paired brow-tip esthetic lines, which represent a smooth and unbroken contour from medial eyebrow to nasal tip on either side, should be followed and outlines when injecting in this area to achieve a straighter and more symmetric midvault [18]. When considering injection strategies, both linear threading and bolus injections are viable techniques for camouflaging midvault twists. It is advisable to start by injecting and defining the brow-tip esthetic line with small linear threads. Once these lines are well established, smaller injections of filler can be used to fill in any contour irregularities. This helps ensure proper straightening occurs while avoiding unnecessary widening of the midvault. In addition to straightening the midvault, an underdeveloped dorsum can be augmented using column injections of small, 90° threads through the dorsum to the radix as described previously in this study [19].

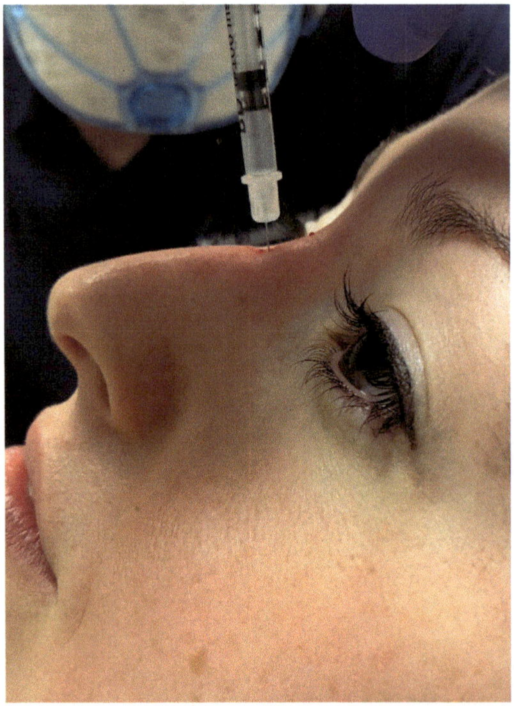

FIG. 6 Vertical injections deep onto bone or periosteum allow precise radix augmentation.

Tip

The tip is a complex structure composed of soft tissue attachments and a cartilaginous framework that influences appearance and function. Injection in this area can often be more challenging due to the 3 dimensional nature and having a clear understanding of a patient's desires can help achieve optimal outcomes. Two key nasal analysis concepts are projection and rotation. Projection is the distance the tip comes out from the face. Rotation is the angle at which the tip is positioned. Rotation of the nasal tip pushes it up and derotation pushes the tip down. The ability to visualize the ideal new tip projection and rotation *before* injecting is a difficult but necessary skill. To find the ideal rotation and projection, the senior author pulls the supratip skin cephalically (upward) to simulate more rotation. Using 2 fingers, the nasal tip can be manipulated in pinching motion to find the ideal projection in the profile view (Fig. 7). These are excellent methods of visualizing the final result and planning the NSR.

To improve tip rotation, filler can be injected into the intercolumellar space or nasal spine (Fig. 8). Injection

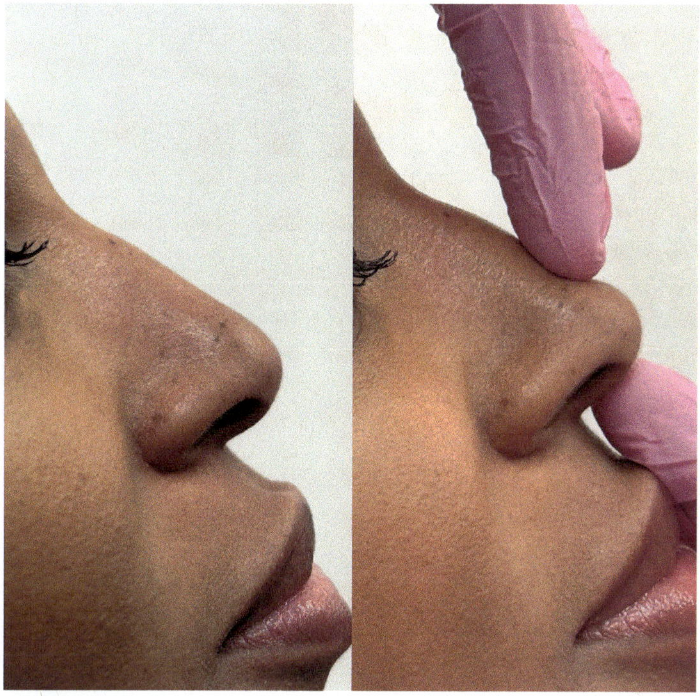

FIG. 7 Using two fingers, the nasal tip can be manipulated in pinching motion to find the ideal projection in the profile view.

into the intercolumellar space increases support to the nasal tip while correcting retracted columella. Similar to a columellar strut graft, injecting in between the medial crura footplates can lengthen the medial tripod, therefore overall increasing the nasolabial angle [7]. During this technique, it is important to hold the membranous septum to decrease filler migration into the nasal cavity and reduce risk of nasal obstruction (Fig. 9). It is important to inject an adequate bolus of filler into this space with volumes of 0.1 to 0.2 cc commonly required. In the appropriate patient, this strategy should be performed prior to injecting material on the tip. Another strategy for tip rotation is injection directly into the inferior border of the nasal spine, subsequently increasing nasolabial angle

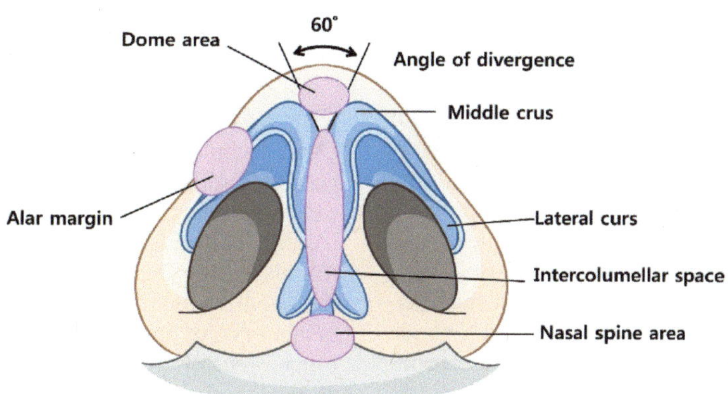

FIG. 8 Commonly injected sites in the tip including the nasal spine, intercolumellar space, interdomal area, and alar margin. (Used with permission from Moon HJ. Injection rhinoplasty using filler. Facial Plast Surg Clin North Am 2018;26(3):323–30. https://doi.org/10.1016/j.fsc.2018.03.006.)

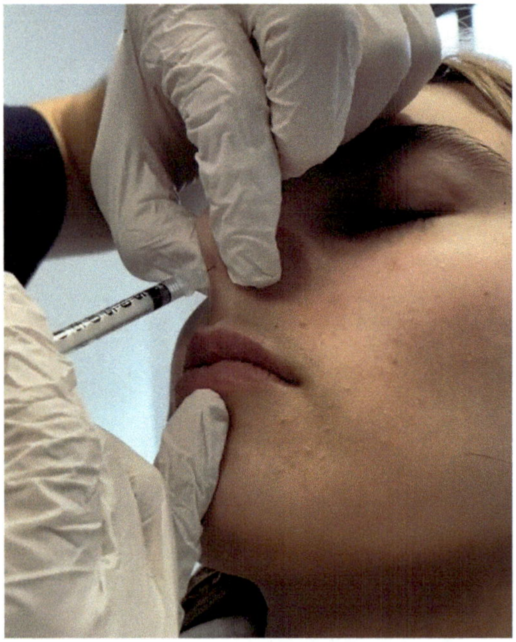

FIG. 9 Similar to a columellar strut graft, injecting in between the medial crura footplates can lengthen the medial tripod, therefore overall increasing the nasolabial angle.

and improving rotation [15]. Prior to starting, it is recommended for the nondominant to pinch the columellar base to maintain midline placement into the submuscular layer [17]. Beyond addressing tip rotation, this technique is also thought to reduce tip retraction while smiling due to its effect on the depressor septi muscle.

Enhancement of the tip and tip projection with fillers can mirror the effect of tip graft placement used in surgical rhinoplasty (Fig. 6). Both infratip and supratip approaches may be utilized to accurately place filler in tip-defining points, resulting in enhanced projection and definition like the effect of shield grafts, onlay tip grafts, or cap grafts (see Fig. 5). The senior author utilizes a 2 handed technique to manipulate the nasal tip into the desired position on profile view, which allows visualization of the ideal location for the new tip defining point (see Fig. 7). Small boluses of filler should be placed on each tip defining point and smoothed. Each additional bolus of filler should be placed only after rechecking the correct tip defining points are being highlighted (Fig. 10). Ideal nasal tip shape is not a single central tip defining point, 2 points exist in close relationship, thus a single central point of injection is to be avoided. One area of caution is injection into the interdomal region (space between the tip cartilages), which may lead to dome splaying and tip widening [7]. The tip should be injected prior to approaching the supratip due to difficulty in predicting amount of projection filler, which may ultimately cause a pollybeak deformity if too much filler is accidently inserted into the tip [15]. The "ideal" location of a new supratip break can be estimated by using the nondominant middle finger to lift the tip cranially while the thumb stabilizes the motion on the dorsum [17]. While the tip is still elevated in the new position, pinching of the domes during injection prevents lateral displacement of filler.

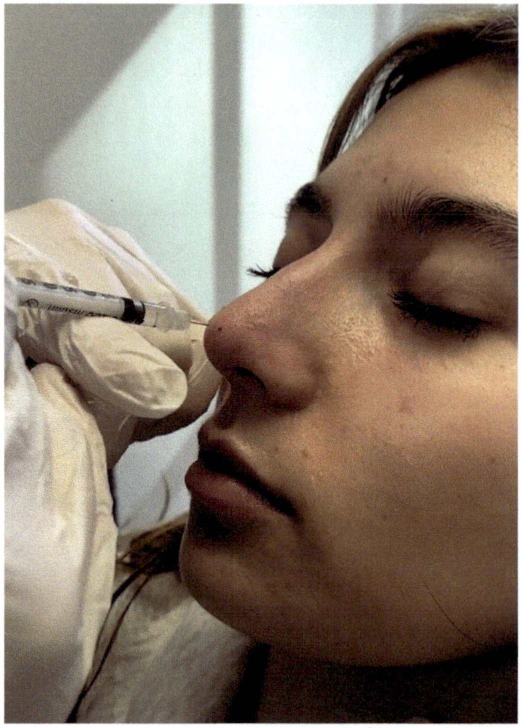

FIG. 10 Small boluses of filler should be placed deep onto perichondrium at each tip defining point and smoothed.

Other Applications

Other techniques include addressing the alar rims and potential improvement of nasal valve collapse. NSR can be used to lower retracted alar rims via vertical columnar threads injected in a retrograde manner into the alar rim with careful downward displacement of the needle. One should imagine the columns of filler being injected in the direction the alar rims need to move. This should be repeated in several locations along the ala and can have similar results to alar rim grafts, strut grafts, or composite grafts. Application of filler in can help with external valve patency, therefore increasing nasal patency. In patients with prior history of rhinoplasty, careful attention is required in this area due to possible compromised or altered blood flow. Other functional applications that have been reported include augmenting the INV, scroll, and nasal sidewall to the level of the perichondrium to improve INV collapse [20].

PROS AND CONS

NSR is a popular alternative to traditional rhinoplasty with several advantages including lower cost, convenience, rapid recovery, lack of general anesthetic, low relative risk profile, and temporary nature. There is also high patient satisfaction associated with the procedure. In a case series of 111 patients undergoing HA augmentation of the tip, columella, and radix/dorsum, 85% of patients were very satisfied at 12 months after treatment [21]. One systematic review including 1600 patients with both HA and CaHa reported nearly 95% patient satisfaction with the results [22]. As with any procedure, patient selection is critical. Indications for NSR can include low radix, mild dorsal hump, underdeveloped dorsum, mild upper and middle vault deformity, decreased tip projection/rotation, alar rim irregularities, alar base deficiency, and small irregularities after rhinoplasty [7].

Patients presenting with severe or extreme forms of deviation, dorsal humps, dynamic collapse, or tip irregularities may not be able to achieve their desired outcomes with NSR. By nature of injection, NSR can only augment and add volume, and patients who require reduction of structures are not good candidates for this procedure. An honest conversation about desired effect and realistic expectations should be held with patients who may benefit from surgical rhinoplasty instead. Patient characteristics should also be considered. Thicker and oilier skin can lead to an increase in postprocedure edema, reducing ability to approximate full effect of filler [15]. Other contraindications include hypersensitivity to filler, pregnancy, active breastfeeding, and bleeding disorders. Patients on anticoagulation, nonsteroidal anti-inflammatory drugs, herbal supplements, and history of nasal implants should be counseled prior to the procedure.

COMPLICATIONS

NSR performed by an experienced clinician is safe with low rates of complications. One systematic review including 8604 patients reported overall rate of all adverse outcomes was 2.52% [23]. Self-limited complications included swelling, erythema, hypersensitivity to filler ingredients, and nodule/lump formation. The most commonly reported complications were bruising in 1.58% and hematoma in 0.13% [23]. Infection rates were also low, with literature reporting rates of 0.04% to 0.07% [23,24]. While the majority of complications is temporary and minor, conservative management, symptom relief, and patient monitoring and reassurance are important to improve patient satisfaction and outcomes.

The most dreaded complication of filler injection is vascular occlusion. The nose is the highest risk area due to rich vascular supply and redundant vessels [25]. Injection in the nasal dorsum, glabella, and nasal sidewall can retrogradely reach the ophthalmic artery and central retinal artery, leading to sudden vision loss. In one of the first retrospective reviews on NSR in 2488 procedures, Rivkin [26] described an overall adverse rate of 7.6%, with 5 cases (0.20%) with ischemic or necrosis issues. Notably, patients with previous surgical rhinoplasty significantly increased the odds of adverse events, likely due to alterations in vasculature. A similar rate was reported in a systematic review with 30 patients developing vessel occlusion (0.35%), 7 with skin necrosis (0.08%), and 8 reports of vision loss (0.09%) [23].

An in-depth understanding of anatomy, use of small blunt cannulas or small needles, and correct depth of placement are critical to prevent vascular events [27]. However, it is important to remain vigilant and be prepared in the event of vascular occlusion. Necessary medications should be easily accessible and within reach during the procedure, as early intervention is necessary to prevent worsening morbidity. Signs of vascular compromise include skin blanching, bruising, slow capillary refill, and skin discoloration (Fig. 7A, B).

Should any of these signs appear, it is important to promptly recognize the event, stop injection, apply hyaluronidase and topical nitropaste under occlusion, provide warm compresses and massage, and give oral aspirin [28]. Hyaluronidase is an enzyme that degrades HA bonds, which can help fragment longer HA chains into smaller particles, therefore helping the pieces pass through the artery more readily [29]. Hyaluronidase should be injected immediately regardless of filler type in high doses (200–300 U) with daily injections until resolution [30]. Evidence for topical nitroglycerin, a vasodilator with systemic risks such as hypotension and dizziness, is inconclusive. While one animal model study using rabbit ears found that application of topical nitroglycerin created more congestion and worsened perfusion, nitroglycerin continues to be recommended by some consensus guidelines [30,31]. Skin necrosis may occur and can be addressed with daily topical wound care, prophylactic antibiotics, and surgical debridement or hyperbaric oxygen therapy as indicated [27,32]. Warm compresses and vigorous massage can encourage blood flow to the area, breaking up embolic material. As a prostaglandin inhibitor, aspirin can reduce platelet aggregation and clot formation. An immediate dose of 300 mg should be given, followed by 75 mg daily until resolution [33].

Accidental intra-arterial injection leading to vision loss requires prompt emergent medical attention. A consensus statement recommends the following protocol: stop treatment immediately, prompt transfer to specialist center with ophthalmology, reduce intraocular pressure with timolol drops, breathe into paper bag to increase CO_2 and dilation, and administer hyaluronidase, sublingual glycerol trinitrate, and aspirin immediately [34]. Ophthalmology workup and management should include full vision test with consideration of intravenous acetazolamide, topical drops, anterior chamber paracentesis, ocular massage, and retrobulbar/peribulbar hyaluronidase injection.

SUMMARY

NSR is a popular alternative to traditional rhinoplasty with the ability to provide similar results without the added risk of general anesthesia or surgery. High affordability, quick recovery times, convenience, and relatively low-risk profile are attractive to patients who desire improvement of mild esthetic defects. A nuanced understanding of nasal anatomy and vasculature is imperative to prevent vascular complications.

CLINICS CARE POINTS

- NSR utilizes filler injection to augment and improve esthetic concerns of the nose.
- HA is the most used material.
- Advantages include low cost, quick recovery times, and convenience without the added risk of general anesthesia.
- Injection techniques closely mirror graft placement in traditional rhinoplasty.
- Vascular compromise leading to blindness is a major complication and requires immediate attention.

DISCLOSURE

Nothing to disclose.

REFERENCES

[1] Naini F, Cobourne M, Garagiola U, et al. Nasofrontal angle and nasal dorsal aesthetics: a quantitative investigation of idealized and normative values. Facial Plastic Surgery FPS 2016;32(4). https://doi.org/10.1055/s-0036-1584234.

[2] Murthy VA, Reddy RR, Pragadeeswaran K. Internal nasal valve and its significance. Indian J Otolaryngol Head Neck Surg 2013;65(Suppl 2). https://doi.org/10.1007/s12070-013-0618-x.

[3] Dibelius G, Hohman MH. *Rhinoplasty tip-shaping surgery. StatPearls.* StatPearls PublishingCopyright © 2024. Treasure Island (FL): StatPearls Publishing LLC.; 2024.

[4] Alfertshofer M, Frank K, Ehrl D, et al. The layered anatomy of the nose: an ultrasound-based investigation. Aesthetic Surg J 2022;42(4). https://doi.org/10.1093/asj/sjab310.

[5] Sobiesk JL, Munakomi S. *Anatomy, Head and neck, nasal cavity. StatPearls.* StatPearls PublishingCopyright © 2024. Treasure Island (FL): StatPearls Publishing LLC.; 2024.

[6] Saban Y, Amodeo CA, Bouaziz D, et al. Nasal arterial vasculature: medical and surgical applications. Arch Facial Plast Surg 2012;14(6). https://doi.org/10.1001/archfacial.2012.202.

[7] Raggio BS, Asaria J. Filler rhinoplasty. *StatPearls.* StatPearls PublishingCopyright © 2024. Treasure Island (FL): StatPearls Publishing LLC.; 2024.

[8] Fundarò SP, Salti G, Malgapo DMH, et al. The rheology and physicochemical characteristics of hyaluronic acid fillers: their clinical implications. Int J Mol Sci 2022; 23(18). https://doi.org/10.3390/ijms231810518.

[9] Gutowski K. Hyaluronic acid fillers: science and clinical uses. Clin Plast Surg 2016;43(3). https://doi.org/10.1016/j.cps.2016.03.016.

[10] Gold M. Use of hyaluronic acid fillers for the treatment of the aging face. Clin Interv Aging 2007;2(3). https://doi.org/10.2147/cia.s1244.

[11] Go BC, Frost AS, Friedman O. Using injectable fillers for midface rejuvenation. Plast Aesthet Res 2021;8:39. https://doi.org/10.20517/2347-9264.2021.35.

[12] Go BC, Frost AS, Friedman O. Using injectable fillers for chin and jawline rejuvenation. World J Otorhinolaryngol Head Neck Surg 2023;9(2). https://doi.org/10.1002/wjo2.93.

[13] Walker K, Basehore BM, Goyal A, et al. Hyaluronic acid. StatPearls. *StatPea*rls PublishingCopyright © 2024. Treasure Island (FL): StatPearls Publishing LLC.; 2024.

[14] Goodman G, Magnusson M, Callan P, et al. A consensus on minimizing the risk of hyaluronic acid embolic visual loss and suggestions for immediate bedside management. Aesthetic Surg J 2020;40(9). https://doi.org/10.1093/asj/sjz312.

[15] Moon H. Injection rhinoplasty using filler. Facial Plast Surg Clin North Am 2018;26(3). https://doi.org/10.1016/j.fsc.2018.03.006.

[16] Becker DG, Pastorek NJ. The radix graft in cosmetic rhinoplasty. Arch Facial Plast Surg 2001;3(2). https://doi.org/10.1001/archfaci.3.2.115.

[17] Segreto F, Marangi GF, Cerbone V, et al. Nonsurgical rhinoplasty: a graft-based technique. Plast Reconstr Surg Glob Open 2019;7(6). https://doi.org/10.1097/GOX.0000000000002241.

[18] Krane NA, Markey JD, Moneta LB, et al. Aesthetics of the nasal dorsum: proportions, light, and shadow. Facial Plast Surg 2017;33(02). https://doi.org/10.1055/s-0037-1598626.

[19] Rivkin A. Non-surgical rhinoplasty using injectable fillers. 2024. Available at: https://www.rejuvenationresource.com/articles/clinical-application-by-anatomic-region/non-surgical-rhinoplasty-using-injectable-fillers. Accessed June 10, 2024.

[20] Mehta U, Fridirici Z. Advanced techniques in nonsurgical rhinoplasty. Facial Plast Surg Clin North Am 2019;27(3). https://doi.org/10.1016/j.fsc.2019.04.008.

[21] Giammarioli G, Liberti A. Non-surgical rhinoplasty technique: an innovative approach for nasal reshaping with hyaluronic acid fillers. J Cosmet Dermatol 2023;22(7). https://doi.org/10.1111/jocd.15669.

[22] Williams L, Kidwai S, Mehta K, et al. Nonsurgical rhinoplasty: a systematic review of technique, outcomes, and complications. Plast Reconstr Surg 2020;146(1). https://doi.org/10.1097/PRS.0000000000006892.

[23] DeVictor S, Ong A, Sherris D. Complications secondary to nonsurgical rhinoplasty: a systematic review and meta-analysis. Otolaryngology-Head Neck Surg (Tokyo) 2021; 165(5). https://doi.org/10.1177/0194599820987827.

[24] Harb A, Brewster C. The nonsurgical rhinoplasty: a retrospective review of 5000 treatments. Plast Reconstr Surg 2020; 145(3). https://doi.org/10.1097/PRS.0000000000006554.

[25] Beleznay K, Carruthers J, Humphrey S, et al. Update on avoiding and treating blindness from fillers: a recent review of the world literature. Aesthetic Surg J 2019; 39(6). https://doi.org/10.1093/asj/sjz053.

[26] Rivkin A. Nonsurgical rhinoplasty using injectable fillers: a safety review of 2488 procedures. Facial Plast Surg Aesthet Med 2021;23(1). https://doi.org/10.1089/fpsam.2020.0291.

[27] Bertossi D, Lanaro L, Dorelan S, et al. Nonsurgical rhinoplasty: nasal grid analysis and nasal injecting protocol. Plast Reconstr Surg 2019;143(2). https://doi.org/10.1097/PRS.0000000000005224.

[28] DeLorenzi C. Complications of injectable fillers, part 2: vascular complications. Aesthetic Surg J 2014;34(4). https://doi.org/10.1177/1090820X14525035.

[29] DeLorenzi C. Transarterial degradation of hyaluronic acid filler by hyaluronidase. Dermatol Surg 2014;40(8). https://doi.org/10.1097/DSS.0000000000000062.

[30] Urdiales-Gálvez F, Delgado NE, Figueiredo V, et al. Treatment of soft tissue filler complications: expert consensus recommendations. Aesthetic Plast Surg 2018;42(2): 498–510. https://doi.org/10.1007/s00266-017-1063-0.

[31] Hwang CJ, Morgan PV, Pimentel A, et al. Rethinking the role of nitroglycerin ointment in ischemic vascular filler complications: an animal model with ICG imaging. Ophthalmic Plast Reconstr Surg 2016;32(2). https://doi.org/10.1097/IOP.0000000000000446.

[32] Hong WT, Kim J, Kim SW. Minimizing tissue damage due to filler injection with systemic hyperbaric oxygen therapy. Arch Craniofac Surg 2019;20(4). https://doi.org/10.7181/acfs.2019.00059.

[33] King M, Walker L, Convery C, et al. Management of a vascular occlusion associated with cosmetic injections. J Clin Aesthet Dermatol 2020;13(1):E53–8.

[34] Walker L, Convery C, Davies E, et al. Consensus opinion for the management of soft tissue filler induced vision loss. J Clin Aesthet Dermatol 2021;14(12):E84–94.

Advances in Cosmetic Surgery 8 (2025) 153–167
ADVANCES IN COSMETIC SURGERY

Advances, Techniques, and Complications Associated with Adjacent Fat Transfer in Lower Blepharoplasty

James J. Law, MD, MSP[a,b], Aretha Zhu, MD[c], Cat N. Burkat, MD[b,*]
[a]Department of Ophthalmology, Lions Eye Institute, Albany Medical College, Albany, NY, USA; [b]Oculoplastics, Orbital, & Cosmetic Facial Surgery, Department of Ophthalmology and Visual Sciences, University of Wisconsin-Madison, 2870 University Avenue, Suite 108, Madison, WI 53705, USA; [c]Institute of Ophthalmology and Visual Science, Rutgers New Jersey Medical School, Newark, NJ, USA

KEYWORDS
• Blepharoplasty • Lower eyelid • Transconjunctival • Transcutaneous • Fat transfer • Fat transposition • Sub-orbicularis oculi fat • Midface rejuvenation

KEY POINTS
- Understand anatomic basics and volumetric changes of the aging midface.
- Provide key preoperative considerations for adjacent fat transfer techniques.
- Discuss the application of adjacent fat transfer techniques and their utility within the various surgical approaches to lower eyelid blepharoplasty along with adjunctive procedures which facilitate a tailored approach to individual anatomy.
- Outline complications relevant to lower blepharoplasty with adjacent fat transfer and offer pearls for avoidance.
- Introduce a reference list for further in-depth study.

INTRODUCTION

In contemporary aesthetic lower blepharoplasty, there has been a trend towards:

1. Volume preservation [1–5], aimed at achieving more durable aesthetic outcomes by anticipating atrophic changes associated with aging, and thus minimizing the risk of eventual hollowing that may be noted with purely subtractive approaches [6].
2. Viewing the lower eyelid and midfacial transition as a single aesthetic unit, recognizing that successful rejuvenation requires addressing areas beyond the lower eyelid in isolation [5,7,8].

These considerations have led to development of techniques directed at a transposition of excess orbital fat to fill, contour, and mask adjacent areas which are deficient in volume, such as the tear trough or palpebromalar groove to approximate a smooth, youthful transition to the midfacial region. A survey of ASOPRS surgeons found that 80% incorporate adjacent fat transfer in their approach to lower blepharoplasty [9]. This article seeks to introduce the facial cosmetic surgeon to techniques in adjacent fat transfer as well as key considerations concerning their application in surgical midfacial rejuvenation.

LOWER EYELID SURGICAL ANATOMY

In performing blepharoplasty involving adjacent fat transfer techniques on the lower eyelids, a firm understanding of the pertinent anatomy and changes that

*Corresponding author. *E-mail address:* cburkat@wisc.edu

https://doi.org/10.1016/j.yacs.2025.02.002
2542-4327/25/ Published by Elsevier Inc.

ABBREVIATIONS

ORL	orbitomalar ligament
SOOF	sub-orbicularis oculi fat

occur with the aging midface is essential for minimizing complications, while maximizing anatomic and aesthetic success [10].

With some individual variation, the lower eyelid margin has a gentle concave contour at the inferior corneal limbus, with its nadir just temporal to the midpupillary line (Fig. 1) [11]. The lower eyelid is divided into the anterior (skin and orbicularis oculi), middle (orbital septum), and posterior lamellae (eyelid retractors or capsulopalpebral fascia, tarsus, and palpebral conjunctiva).

Apart from a subciliary prominence or "pretarsal roll", which is formed by tonal contraction of the pretarsal orbicularis [12], the lower eyelid volume is chiefly constituted by 3 retro-septal fat pads. The inferior oblique divides the medial and central fat pads [13], while Clifford's ligament, an arcuate expansion of Lockwood's ligament extending from the retractors to the lateral infraorbital rim, divides the central and lateral fat pads [14]. In addition to being a check ligament for the inferior rectus and inferior oblique, the arcuate expansion maintains lateral support to the eyelid by preventing backwards displacement of Lockwood's ligament [15]. The lateral fat pad may be subdivided into an anterior and posterior component, with the anterior portion extending over into the recess of Eisler where the orbital septum inserts 2 mm outside the inferolateral orbital rim [16].

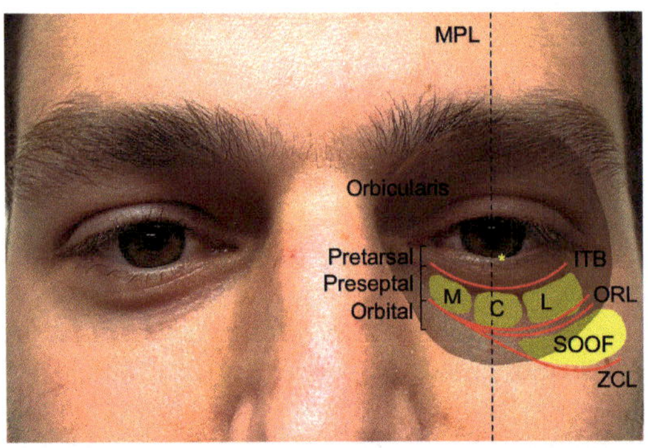

FIG. 1 Youthful lower eyelid in frontal view. Annotated on the left side by an asterisk is the nadir of marginal contour, occurring just lateral to the midpupillary line (MPL). Also illustrated are the inferior tarsal border (ITB), orbicularis retaining ligament (ORL, which laterally is constituted by upper and lower lamellae), and zygomatic cutaneous ligament (ZCL). Three retro-septal fat pads—medial (M), central (C), and lateral (L, with extension into the recess of Eisler)—are also shown along with the SOOF. The orbicularis can be divided into pretarsal, preseptal, and orbital portions according to the structures it overlies. (*Data from* Golan S, Levine B, Lelli GJ. Lower eyelid blepharoplasty. J Opthalmol Clin Res. 2019 Mar;3:1–4.)

The lower eyelid is suspended by the bilaminar orbicularis (or orbital) retaining ligament (ORL, also orbitomalar ligament), which is continuous with the lateral orbital thickening laterally and the orbital septum superiorly [17], and which indirectly secures the deep orbicularis and overlying skin to the orbital rim, providing major osteo-cutaneous support to the midface [8,18,19]. The ORL also constitutes the superior border of the sub-orbicularis oculi fat (SOOF), which is deep to the orbital orbicularis and confined inferiorly by the zygomatico-cutaneous ligament [20]. The lateral fibro-fatty SOOF is continuous with the inferior temporal compartment of the midface via the temporal tunnel, whereas its medial aspect extends 2 mm to 4 mm medial to the midpupillary line [14,21]. It provides a supportive buttress to the midface in addition to contributing to volume [22]. These fatty and ligamentous structures within the youthful midface are depicted in Fig. 1.

The undesirable appearance of "(under) eye bags", or lower eyelid steatoblepharon, is due to herniation and/or expansion of the orbital fat pads against an attenuated orbital septum and orbicularis (Fig. 3) [23,24]. Excessive steatoblepharon creates a step-off between palpebral and malar skin, expanding apparent eyelid height [23,25]. The development of dermatochalasis, hyperpigmentation, and rhytidosis also contributes to increased eyelid prominence [2,26]. These changes exacerbate the "tear trough deformity", which Flowers attributed to poor development of the infraorbital malar complex, descent of aging malar tissues, volume loss of facial tissues, and a muscular defect between the inferomedial orbital orbicularis and levator labii superioris (angular head) [27].

The orbital rim hollow is constituted medially by the tear trough hollow and laterally by the palpebromalar groove; it is bounded superiorly by the orbital fat pads and inferiorly by the SOOF and malar fat pads (Fig. 2) [28–30]. Other areas where there is close association of skin to underlying bony or ligamentous support similarly give rise to hollows that become more apparent as surrounding soft tissues age [31]. Other hollows have been described around the orbital rim (see Fig. 2).

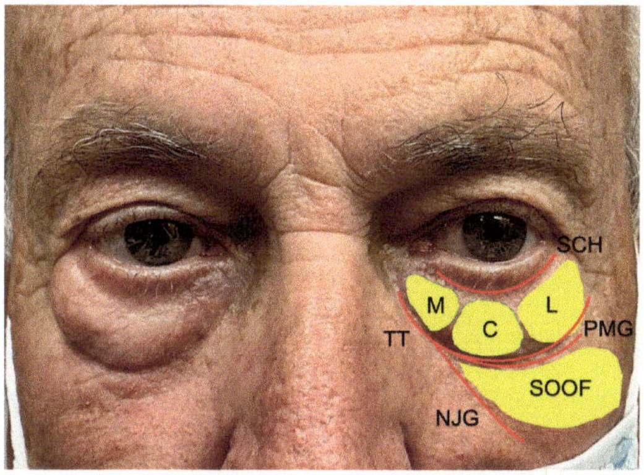

FIG. 2 Frontal view of a patient whose midface anatomy is demonstrative of significant steatoblepharon and hollows. As is annotated on the left side, volume expansion results in prominence of the medial (M), central (C), and lateral (L) fat pads. Similarly, SOOF volume also expands as it descends along with the midface. Hollows, such as that of the septal confluence (SCH), tear trough (TT), palpebromalar groove (PMG), and nasojugal groove (NJG) also become increasingly apparent around areas of ligamentous anchoring. (*Data from* [28–30])

1. Superiorly lies the septal confluence or eyelid crease hollow, formed by the convergence of the retractors, orbital septum, and tarsal plate [28,30].
2. Inferiorly, the "nasojugal fold/groove" is found at the inferior orbital orbicularis and extends from the tear trough laterally at an oblique angle [32,33].
3. The zygomatic hollow or "midcheek groove" overlies the medial zygomatico-cutaneous ligament and extends from the tear trough obliquely between the levator labii superioris and zygomatic muscles [28].

These hollows and their intervening convexities or "mounds" often constitute a "double convex deformity" of the lower eyelid, wherein prolapsed orbital fat forms the superior convexity, a hollowed inferior orbital rim the concavity, and the malar mound the inferior convexity [34].

A negative orbital vector occurs where inferior orbital rim is located more posteriorly than the cornea and is considered unaesthetic, giving the appearance of "bulging eyes" [35]. Conversely, a positive orbital vector is associated with "deeper-set eyes". Festoons—cascades of lax skin and orbital orbicularis sometimes also containing herniated fat and edema—may occur between orbicularis retaining and zygomatico-cutaneous ligaments [36]. Their extent is always inferior to the orbital rim, as opposed to prominence of the fat pads above (see Fig. 3).

PREOPERATIVE CONSIDERATIONS FOR ADJACENT FAT TRANSFER

Each patient should be carefully evaluated to determine the best surgical approach—detailed preoperative assessment must consider ophthalmic and systemic history, including past surgical interventions, and involve individualized discussion of the expected outcomes and limitations of surgery. Reference photos are helpful in this regard, and comprehensive photographic documentation in standardized reference frames (Fig. 4A, B) for both preoperative and postoperative states is critical (Fig. 4C,D) [37]. Various grading systems have been proposed for the tear trough deformity (Table 1) [26,38,39] and steatoblepharon (Table 2) [26,40]; these provide a helpful algorithmic basis for clinical assessment of patient eligibility for various lower blepharoplasty techniques.

The 2 main approaches for lower blepharoplasty are:

1. Transconjunctival approach—avoids the potential for visible scars due to dissection from the posterior eyelid/conjunctival fornix.
2. Transcutaneous approach—is performed through an external skin incision below the lash line. Whereas visibility may be better in this approach, iatrogenic orbicularis muscle injury can result in postoperative muscle atony, retraction, and ectropion [41]. Many studies have also demonstrated a higher risk of lower eyelid malposition due to manipulation of the orbital septum [42–44].

In a 2018 survey, the transconjunctival approach was more popular for lower blepharoplasty, utilized by 96% of respondents, versus 82% who employed the transcutaneous approach, 51% used both approaches [9]. Although the transconjunctival approach is often preferred over the transcutaneous approach, both can afford excellent results for lower blepharoplasty with adjacent fat transfer when performed properly; thus individualization for each patient may warrant different techniques [45].

Generally, young patients with minimal skin excess or textural changes would benefit from a transconjunctival approach, while older patients are more amenable to a transcutaneous approach to include excision of redundant skin [46]. A combination of anterior and posterior approaches can also be performed, and in some cases, skin resurfacing with ablative lasers can replace skin excision and augment outcomes [47].

Adjacent fat transfer techniques may be employed regardless of chosen approach to lower blepharoplasty, and are most applicable for patients in whom there is both steatoblepharon as well as hollowing at the tear trough and/or palpebromalar groove; in effect, volume

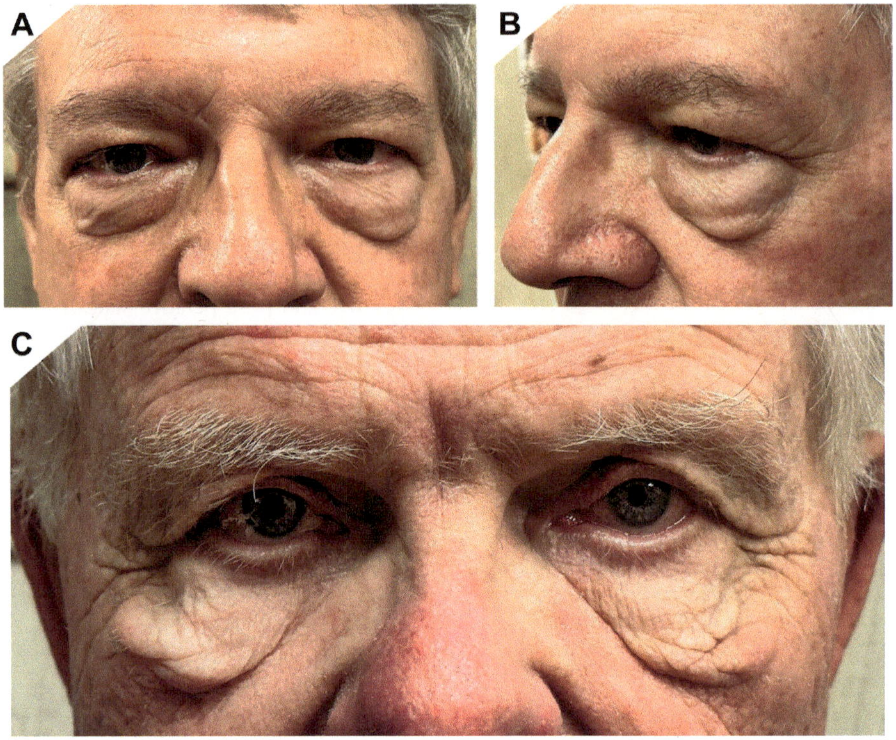

FIG. 3 Festoons. (*A*) Frontal and (*B*) oblique views of this patient depict a unilateral festoon of the left lower eyelid/midface in addition to the significant lower eyelid fat pads. Festoons always extend below the level of the inferior orbital rim, in contrast to steatoblepharon alone, as may be seen on the right side. (*C*) In the frontal view of another patient, prominent festoons and skin laxity are seen bilaterally, extending well below the inferior orbital rim.

may be borrowed from the former areas where it is in excess to fill in relative voids of the latter.

Subtractive lower blepharoplasty without fat transposition could be considered sparingly in young patients with isolated fat prominence and limited to no skin redundancy or midfacial ptosis [2,6]. In such patients, a transconjunctival incision avoids the potential for a visible scar; as the midface has not yet descended and exposed the inferior orbital rim, transposition of fat is less needed. However, for most patients, a purely subtractive approach can result in a hollowed or skeletonized appearance that may appear more aged, as it accentuates any shadows in the lower eyelids [48]. This is particularly noticeable in patients with thinner skin, naturally dark shadows, or prominent lower eyelid vessels in whom removing additional fat through subtractive surgery can exacerbate the issue. In contrast, adding volume to the lower eyelid and over the orbital rim can improve the hollowed and shadowed appearance of the tear trough [49].

The appearance of festoons can generally be improved through lower blepharoplasty with adjacent fat transfer, which is more forgiving than a purely subtractive approach in smoothing of the lid cheek junction. Ancillary procedures such as a midface lift or direct excision may be considered along with other noninvasive techniques including ablative laser resurfacing or chemical peels [50,51].

Cheek projection and vector of the orbital rim and malar eminence in relation to the anterior-most aspect of the cornea and lower eyelid margin should be noted, and the relative position of the ocular apex documented via exophthalmometry. A negative vector may require inferior orbital rim/malar augmentation, or additional vertical support to the lower eyelid with an implant in order to decrease risk of eyelid retraction following blepharoplasty [35]. Distribution of fat across the inferior orbital rim during lower blepharoplasty may help augment volume where it is deficient and thereby improve the apparent orbital vector.

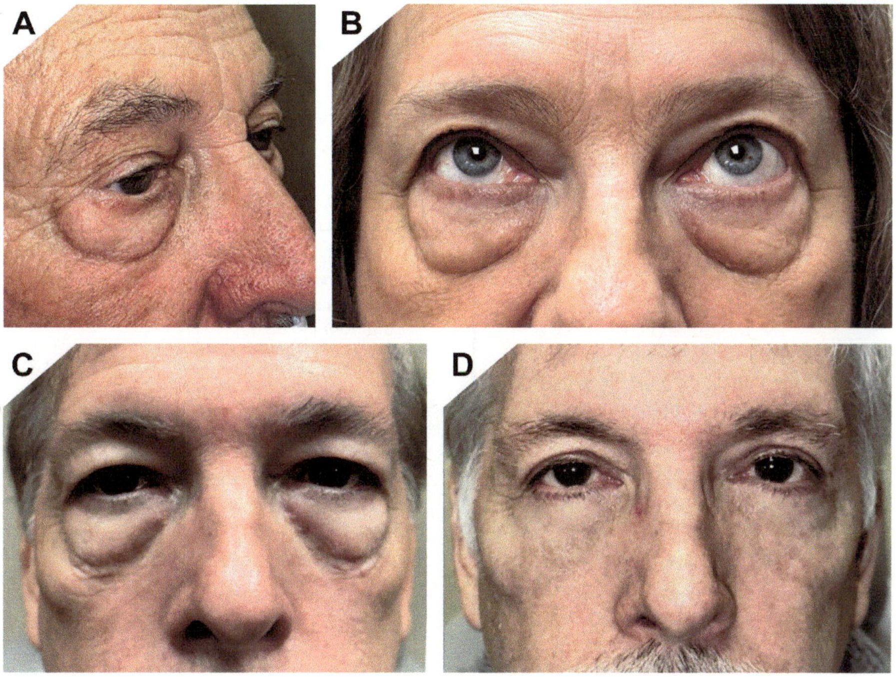

FIG. 4 Clinical photos demonstrating tear trough. (*A*) An oblique view of a patient with prominent tear trough and palpebromalar hollows better captures their three-dimensional appearance. (*B*) In frontal view, with this patient in upgaze, fat pads are more pronounced, and skin pinch testing may be performed. The patient in (*C*) has prominent steatoblepharon of the lower eyelids as well as dermatochalasis with hooding of the upper eyelids. He was determined to be a good candidate for bilateral upper blepharoplasty and lower blepharoplasty, with the latter being done via a transcutaneous approach with fat repositioning to mask the orbital rim hollow; the patient's postoperative appearance is shown in (*D*).

Eyelid margin malpositions such as ectropion or entropion should be considered when planning an approach to lower blepharoplasty as concurrent repair can enhance the aesthetic outcome and guard against complications such as lid retraction.

Relative contraindications for lower blepharoplasty with fat transposition include preexisting lower eyelid retraction and/or cicatricial change as well as excessive hollowing, suggesting insufficient orbital fat volume, in which case augmentation techniques rather than adjacent fat transfer should be considered. Absolute contraindications include inflammatory conditions of the orbit which involve the fatty tissues, such as active thyroid eye disease, which may complicate healing and increase risk of postoperative inflammation. Dry eye syndrome should be optimized prior to proceeding with surgery.

SURGICAL TECHNIQUES

Lower eyelid blepharoplasty is safely performed under local anesthesia with oral sedatives or under monitored anesthesia. General anesthesia may be considered if excessive traction on fat pads is uncomfortable, if the patient is highly anxious, or if minimizing the volume of local analgesics to limit anatomic distortion is desired [2].

Transconjunctival Approach

A mixture of 1% lidocaine and 0.25% bupivacaine with 1:100,000 epinephrine is injected into the inferior fornix, skin, and fat pads to ensure adequate anesthesia and hemostasis without excessive anatomic distortion. Conjunctiva is incised with Westcott scissors, monopolar cautery, or CO_2 laser in an arcuate fashion below the inferior tarsal border [52]. Since the initial description of this approach by Bourguet in 1924 and its later popularization by Tessier [53,54], various modifications have led to 2 contemporary modes by which the infraorbital fat pads may be accessed:

1. Preseptal (2 mm–4 mm inferior to the tarsus), which initiates the dissection plane anterior to the orbital septum, which is then opened over each fat pad (Fig. 5).

TABLE 1
Tear-trough deformity grading schemes

Grading/System	Description
Barton et al, [41] 2004	
Grade 0	Absence of medial/lateral lines demarcating arcus marginalis/orbital rim; smooth, youthful contour without a transition zone at orbit-cheek junction
Grade I	Mild, subtle presence of a medial line or shadow; smooth lateral transition of orbit-cheek junction
Grade II	Moderate prominence of a visible demarcation of orbit-cheek junction, extending medial to lateral
Grade III	Severe demarcation of orbit-cheek junction; obvious step between orbit and cheek
Hirmand [42] 2010	
Class I	Volume loss limited medially to tear trough; may have mild flattening extending to central cheek
Class II	Volume loss in lateral infraorbital area in addition to medial orbit; may have moderate volume deficiency in medial cheek, flattening of central upper cheek
Class III	Full depression circumferentially along orbital rim; associated with more advanced volume deficiency in medial and central cheek, malar eminence
Sadick et al, [35] 2007[a]	
Tear trough depth	Each mm of depth=one point
Hyperpigmentation	I: No hyperpigmentation II: Mild III: Moderate IV: Intense/deep
Prolapse of nasal fat pad/pockets	I: Mild II: Moderate III: Severe
Rhytidosis[b]	I: Mild II: Moderate III: Advanced IV: Severe

(continued on next page)

TABLE 1 (*continued*)

[a] Sadick et al.'s tear trough rating score is the additive total of each component.
[b] Rhytidosis graded according to Glogau scale.
Data from [26,38,39].

2. Postseptal (6 mm–7.5 mm inferior to the tarsus), which avoids violation of the septum by incising directly from the conjunctiva and retractors into the fat pads [55].

Exposure of the forniceal space and fat pads may be enhanced with the use of a retractor (eg, Desmarres, Senn, or malleable) or traction sutures placed in the conjunctival/retractor layer pulled upwards over the globe (see Fig. 5) [56]. Conjunctival pocket incisions should be avoided in favor of a longer continuous incision as they may limit visibility during fat repositioning.

Once accessed, gentle retropulsion of the globe prolapses the fat pads, which may be further exposed with forceps by light traction. During dissection, care must be taken to avoid disruption of the intervening inferior oblique muscle or arcuate expansion [13,15], though the latter is sometimes lysed to allow access to the posterior "Putterman" fat pad which can account for residual temporal fullness [57]. The exposed fat pads can then be transposed to shift their volume to conceal undesired hollows with or without partial reduction.

Fat reduction

Often, some fat excision is necessary in shaping pedicles prior to transposition in facilitating optimal contour, though a minority of surgeons prefer to preserve all fat in performing a transposition [9]. While the amount

TABLE 2
Steatoblepharon grading scheme

Steatoblepharon grading	Description
+2	Very prominent fat pads
+1	Mildly noticeable fat pads
0	Absence of all 3 fat pads
−1	Hollowing of periorbital fat

Data from [24,26,40].

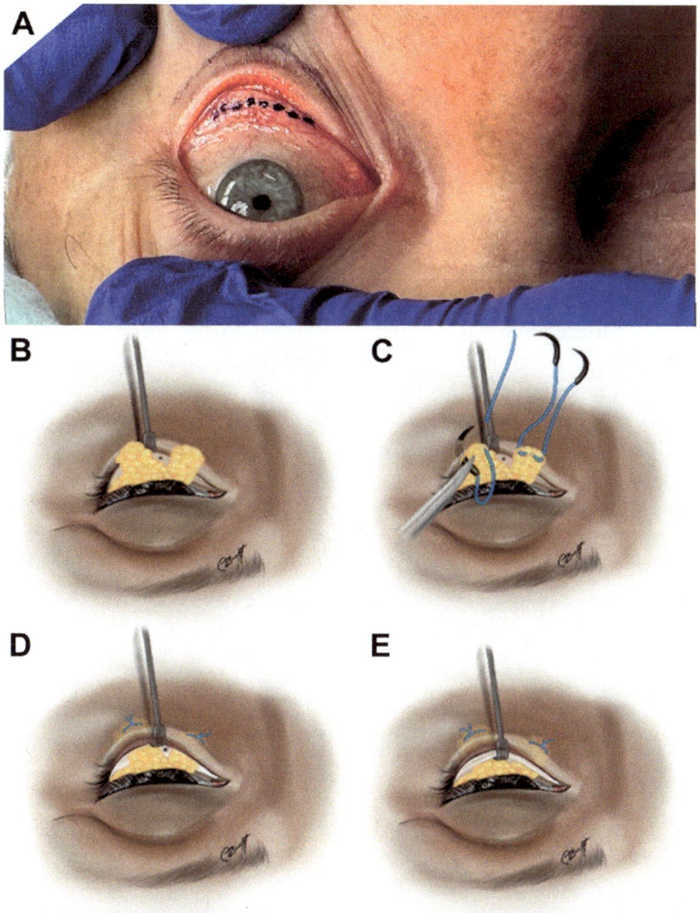

FIG. 5 Transconjunctival approach with fat repositioning. (*A*) Surgeon's view of incisional marking approximately 2 mm inferior to the inferior border of the tarsus. Fat pads are dissected, fashioned into (*B*) pedicles and (*C*) loosely imbricated with polypropylene sutures, then transposed across the inferior orbital rim. (*D*) Preperiosteal fat repositioning is demonstrated with externalization of sutures below the tear trough, versus (*E*) a subperiosteal fat repositioning; the periosteum observed as a thin white layer. (*Illustrations by Cat N. Burkat, MD FACS. Data from* [6,56,71,72].

of excess fat varies in each patient, we prefer to utilize all of the fat when possible to optimally drape the entire medial to lateral orbital rim. Meticulous hemostasis during fat pad manipulation and before closure is critical to avoid retrobulbar hemorrhage. Cross-clamping with a hemostat in conjunction with application of cautery may be beneficial. Intermittent external inspection of the lower eyelid helps prevent excessive fat removal which would exacerbate a tear-trough hollow.

Fat repositioning

Fat pedicles are draped across the inferior orbital rim, reducing its prominence and providing a more youthful contour by smoothing the hollowed transition point (see Fig. 5) [5]. The pedicles, either whole or sparingly reduced, are transposed over the inferior orbital rim into prezygomatic and premaxillary spaces created within one of a few midfacial dissection planes.

1. Supraorbicularis plane (less commonly used): where pedicles are tucked in between skin and orbicularis [58,59].
2. Suborbicularis plane: where fat is tucked into a pocket fashioned below the orbital orbicularis. While posing a higher risk of injury to vascular structures, it allows more direct access to release the ORL and arcus marginalis, providing access

into premaxillary and prezygomatic spaces, which is useful in correcting contour issues of the tear trough and lid-cheek junction [33,60–62].

3. Preperiosteal/intra-SOOF plane: where fat pedicles are thought to thrive from placement adjacent to, or within, the SOOF due to the vascularity of this space [63]. Though denervation of the orbicularis (whose terminal innervation rises through SOOF) and resulting ectropion can be a concern [64], this complication may be avoided by a limited dissection 8 mm to 12 mm below the inferior orbital rim and away from the "critical zone", a circular area of 0.5 cm radius, with its center located 2.5 cm inferolateral 30° to the lateral canthus [47].
4. Subperiosteal plane: accessed by incision of the arcus marginalis below inferior orbital rim, followed by elevation of periosteum via Freer or Cottle elevator to fashion a pocket extending approximately 15 mm inferiorly. While potentially providing better outcomes relating to contour and postoperative edema/ecchymosis as it is a relatively avascular plane, it risks disrupting the infraorbital nerve [29,41,65].

Studies have demonstrated similar aesthetic results with either supra or sub-periosteal fat transpositioning [65].

An ORL release may be performed in conjunction within any of the above dissection planes. Either a monolamellar or bilamellar lysis may be performed depending on the extent of the tear trough deformity as suggested by Rohrich and colleagues [66]. With one of a variety of instruments such as monopolar cautery, scalpel, or CO_2 laser, the ligamentous attachment of the ORL is first incised, and the ligamentous attachments released proceeding from medial to lateral with a Freer or Cottle elevator [67,68]. Dissection should be caried out within a "safe zone" described by Choi and Kim as bounded 9.4 mm from medial canthus line, 3 mm from the lateral canthal crease, and 6.0 mm from the eyelid margin to avoid damage to the palpebral branch trunks where they cross the orbital rim [69,70]. It is recommended that if electrocautery is used in dissection, the device tip should be directed deeper toward the bone (rather than parallel to the skin surface) to limit exposure of nervous tissue to injury from radiant heat [70].

It is critical to release all septal attachments from the base of the fat pedicle in order to avoid lower eyelid traction. The fat pedicle should be freely mobile with absolutely no lower eyelid pulling when the fat is transposed inferiorly. Pedicles can be transposed directly over the orbital rim or shifted medially or laterally as needed to volumize any areas of deficiency; placement within each individual eyelid may vary depending on the specific areas of volume deficiency, and according to how eyelid-midface contour might best be improved. The fat pads may also be variably debulked or excised prior to transposition as pedicles. Most surgeons also prefer debulking the lateral fat pad, while repositioning only the medial and central pads. Others may transpose all 3: for instance, one fat pedicle can be draped over the medial-most orbital rim, another placed inferiorly and medial to the infraorbital foramen, with the final fat pedicle directed laterally. By transposing multiple pedicles in different vectors, optimal effacement can be achieved.

Fat pedicles are secured to their desired location with sutures via external, internal, or combined methods of fixation (see Fig. 5) [6,71,72].

- In external fixation, sutures are typically placed temporarily; they are first introduced through the skin at a point below the ORL into a sub-orbicularis/subperiosteal pocket, then engaged apically through the fat pedicle and returned full thickness through skin to quilt it into place [6,71,73]. Alternatively, a double-armed suture allows both needles to travel from pedicle to skin, thus only passing away from the globe.
- With internal fixation techniques, transposed fat is either secured subcutaneously or to other structures within the dissection plane, such as periosteum [63,64].
- As there is some thought that transposed fat is prone to retract back into the orbit, combination internal/external fixation may be used to provide a dual means of secure fixation [72].

As exposure via the transconjunctival approach is often limited, especially with tight eyelids, a small needle is recommended. The use of permanent sutures, which are removed the following week, is favored by the authors due to their lower potential to cause an inflammatory reaction, or cyst, or granuloma formation.

Fat transposition may be performed even in patients without excess infraorbital fat, such as those who have had prior reduction, or in younger patients, so long as there is sufficient fat volume present [72]. The interposition of a fatty spacer over the orbital rim, whether it be a fat pedicle or free fat graft introduced from another site (such as concurrent upper blepharoplasty or face lift) is thought to permit sustained effacement of the tear trough deformity by preventing readherence of released ligaments [72,74]. The long-term durability of transposition techniques has yet to be conclusively determined in the literature [72].

At closure, some surgeons may prefer securing the retractor layer and/or conjunctiva with 1 to 2 fine sutures such as 6-0 (fast, plain, or chromic) gut or 7-0 polyglactin; buried placement minimizes postoperative discomfort. It is also acceptable for the incised conjunctival edges to simply be apposed to avoid overlapping without suture closure. While a sutureless method confers the benefit of providing an outlet of any fluid buildup, it also permits entry of foreign materials such as ointment or ophthalmic lubricant [75]. We typically place 1 to 2 sutures to close the inferior retractor layer only. Instructions for the application of topical ointments such as erythromycin, tobramycin, or neomycin-polymyxin-dexamethasone should be reviewed.

Transcutaneous Approach

Skin marking

Transcutaneous lower eyelid blepharoplasty is performed through a subciliary incision about 1 mm to 2 mm below the lash line extending 4 mm to 5 mm from the lateral canthus (Fig. 6) following administration of local anesthetic to the skin, orbicularis, and fat pads [76].

Skin-muscle flap

The conventionally used skin-muscle flap technique involves elevation of skin and preseptal orbicularis as a single flap, and should be used in patients with both muscle and skin laxity [77,78]. Release of the ORL and orbicularis is then performed [66,68,76,77], and the periosteum or SOOF divided to permit access to one of the previously outlined midfacial planes where fat pedicles may be placed.

Skin-only flap

A skin-only technique can be beneficial in certain patients who have excessive rhytidosis [1]. As this method does not violate the orbicularis, it minimizes risk of muscle denervation and postoperative edema [78]. The "pinch blepharoplasty" technique, which is even more conservative, avoids any undermining of skin and can reduce risk of lower lid malposition [79]. It is often combined with transconjunctival fat removal and/or laser resurfacing, avoiding septal violation. While specialized instruments for skin pinching (eg, Green fixation clamp) can be used, a curved hemostat will suffice.

Orbicularis muscle flap

Though resection of the orbicularis can be performed [80], current trends are toward muscle preservation [66], as retained muscle can be repositioned or redraped to improve midface smoothing in conjunction with fat transposition [81,82]. Other variations include creation of a preseptal orbicularis flap with suspension of muscle to lateral orbital rim to augment vertical eyelid support [83–85].

Accessing and repositioning orbital fat

It is important to stay superficial to the orbital septum during the above dissection and only incise it just above the orbital rim to access fat. This preserves the septal span and overlying preseptal orbicularis (especially in the skin-only flap approach), greatly minimizing the risk of lower eyelid retraction. Opening the septum below the tarsus or in the middle of the eyelid will increase the risk of retraction. Once the fat pads are exposed, they may be repositioned and secured previously described above. A septal reset technique, as described by Hamra, which involves fat repositioning over the infraorbital rim into a subperiosteal pocket, followed by reattachment of the septum to improve structural support [86]. A "septal window" may also be created to allow for additional manipulation and removal of the lateral fat pad after septal reset [87]. Skin closure either with suture (typically either 6–0 gut or 6–0 polypropylene) or tissue adhesive is performed after excision of excess skin and addressing canthal position [7,88–91].

Adjunctive Procedures

If there is a paucity of transposable fat, or in instances where the patient is asthenic with a paucity of orbital fat, adjunctive procedures may be necessary. These include:

- Liposculpture via (micro) autologous or minced fat grafting [74,92–94]
- Midface lifting [95]
- SOOF lifting [60,66]
- Tear trough implants [27]
- Soft tissue dermal filler injections (such as hyaluronic acid) [93,96–98]

The surgeon and patient should be able to determine whether these procedures are necessary prior to the surgery. In such cases, it especially behooves the surgeon to use a preservation approach rather than removing any fat.

POSTOPERATIVE CARE

Patients should be evaluated initially for development of hematoma or other postoperative bleeding; a brief visual and pupillary assessment is also recommended. Postoperative patching may be performed, although this may be forgone in preference of frequent and hygienic application of cold compresses to minimize

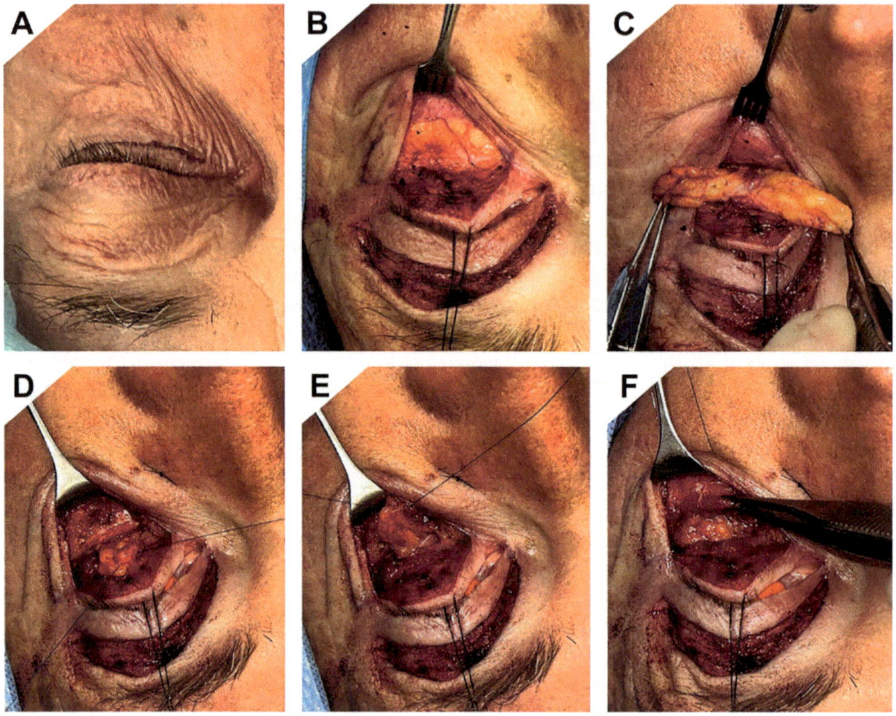

FIG. 6 Transcutaneous lower blepharoplasty. (*A*) Surgeon's view demonstrating incisional marking. Traction is achieved with a silk suture at the margin and a dissection performed in the preseptal plane to orbital rim. (*B*) Retro-septal fat pads are seen behind the septum, which is then carefully opened at the orbital rim/arcus marginalis to minimize retraction. (*C*) The inferior oblique muscle is seen between the medial and central fat pedicles. (*D*) Fat pads are imbricated with a double-armed polypropylene suture and (*E*) transposed across the inferior orbital rim in a preperiosteal plane, with care being taken to avoid the infraorbital nerve. (*F*) Sutures are externalized below the tear trough and will be removed 1 week postoperatively.

inconvenience and/or discomfort. Appropriate wound hygiene, topical ointments, and ocular surface lubrication (with artificial tears) should be administered along with analgesia as needed. Head elevation for 1 week may aid in resolution of ecchymosis and edema. Return precautions for pain, bleeding, or vision changes should be discussed. Suture removal is typically performed 5 to 7 days postoperatively.

COMPLICATIONS

Many of the complications which might occur in lower blepharoplasty employing fat transfer/repositioning techniques are similar to those described for subtractive lower blepharoplasty, including corneal abrasions, globe perforations, orbital hematoma, infections, scarring, diplopia, or eyelid malpositions and are described in elsewhere in the literature [99,100].

Chemosis occurs fairly commonly following lower blepharoplasty (2%–84.6%) due to a combination of lymphatic disruption as well as an inflammatory reaction to surgical trauma [66,67,101,102]. When the ORL is released to permit adjacent fat transfer, chemosis has been reported to occur more frequently (84.6% vs 59.3%), and with greater tendency to persist beyond 3 weeks, as opposed to when the ORL is left intact [67]. Postoperative chemosis is also more likely if a transconjunctival approach is used, if dissection is made using radiofrequency ablation (vs sharp dissection with cautery) [14]. Conservative remedies including lubrication, cool compresses, and head elevation are beneficial, while topical steroidal ointments can be included if chemosis is persistent. Oral steroids and eye patching may be considered in cases of particularly stubborn edema [103]. While incision and drainage of the chemosis with scissors in the office has been described, recurrence of chemosis is not uncommon.

Diplopia may be more common following lower blepharoplasty with adjacent fat transfer. Though this is typically due to postsurgical edema, strabismus from injury to the extraocular muscles during lower eyelid can also result from iatrogenic shifting or scarring of the muscle pulley (or muscle septa) and cause transient or even permanent diplopia [104–106]. Although the inferior oblique is most commonly affected, involvement of the inferior rectus has also been noted [106–110]. In 1 study, 23.2% of respondents (86/371) reported at least 1 patient with persistent diplopia following lower blepharoplasty [111]. Most patients (73%) had complete resolution of diplopia, although diplopia was persistent in primary gaze for 8% and in gazes other than primary in 19% of patients [111]. While prism glasses and extraocular muscle surgery may help address diplopia in primary gaze, successful treatment is challenging. Should strabismic diplopia be suspected postoperatively, prompt intervention should be undertaken via lysis of bolster sutures, while motility exercises and intermittent eyelid massage can also be considered.

Compromise of the blood supply to a transposed fat pad either by excessive cautery, overzealous debulking, or strangulation by overly tightened sutures can lead to fat necrosis and granuloma formation (Fig. 7). Though often persistent as later complications, fat granulomas may be seen earlier in the postoperative period and can be difficult to resolve, although oral or injected steroids may be considered. Conversely, transposed fat may migrate or retract back into the orbit if not sufficiently anchored at their premaxillary and/or premaxillary targets. Care should be taken to ensure that fat pedicles are properly fixated after being draped across the inferior orbital rim. Moreover, use of the septal reset technique limits unpredictable postoperative fat migration via securement of transposed pedicles to preperiosteal fat [41,86].

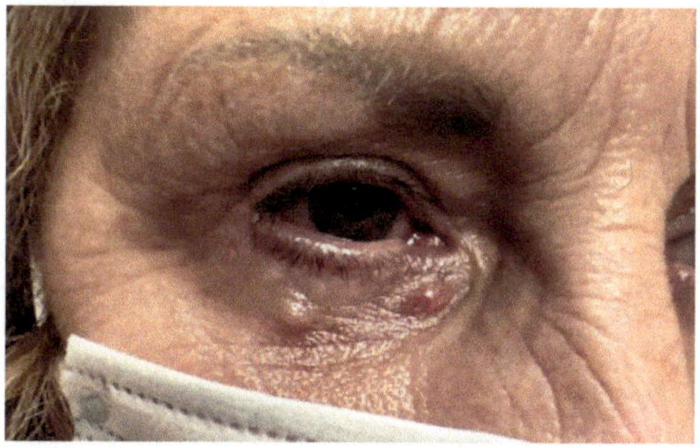

FIG. 7 Fat granuloma. Appearing as firm nodules in an oblique view of this patient, fat granulomas may occur as a result of fat inflammation and/or necrosis, which can manifest if pedicular blood supply is compromised.

Overly aggressive fat reduction may exacerbate hollowing, especially as volume loss continues with age; efforts should therefore be made to remove fat as sparingly as possible when fashioning fat pedicles. Conversely, residual steatoblepharon may be apparent with insufficient fat reduction, inaccurate pedicle transposition, or continued anterior bulging through an open septum. Pseudo-steatoblepharon may also occur due to dermal fillers or consequent edema, if these are used for volume augmentation [112]. Finally, hypertrophic scars or dermal pigmentation may persist in the late postoperative period, particularly in areas where bolster sutures were formerly secured.

Atrophy (seen as flattening, usually medially) of the subciliary or pretarsal orbicularis along with a degree of eyelid malposition (typically a subtle increase scleral show, though possibly leading to lagophthalmos and worsened ocular surface disease) may occur with iatrogenic injury to the lower palpebral trunks during ORL release and can account for postoperative asymmetry. Though this complication is best prevented by careful dissection taking place within the "safe zone" as previously described, various techniques, such as augmentation via hyaluronic acid filler, microautologous fat grafting, or surgical means may be employed to restore the eyelid contour [12,113].

Injury to the infraorbital nerve may occur especially with deeper dissection within the subperiosteal plane in up to 17.7% of patients [114]. Though the consequent numbness is typically transient with patients recovering sensation within 6 months following surgery, careful dissection should be undertaken with sparing use of electrocautery and gentle retraction (such as with a cold light retractor) to prevent such injuries in its vicinity. Should a supraperiosteal dissection plane be chosen, the levator labii superioris muscle, which directly overlies the infraorbital nerve, should be left intact to serve as a protective floor of the fashioned premaxillary space [62].

SUMMARY

Adjacent fat repositioning should be considered over a purely subtractive approach for lower blepharoplasty in patients with tear trough or palpebromalar hollows abutting significant steatoblepharon. These surgical nuances to utilize existing healthy fat pedicles to volumize the tear trough, with or without concurrent midface lifting, allows for optimal harmonious rejuvenation of the midfacial area.

CLINICS CARE POINTS

- An in-depth, individualized discussion of patient goals and expectations should be conducted prior to surgery, such that a shared understanding of attainable outcomes is reached by both patient and surgeon.
- In considering an approach to lower blepharoplasty, factors such as skin and/or muscle redundancy, ligamentous hollowing, fat volume status, orbital vector, horizontal eyelid tension, and eyelid margin position should be considered.
- Judicious management of fat volume is essential in the avoidance of under- or overcorrection of steatoblepharon, which can be difficult to rectify; care must also be taken to maintain an adequate blood supply with any fat manipulation.
- Fat pedicles may be variably debulked and transposed toward different vectors to achieve optimal effacement of hollows can be achieved.

PROPRIETARY INTEREST STATEMENT

The authors have no pertinent financial relationships to disclose.

DISCLOSURE

Financial support - This work was supported by an unrestricted grant from Research to Prevent Blindness, Inc, United States, to the University of Wisconsin-Madison Department of Ophthalmology and Visual Sciences.

REFERENCES

[1] Miotto GC, Shauly O, Menon A. Lower eyelid blepharoplasty with volume preservation using the skin flap. Aesthet Surg J Open Forum 2023;5:ojad074.

[2] Bhattacharjee K, Ghosh S, Ugradar S, et al. Lower eyelid blepharoplasty: an overview. Indian J Ophthalmol 2020; 68(10):2075–83.

[3] Davison SP, Iorio ML, Oh C. Transconjunctival lower lid blepharoplasty with and without fat repositioning. Clin Plast Surg 2015;42(1):51–6.

[4] Hamra ST. The role of orbital fat preservation in facial aesthetic surgery. A new concept. Clin Plast Surg 1996; 23:17–28.

[5] Hamra ST. Arcus marginalis release and orbital fat preservation in midface rejuvenation. Plast Reconstr Surg 1995;96(2):354–62.

[6] Hidalgo DA. An integrated approach to lower blepharoplasty. Plast Reconstr Surg 2011;127:386–95.

[7] Murri M, Hamill EB, Hauck MJ, et al. An update on lower lid blepharoplasty. Semin Plast Surg 2017; 31(1):46–50.

[8] Lucarelli MJ, Khwarg SI, Lemke BN, et al. The anatomy of midfacial ptosis. Ophthalmic Plast Reconstr Surg 2000;16(1):7–22.

[9] Kossler AL, Peng GL, Yoo DB, et al. Current trends in upper and lower eyelid blepharoplasty among American society of ophthalmic plastic and reconstructive surgery members. Ophthalmic Plast Reconstr Surg 2018;34(1): 37–42.

[10] Mojallal A, Cotofana S. Anatomy of lower eyelid and eyelid-cheek junction. Ann Chir Plast Esthet 2017; 62(5):365–74.

[11] Golan S, Levine B, Lelli GJ. Lower eyelid blepharoplasty. J Opthalmol Clin Res 2019;3:1–4.

[12] Wang D, Huang X, Zhou Y, et al. Cosmetic augmentation of lower-lid pretarsal roll with injection of autologous fat for Asians. J Plast Reconstr Aesthet Surg 2023; 87:46–53.

[13] Mowlavi A, Neumeister MW, Wilhelmi BJ. Lower blepharoplasty using bony anatomical landmarks to identify and avoid injury to the inferior oblique muscle. Plast Reconstr Surg 2002;110(5):1318–22 [discussion: 1323-4].

[14] Hwang K. Surgical anatomy of the lower eyelid relating to lower blepharoplasty. Anat Cell Biol 2010;43(1): 15–24.

[15] Dutton JJ. Atlas of clinical and surgical anatomy. Philadelphia, PA, United States: WB Saunders; 1994. p. 95–6.

[16] Bartley GB, Gerber TC. Eisler and his pocket. Am J Ophthalmol 2006;141(2):417–8.

[17] Muzaffar AR, Mendelson BC, Adams WP Jr. Surgical anatomy of the ligamentous attachments of the lower lid and lateral canthus. Plast Reconstr Surg 2002; 110(3):873–84 [discussion: 897-911].

[18] Kikkawa DO, Lemke BN, Dortzbach RK. Relations of the superficial musculoaponeurotic system to the orbit and characterization of the orbitomalar ligament. Ophthalmic Plast Reconstr Surg 1996;12(2):77–88.

[19] Pessa JE, Garza JR. The malar septum: the anatomic basis of malar mounds and malar edema. Aesthet Surg J 1997;17(1):11–7.

[20] Cotofana S, Schenck TL, Trevidic P, et al. Midface: clinical anatomy and regional approaches with injectable fillers. Plast Reconstr Surg 2015;136(5 Suppl):219S–34S.

[21] O'Brien JX, Ashton MW, Rozen WM, et al. New perspectives on the surgical anatomy and nomenclature of the temporal region: literature review and dissection study. Plast Reconstr Surg 2013;131(3):510–22.

[22] Andretto Amodeo C, Casasco A, Icaro Cornaglia A, et al. The suborbicularis oculi fat (SOOF) and the fascial planes: has everything already been explained? JAMA Facial Plast Surg 2014;16(1):36–41.

[23] Coban I, Derin O, Sirinturk S, et al. Anatomical basis for the lower eyelid rejuvenation. Aesthetic Plast Surg 2023;47(3):1059–66.

[24] Shah M, Lee G, Lefebvre DR, et al. A cross-sectional survey of the association between bilateral topical prostaglandin analogue use and ocular adnexal features. PLoS One 2013;8(5):e61638.

[25] Lim WK, Rajendran K, Choo CT. Microscopic anatomy of the lower eyelid in asians. Ophthalmic Plast Reconstr Surg 2004;20(3):207–11.

[26] Sadick NS, Bosniak SL, Cantisano-Zilkha M, et al. Definition of the tear trough and the tear trough rating scale. J Cosmet Dermatol 2007;6(4):218–22.

[27] Flowers RS. Tear trough implants for correction of tear trough deformity. Clin Plast Surg 1993;20:403–15.

[28] Goldberg RA. The three periorbital hollows: a paradigm for periorbital rejuvenation. Plast Reconstr Surg 2005; 116(6):1796–804.

[29] Stutman RL, Codner MA. Tear trough deformity: review of anatomy and treatment options. Aesthet Surg J 2012; 32(4):426–40.

[30] Naik MN. Hills and valleys: understanding the under-eye. J Cutan Aesthet Surg 2016;9(2):61–4.

[31] Naik MN, Honavar SG, Das S, et al. Blepharoplasty: an overview. J Cutan Aesthet Surg 2009;2(1):6–11.

[32] Duke Elder S, Wybar KC. The eyelids. In: Duke Elder S, editor. System of Ophthalmology: anatomy of the visual system. St Louis, MO, United States: C V Mosby CO; 1961.

[33] Loeb R. Nasojugal groove leveling with fat tissue. Clin Plast Surg 1993;20:393–400.

[34] Goldberg RA, Edelstein C, Balch K, et al. Fat repositioning in lower eyelid blepharoplasty. Semin Ophthalmol 1998;13(3):103–6.

[35] Mommaerts MY. Definitive treatment of the negative vector orbit. J Craniomaxillofac Surg 2018;46(7): 1065–8.

[36] Kpodzo DS, Nahai F, McCord CD. Malar mounds and festoons: review of current management. Aesthet Surg J 2014;34(2):235–48.

[37] Ong CT, Yap JF, Wai YZ, et al. A review of oculoplastic Photography: a Guide for clinician Photographers. Cureus 2016;8(8):e733.

[38] Barton FE Jr, Ha R, Awada M. Fat extrusion and septal reset in patients with the tear trough triad: a critical appraisal. Plast Reconstr Surg 2004;113(7):2115–21 [discussion: 2122-3].

[39] Hirmand H. Anatomy and nonsurgical correction of the tear trough deformity. Plast Reconstr Surg 2010;125(2): 699–708.

[40] Jo SJ, Kim HS, Park JT, et al. Assessment of age- and sex-related changes in baggy lower eyelids using a novel objective image analysis method: orbital gray scale analysis. J Cosmet Dermatol 2018;17(5):874–80.

[41] Hwang K, Lee DK, Lee EJ, et al. Innervation of the lower eyelid in relation to blepharoplasty and midface lift: clinical observation and cadaveric study. Ann Plast Surg 2001;47(1):1–5 [discussion: 5-7].

[42] Williams KJ, Allen RC. Eyelid malposition after blepharoplasty: an ounce of prevention. Semin Plast Surg 2021; 35(2):72–7.

[43] Schwarcz R, Fezza JP, Jacono A, et al. Stop blaming the septum. Ophthalmic Plast Reconstr Surg 2016;32(1): 49–52.

[44] Yaremchuk MJ. Restoring palpebral fissure shape after previous lower blepharoplasty. Plast Reconstr Surg 2003;111(1):441–50 [discussion: 451-452].

[45] Collar RM, Lyford-Pike S, Byrne P. Algorithmic approach to lower lid blepharoplasty. Facial Plast Surg 2013;29(1):32–9.

[46] Griffin RY, Sarici A, Ozkan S. Treatment of the lower eyelid with the CO2 laser: transconjunctival or transcutaneous approach? Orbit 2007;26(1):23–8.

[47] Guo L, Bi H, Xue C. Comprehensive considerations in blepharoplasty in an Asian population: a 10-year experience. Aesthetic Plast Surg 2010;34:466–74.

[48] Putterman AM. Eyelid circles: fat excision versus repositioning. Ophthalmic Plast Reconstr Surg 2023;39(6): 647–8.

[49] Etman AG, Badawy MS, Setta HS, et al. Evaluation of fat excision versus sparing in lower blepharoplasty using orbital gray scale analysis. Plast Reconstr Surg Glob Open 2022;10(9):e4530.

[50] Newberry CI, Mccrary H, Thomas JR, et al. Updated management of malar edema, mounds, and festoons: a systematic review. Aesthet Surg J 2020;40(3):246–58.

[51] Chon BH, Hwang CJ, Perry JD. Treatment options for lower eyelid festoons. Facial Plast Surg Clin North Am 2021;29(2):301–9.

[52] Rokhsar CK, Ciocon DH, Detweiler S, et al. The short pulse carbon dioxide laser versus the Colorado needle tip with electrocautery for upper and lower eyelid blepharoplasty. Lasers Surg Med 2008;40(2):159–64.

[53] Bourguet J. Les hernies graisseuses de l'orbite: Notre traitement chirurgical. Bull Acad Med (Paris) 1924;92: 1270–1.

[54] Tessier P. The conjunctival approach to the orbital floor and maxilla in congenital malformation and trauma. J Maxillofac Surg 1973;1(1):3–8.

[55] Undavia S, Briceño CA, Massry GG. Quantified incision placement for postseptal approach transconjunctival blepharoplasty. Ophthal Plast Reconstr Surg 2016;32(3): 191–4.

[56] Massry GG, Nassif PS. Transconjunctival lower lid blepharoplasty with and without fat repositioning. In: Hartstein ME, Holds JB, Massry GG, editors. Pearls and pitfalls in cosmetic oculoplastic surgery. New York, NY United States: Springer; 2008.

[57] Putterman AM. The mysterious second temporal fat pad. Ophthalmic Plast Reconstr Surg 1985;1(2):83–6.

[58] Majidian M, Kolli H, Moy RL. Transconjunctival lower eyelid blepharoplasty with fat transposition above the orbicularis muscle for improvement of the tear trough deformity. J Cosmet Dermatol 2021;20(9):2911–6.

[59] Reed DS, Nakra T. Re: "Transconjunctival lower eyelid blepharoplasty with fat transposition above the orbicularis muscle for improvement of the tear trough deformity". J Cosmet Dermatol 2022;21(8):3611–2.

[60] Freeman MS. Transconjunctival sub-orbicularis oculi fat (SOOF) pad lift blepharoplasty: a new technique for the effacement of nasojugal deformity. Arch Facial Plast Surg 2000;2(1):16–21.

[61] Wong CH, Mendelson B. Facial soft-tissue spaces and retaining ligaments of the midcheek: defining the premaxillary space. Plast Reconstr Surg 2013;132(1): 49–56.

[62] Gu J, Duan R, Wei B, et al. Internal fixation of redistributed orbital fat in transconjunctival lower eyelid blepharoplasty. Plast Reconstr Surg 2024;153(4):722e–5e.

[63] Mohadjer Y, Holds JB. Cosmetic lower eyelid blepharoplasty with fat repositioning via intra-SOOF dissection: surgical technique and initial outcomes. Ophthalmic Plast Reconstr Surg 2006;22(6):409–13.

[64] Ramirez OM, Santamarina R. Spatial orientation of motor innervation to the lower orbicularis oculi muscle. Aesth Plast Surg 2000;20:107–13.

[65] Yoo DB, Peng GL, Massry GG. Transconjunctival lower blepharoplasty with fat repositioning: a retrospective comparison of transposing fat to the subperiosteal vs supraperiosteal planes. JAMA Facial Plast Surg 2013;15:176–81.

[66] Rohrich RJ, Ghavami A, Mojallal A. The five-step lower blepharoplasty: blending the eyelid-cheek junction. Plast Reconstr Surg 2011;128(3):775–83.

[67] Chan NJ, Nazemzadeh M, Hartstein ME, et al. Orbicularis retaining ligament release in lower blepharoplasty: assessing efficacy and complications. Ophthalmic Plast Reconstr Surg 2018;34(2):155–61.

[68] Schiller JD. Lysis of the orbicularis retaining ligament and orbicularis oculi insertion: a powerful modality for lower eyelid and cheek rejuvenation. Plast Reconstr Surg 2012;129:692e700e.

[69] Choi Y, Kang HG, Nam YS, et al. Facial nerve supply to the orbicularis oculi around the lower eyelid: anatomy and its clinical implications. Plast Reconstr Surg 2017; 140(2):261–71.

[70] Choi Y, Kim IB. Avoiding pretarsal denervation in lower blepharoplasty incisions: refined pretarsal motor nerve anatomy. Plast Reconstr Surg 2024;154(1):81–93.

[71] Goldberg RA. Transconjunctival orbital fat repositioning: transposition of orbital fat pedicles into the subperiosteal pocket. Plast Reconstr Surg 2000;105:743–8 [discussion: 749-51].

[72] Chen J, Wu Y, Wang Y, et al. Transconjunctival fat repositioning blepharoplasty: is excess fat herniation a prerequisite? Plast Reconstr Surg 2024;153(5):1039–46 [discussion: 1047-8].

[73] Wong CH, Mendelson B. Extended transconjunctival lower eyelid blepharoplasty with release of the Tear Trough ligament and fat redistribution. Plast Reconstr Surg 2017;140(2):273–82.

[74] Cheng CY, Lin TM, Chang SL, et al. Transcutaneous lower eyelid blepharoplasty with micro-autologous fat transplantation harvested from orbital fat pads for lower eyelid aging treatment. J Plast Reconstr Aesthet Surg 2024;93:111–3.

[75] Belinsky I, Patel P, Charles NC, et al. Ointment granulomas following sutureless transconjunctival blepharoplasty: diagnosis and management. Ophthalmic Plast Reconstr Surg 2015;31(4):282–6.

[76] Drolet BC, Sullivan PK. Evidence-based medicine: blepharoplasty. Plast Reconstr Surg 2014;133(5):1195–205.

[77] Hashem AM, Couto RA, Waltzman JT, et al. Evidence-Based medicine: a graded approach to lower lid blepharoplasty. Plast Reconstr Surg 2017;139(1):139e–50e.

[78] de Castro CC. A critical analysis of the current surgical concepts for lower blepharoplasty. Plast Reconstr Surg 2004;114(3):785–93 [discussion: 794-6].

[79] Kim EM, Bucky LP. Power of the pinch: pinch lower lid blepharoplasty. Ann Plast Surg 2008;60(5):532–7.

[80] Bernardi C, Dura S, Amata PL. Treatment of orbicularis oculi muscle hypertrophy in lower lid blepharoplasty. Aesthetic Plast Surg 1998;22(5):349–51.

[81] Hamra ST. Repositioning the orbicularis oculi muscle in the composite rhytidectomy. Plast Reconstr Surg 1992; 90(1):14–22.

[82] McCord CD Jr, Codner MA, Hester TR. Redraping the inferior orbicularis arc. Plast Reconstr Surg 1998;102(7): 2471–9.

[83] Lee H, Shin H, Baek S. Effects of orbicularis oculi flap suspension on transcutaneous lower blepharoplasty. J Craniofac Surg 2024;35(1):46–8.

[84] Carriquiry CE, Seoane OJ, Londinsky M. Orbicularis transposition flap for muscle suspension in lower blepharoplasty. Ann Plast Surg 2006;57(2):138–41.

[85] Little JW, Hartstein ME. Simplified muscle-suspension lower blepharoplasty by orbicularis hitch. Aesthet Surg J 2016;36(6):641–7.

[86] Hamra ST. The role of the septal reset in creating a youthful eyelid-cheek complex in facial rejuvenation. Plast Reconstr Surg 2004;113(7):2124–41 [discussion: 2142-4].

[87] Tran BNN, Luthringer M, Reed L, et al. Addition of "septal window" to lower blepharoplasty for the management of fat of the lower eyelids. Ann Plast Surg 2022;88(3 Suppl 3):S214–8.

[88] Mommaerts MY, Beirne JC, Jacobs WI, et al. Use of fibrin glue in lower blepharoplasties. J Craniomaxillofac Surg 1996;24(2):78–82.

[89] McCord CD, Boswell CB, Hester TR. Lateral canthal anchoring. Plast Reconstr Surg 2003;112(1):222–37 [discussion: 238-9].

[90] Reggie SN, Ho TC, Buchanan AG, et al. Simple incisionless temporary stabilization: an adjunct to lower blepharoplasty. Aesthet Surg J Open Forum 2024;6:ojae014.

[91] Jelks GW, Glat PM, Jelks EB, et al. The inferior retinacular lateral canthoplasty: a new technique. Plast Reconstr Surg 1997;100:1262–70 [discussion: 1271].

[92] Tonnard PL, Verpaele AM, Zeltzer AA. Augmentation blepharoplasty: a review of 500 consecutive patients. Aesthet Surg J 2013;33(3):341–52.

[93] Glasgold M, Lam SM, Glasgold R. Volumetric rejuvenation of the periorbital region. Facial Plast Surg 2010; 26(3):252–9.

[94] Marten T, Elyassnia D. Facial fat grafting: why, where, how, and how much. Aesthetic Plast Surg 2018;42(5): 1278–97.

[95] Cheng AM, Chuang AY, Wei YH, et al. Supraperiosteal fat repositioning with midface lift in lower eyelid blepharoplasty: an 18-year experience. Graefes Arch Clin Exp Ophthalmol 2024;262(7):2291–8.

[96] Donath A, Glasgold R, Meier J, et al. Quantitative evaluation of volume augmentation in the tear trough with a hyaluronic acid-based filler: a 3-dimensional analysis. Plast Reconstr Surg 2010;125:1515–22.

[97] Jiang J, Wang X, Chen R, et al. Tear trough deformity: different types of anatomy and treatment options. Postepy Dermatol Alergol 2016;33(4):303–8.

[98] Hamed-Azzam S, Burkat C, Mukari A, et al. Filler migration to the orbit. Aesthet Surg J 2021;41(6):NP559–66.

[99] Lelli GJ Jr, Lisman RD. Blepharoplasty complications. Plast Reconstr Surg 2010;125(3):1007–17.

[100] Patipa M. The evaluation and management of lower eyelid retraction following cosmetic surgery. Plast Reconstr Surg 2000;106(2):438–53 [discussion: 454-9].

[101] Di Maria A, Barone G, Gaeta A, et al. Persistent conjunctival chemosis after lower lid blepharoplasty: a comparison of different surgical techniques. J Clin Med 2024; 13(7):2093.

[102] Shao C, Fu Y, Lu L, et al. Dynamic changes of tear fluid after cosmetic transcutaneous lower blepharoplasty measured by optical coherence tomography. Am J Ophthalmol 2014;158(1):55–63.e1.

[103] Levine MR, Davies R, Ross J. Chemosis following blepharoplasty: an unusual complication. Ophthalmic Surg 1994;25:593–6.

[104] Lee HJ, Rhiu S, Oh DE, et al. Transient inferior oblique muscle palsy following transconjunctival lower lid blepharoplasty. Kosin Medical Journal 2018;33(2):208–14.

[105] Shin SY, Demer JL. Location and gaze-dependent shift of inferior oblique muscle position: anatomic contributors to vertical strabismus following lower lid blepharoplasty? Investig Ophthalmol Vis Sci 2015;56(4):2408–15.

[106] Ghabrial R, Lisman RD, Kane MA, et al. Diplopia following transconjunctival blepharoplasty. Plast Reconstr Surg 1998;102(4):1219–25.

[107] Alfonso E, Levada AJ, Flynn JT. Inferior rectus paresis after secondary blepharoplasty. Br J Ophthalmol 1984; 68(8):535–7.

[108] Harley RD, Nelson LB, Flanagan JC, et al. Ocular motility disturbances following cosmetic blepharoplasty. Arch Ophthalmol 1986;104(4):542–4.

[109] Goldberg RA, Yuen VH. Restricted ocular movements following lower eyelid fat repositioning. Plast Reconstr Surg 2002;110(1):302–5 [discussion 306-8].

[110] Syniuta LA, Goldberg RA, Thacker NM, et al. Acquired strabismus following cosmetic blepharoplasty. Plast Reconstr Surg 2003;111(6):2053–9.

[111] Becker BB. Diplopia following lower blepharoplasty. J AAPOS 2020;24(6):363.e1–4.

[112] Soares DJ, Zuliani GF. Orbital post-septal hyaluronic acid: an iatrogenic etiology compounding lower eyelid steatoblepharon. JPRAS Open 2022;34:173–7.

[113] Jeon YR, Rah DK, Lew DH, et al. Pretarsal augmented lower blepharoplasty. Plast Reconstr Surg 2016;138(1): 74–82.

[114] Zhang H, Liu C, Peng C, et al. Blending of the eyelid-cheek junction and removal of protruding fat: an intraoral approach to blepharoplasty of the lower eyelid. Br J Oral Maxillofac Surg 2009;47:541–4.

Advances in Cosmetic Surgery 8 (2025) 169–176
ADVANCES IN COSMETIC SURGERY

Aging Rhinoplasty

Grace C. Keane Tahmaseb, MD[a], Alexandra M. Keane, MD[a], Samuel J. Lin, MD, MBA[b], Trina G. Ebersole, MD[c,*]

[a]Division of Plastic and Reconstructive Surgery, Department of Surgery, Washington University, 660 South Euclid Avenue Campus Box 8238, St Louis, MO 63110, USA; [b]Division of Plastic Surgery, Beth Israel Deaconess Medical Center, Harvard Medical School, 330 Brookline Avenue, SCG 03, Boston, MA 02215, USA; [c]Division of Plastic and Reconstructive Surgery, Department of Surgery, Washington University, 1020 North Mason Road, Suite 110, Saint Louis, MO 63141, USA

KEYWORDS

• Aging rhinoplasty • Elderly • Tip ptosis • Tip rotation • Tip projection • Dorsal hump

KEY POINTS

- Rhinoplasty in the aging population requires deep understanding of the attenuation of the underlying anatomic framework with time.
- Careful patient selection is of utmost importance, which can be parsed out in the initial patient interview.
- Primary surgical maneuvers address tip ptosis, the main aesthetic concern in this patient population.
- Nasal airway obstruction is common, which may be addressed by some combination of septoplasty, inferior turbinate reduction, internal and external nasal valve stabilization, and tip support.

INTRODUCTION: NATURE OF THE PROBLEM

The aging nose presents a particularly difficult challenge to the rhinoplasty surgeon. In 2023, there were over 40,000 rhinoplasties performed in the United States according to the Aesthetic Society Procedural Statistics [1]. Of those, 14.9% and 4.2% were performed on patients in the 51 to 64 and 65+ age range, respectively, an increase in both overall volume and proportion from 2019. The nasal infrastructure undergoes well-described anatomic changes as the face ages, and these must be addressed with particular surgical techniques.

The structural framework of the nose is composed of paired nasal bones, upper lateral cartilages, and lower lateral cartilages. The lower lateral cartilages form the nasal tip, which can be divided into the medial, middle, and lateral crural cartilages. The integrity of the nasal tip relies on the ligamentous attachments of the scroll area, connecting the caudal border of the upper lateral cartilages to the cephalic border of the lower lateral cartilages.

The main aesthetic concerns specific to this population include tip ptosis and gradual nasal lengthening due to changes in skin quality, weakening of the cartilaginous structures, and remodeling of the underlying bony framework [2–6]. In the younger patient, the face can be divided into thirds by drawing horizontal lines at the menton, nasal base, and brow. The aging face undergoes subcutaneous fatty resorption, orbicularis oculi atrophy, midface volume loss, and maxillary alveolar hypoplasia resulting in shortening of the lower third and relative lengthening of the upper and middle third of the face [6]. These aesthetic changes can be corrected with tip rotation and projection [2–6]. Elderly patients may also present with functional concerns, including nasal airway obstruction due to either longstanding internal valve collapse, or newly developed external valve collapse secondary to lateral nasal wall

*Corresponding author. *E-mail address:* trinaebersole@wustl.edu

https://doi.org/10.1016/j.yacs.2024.12.003

collapse [2]. Nasal tip ptosis may simply cause nasal airway obstruction over time that patients will note on their own. These patients may require extra intervention to stabilize the lower lateral cartilages to improve their functional and aesthetic concerns or nasal tip rotation.

Skin and Subcutaneous Tissue

With time, the epidermis and dermis thin, dermal collagen levels decrease, and elastin and fibrillin become more disorganized [2]. Lifelong sun exposure further compounds the effects of aging, resulting in decreased skin elasticity and rhytid formation [2,7]. Aging of the skin of the nose, specifically, exhibits increased density of sebaceous glands, most notably in males [2,7]. At its most extreme, this can lead to rhinophyma. However, even a slight increase in sebaceous glands can result in the appearance of increased thickness of the nasal alae and tip. This increases the weight of the nasal tip and contributes to tip ptosis. The combination of decreased skin elasticity, midface volume loss, and increased density of sebaceous glands require more pronounced change to the nasal framework to change the nasal appearance.

Cartilage Changes

Many elderly patients complain of tip deprojection and underrotation largely as a result of structural changes to the cartilaginous nasal tip complex and the effects of aging/gravity. Tip rotation is defined as the movement of the nasal tip in reference to the upper lip. The ideal angle varies with societal norms and gender, but is typically within 95 to 115° for women and 90 to 95° for men [3]. Tip projection is defined as the horizontal distance from the alar crease to the nasal tip on lateral view. Several metrics have sought to define the ideal tip projection: the Goode ratio defines the ideal ratio of tip projection to nasal length as 0.55:1; Simon's method states tip projection should be equivalent to the length of the upper lip; and Lanser's ratio describes the nose as a right triangle with the proportion of projection: height: length equivalent to 3:4:5 [8].

There is weakening of the intracrural ligament resulting in loss of medial crura tip support and derotation over time, a major contributor to tip ptosis [2,3,6,9]. Age-related maxillary alveolar hypoplasia leads to spreading of the medial crural foot plates and columellar shortening, further destabilizing the nasal tip [2,6]. Additionally, attenuation of the ligamentous attachments of the scroll area, connecting the upper and lower lateral cartilages, contributes to the changes associated with the aging nose [2]. This results in downward migration of the lower lateral cartilages, contributing to loss of tip support and external nasal valve collapse.

Nasal Dorsum

One must assess whether a dorsal hump is a long-standing nasal characteristic or newly developed aesthetic concern [2,3]. As a result of age-related tip ptosis and nasal lengthening, the illusion of a prominent dorsal hump may present due to the appearance of nasal convexity. In many cases, this is resolved by addressing tip ptosis. Therefore, one should start with surgical maneuvers to rotate and project the nasal tip before pursuing dorsal hump reduction. This can be assessed preoperatively by holding the tip in desirable location and visualizing whether dorsal hump persists [3].

Airway Concerns

In addition to nasal aesthetics, many elderly patients have a combination of functional complaints as well. Patients may present with long-standing nasal airway obstruction due to internal or external nasal valve collapse, septal abnormalities, or inferior turbinate hypertrophy. Additionally, aging itself affects nasal airway mechanics. Tip ptosis alters airflow within the nasal vault and produces obstructive symptoms by shunting air flow superiorly [2,4,6]. Internal nasal valve collapse may worsen secondary to age-related separation of upper and lower lateral cartilages [2–6]. External nasal valve collapse may result due to a combination of tip ptosis and lateral nasal wall collapse [2,4,6]. Many of the age-specific airway concerns can be addressed with tip rotation and projection, which will be discussed in a later section.

Skeletal Remodeling

The facial skeleton undergoes well-defined differential craniofacial growth throughout adulthood. The horizontal position between the sella nasion line to the pyriform on lateral view has shown to increase with age, indicating midface retrusion [10]. This leads to alar base recession and tip support attenuation. The pyriform also remodels cephalad, causing the alar base to be pulled superiorly and nasal tip to rotate inferiorly. The effect is an elderly appearing nose with an alar base that lies above the columella and nasal tip. Age-related maxillary alveolar hypoplasia results in spreading of the medial crural footplates and columellar shortening, further attenuating tip support mechanisms [6]. Lastly, the nasal bones become increasingly fragile with age.

Therefore, osteotomies should be done with extreme care, or avoided altogether [2].

SURGICAL TECHNIQUE

Preoperative Planning

Patients should be evaluated preoperatively with a complete medical history and focused physical examination. In the patient interview, one should tease out motivation for pursuing rhinoplasty. The ideal patient is realistic and secure, understands the limitations of rhinoplasty in the aging person, and lists specific concerns about their nasal appearance. In our practice, we ask patients to verbalize their concerns about their nose, in order of importance. If they are unable to verbalize specific complaints, surgical intervention should be avoided. Patients may present with aesthetic or functional chief complaints. If the patient has long-standing aesthetic concerns, expectations should be tempered, as these issues are more difficult to address due to age-related changes to the nasal framework. Recent changes in financial status are common in this cohort, such as career change or promotion, retirement, or inheritance. These patients tend to be good candidates for surgery, demonstrating high postoperative satisfaction rates [2]. Patients in this age group may pursue surgery because of a recent life stressor, such as divorce or death of a loved one. This should be recognized, and aesthetic surgery delayed until any grief or stress has completely resolved.

Medical comorbidities are more common in the elderly population and should be carefully assessed to determine if a patient is a surgical candidate. Hypertension should be properly medically managed to prevent risk of postoperative bleeding. Ideally, diabetic patients should be well controlled to decrease wound healing complications and infection risk. Patients with a history of cardiovascular disease or stroke need to obtain surgical clearance from their cardiologist and primary care physician. A complete list of medications should be assessed. Any anticoagulants should be stopped before surgery after receiving medical clearance. Patients unable to stop anticoagulation therapy in the perioperative period should not be considered a surgical candidate. Lastly, specific nasal history should be obtained, including any previous nasal trauma, allergies or sinus pathology, or nasal surgeries.

The physical examination should include a complete head and neck examination, as head and neck malignancies are more common in the elderly population. A complete external aesthetic nasal analysis is then performed to define nasal deformities, paying close attention to the patient's specific aesthetic complaints. An internal examination is performed to evaluate the integrity of the internal nasal valve, inferior turbinate hypertrophy, or septal deviation. Standard photographs should be taken and reviewed with the patient, permitting a genuine discussion of any surgical limitations to their concerns. If jointly realistic results are defined and agreed upon between patient and surgeon, an operative plan can be devised.

Preparation and Patient Positioning

The patient is positioned supine on the operating table. Following endotracheal intubation, the table is turned either 90 or 180° with the endotracheal tube extended off the foot of the bed. The skin is prepped with povidone-iodine solution before draping. Surgical techniques are detailed in Table 1.

Procedural Approach

Incision and soft tissue dissection

An open or closed rhinoplasty is performed in standard fashion. For an open rhinoplasty, bilateral marginal incisions along the caudal edges of the lower lateral cartilages are completed and connected medially at the narrowest part of the columella using an inverted-V or stairstep incision. The soft tissue envelope is carefully elevated to maintain ligamentous attachments between the upper and lower lateral cartilages.

Septoplasty and cartilage harvest

Septoplasty and cartilage harvest can be achieved through an open approach or through a modified Killian or hemitransfixion incision if closed rhinoplasty is performed. The septal cartilage can become calcified over time, rendering it unusable for grafting purposes [6]. Alternate sources of autologous graft may be required and should be discussed with the patient preoperatively, including auricular and rib cartilage. Excessive septal cartilage harvest is avoided in the elderly to avoid perforation of the thinned mucoperichondrial flaps and destabilization of the dorsum and tip [6].

Addressing tip ptosis and support

Nasal tip deprojection and derotation is the hallmark of the aging nose. Tip projection and rotation can be explained by envisioning the nasal tip complex as a tripod, with the paired lateral crura as the superior tripod legs and the medial crural foot plate as the inferior tripod leg. Surgical maneuvers to alter one leg of this construct serve to affect tip projection and rotation.

TABLE 1
Aging Rhinoplasty Surgical Techniques

Surgical Maneuver	Technique	Result
Medial crura-septal fixation suture	• Permanent suture adjusting the medial crura superiorly on the septum	• Tip rotation upwards
Septal extension graft	• Graft to the caudal or dorsal septum extended between lower lateral cartilages	• Augmented tip support • Increased tip projection and rotation
Columellar strut graft	• Sturdy segment of cartilage graft (5 mm x 20 mm) • Sutured in pocket between medial crural foot plates down to anterior nasal spine	• Augmented tip support • Increased tip projection and rotation
Premaxillary graft	• Diced or crushed cartilage graft in pocket at base of columella • Reserved primarily for edentulous patients	• Augmented tip support • Increased tip projection and rotation
Lateral crural steal	• Interdomal mattress suture to advance lateral crura onto the medial crura	• Increased tip projection and rotation
Lateral crural overlay	• Divide lateral crura at midsection • Overlap distal and proximal ends	• Increased tip rotation • Decreased or maintained tip projection
Alar cephalic trim	• Conservative cephalic alar trim • Maintain at least 6–8 mm rim strip	• Increased tip rotation • Address wide lateral crura
Onlay Tip raft	• Oval or trapezoidal onlay tip graft (4 mm x 9 mm) • Position in a pocket dissected over domes	• Increased tip projection • Augmented tip support
Dorsal Hump Reduction	• Limited dorsal hump reduction • Dorsal hump <3 mm—simple rasping • Dorsal hump >3 mm—submucous tunnel to separate the upper lateral cartilages from septum before rasping	• Decrease nasal height
Nasal bone osteotomies	• Should be done with extreme caution or avoided altogether	
Lateral Crural Strut Grafts	• Segment of cartilage graft (3 mm x 15 mm) • Placed on deep surface of lateral crura	• Stabilizes external nasal valve • Improves alar rim retraction

Columellar strut grafting. The structural integrity of the medial crural foot plate is commonly compromised in the aged nose. This is due to both the loss of the intracrural ligament support and age-related maxillary alveolar hypoplasia. This can be addressed with either a columellar strut graft sutured between the medial crural foot plates or with a medial crura-septal fixation suture (detailed below) [3]. With columellar strut grafting, a sturdy segment of cartilage graft measuring 20 mm x 5 mm is typically adequate. The graft is secured in a pocket dissected between the medial crural segments down to the anterior nasal spine. In patients with loss of bony support due to maxillary alveolar hypoplasia, an additional premaxillary graft can be placed in the surgical pocket at the base of the columella. One can better determine the contribution of the lateral crura to tip ptosis once these maneuvers are performed.

Medial crura-septal fixation suture. This technique fixates the medial crura superiorly on the septum to improve tip rotation and adjust the tip position cephalad. When this is performed, a columellar strut graft is not required. We believe this fixation technique, done with a permanent suture, gives a more reliable tip position postoperatively compared to other grafting techniques used to address tip rotation.

Lateral crura manipulation. Following columellar strut grafting or medial crura-septal fixation suture, surgical manipulation of the lateral crura is chosen based on whether the tip requires more or less projection and rotation. To increase projection and rotation, lateral crural steal is used. This involves placing an interdomal mattress suture to advance the lateral crura onto the medial crura [3]. By contrast, if maintained or decreased tip projection is desired, a lateral crural overlay is employed. With this, the lateral crura are divided at their midsection and the distal and proximal ends are secured in overlapped position [3].

Alar cephalic trim. For wide lateral crura and to increase tip rotation, cephalic trim may be performed. Care should be taken to preserve 6-8 mm of lateral crura to maintain tip support [2,3].

Tip graft. Following the previous surgical maneuvers, a tip graft can be used to support the nasal tip complex. The graft is curated from septal cartilage and sutured to the caudal border of the medial crura. This can reshape nasal contour and provide slight increase in nasal projection and rotation [4].

Addressing the nasal dorsum

Once tip ptosis is addressed with the above surgical manipulations, any remaining prominent nasal dorsum is addressed. If necessary, component nasal hump reduction maintaining the periosteal attachments to the nasal sidewalls can be performed. Care should be taken not to over-resect the nasal dorsum to prevent open roof deformity. Simple rasping can be performed for small nasal hump reductions with care to resect both the bony and cartilaginous hump. The skin quality of the nasal dorsum thins throughout adulthood producing contour abnormalities, which can be addressed with onlay grafts or allografts [2]. Osteotomies should be undertaken with an abundance of caution, or avoided all together, due to nasal bone fragility with age [6].

Addressing the airway

Many patients present with obstructive symptoms owing to a multitude of factors. Any altered nasal airflow from tip ptosis is addressed with tip rotation and projection. If internal nasal valve collapse is noted, spreader grafts fabricated from autologous cartilage are placed in typical fashion. Inferior turbinate hypertrophy is addressed with outfracture. In the case of true external valve collapse, lateral crural strut grafts or alar batten grafts can be employed to stabilize the external valve on inspiration.

Immediate Postprocedural Care

At the end of the surgical case, internal nasal stents are secured to the nasal septum. An external dressing can be applied as well for extra protection. These remain in place until postoperative day 5 to 7, at which point the patient returns to clinic for their first postoperative

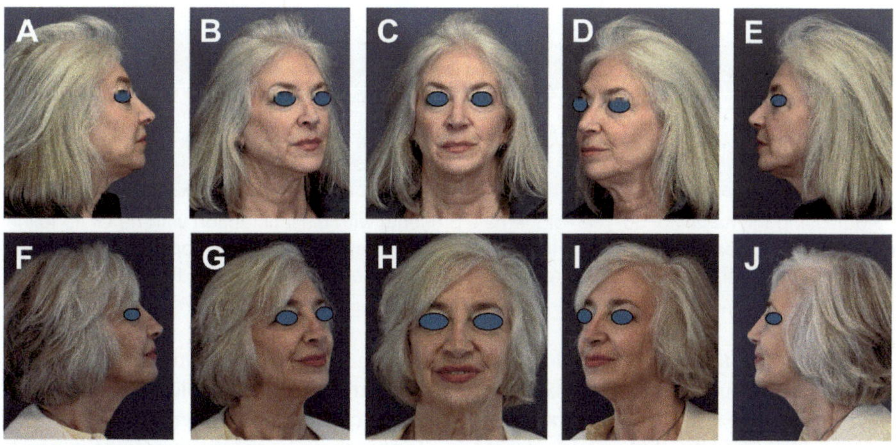

FIG. 1 **(A–J)** Addressing the nasal tip and dorsum. An elderly female, who previously underwent open rhinoplasty, underwent revision open rhinoplasty to address both functional and cosmetic concerns. For function, revision septoplasty, turbinate reduction, spreader grafting, and septal perforation repair were performed. For aesthetics, the following maneuvers were performed: removal of prior columellar strut graft, medial caudal resection, centralization of the nasal tip from right to left, right cephalic trim, right alar rim graft, medial crura-septal fixation suture, and dorsal only graft. Postoperatively, she noted improvement in functional concerns and improved nasal tip and dorsal aesthetics.

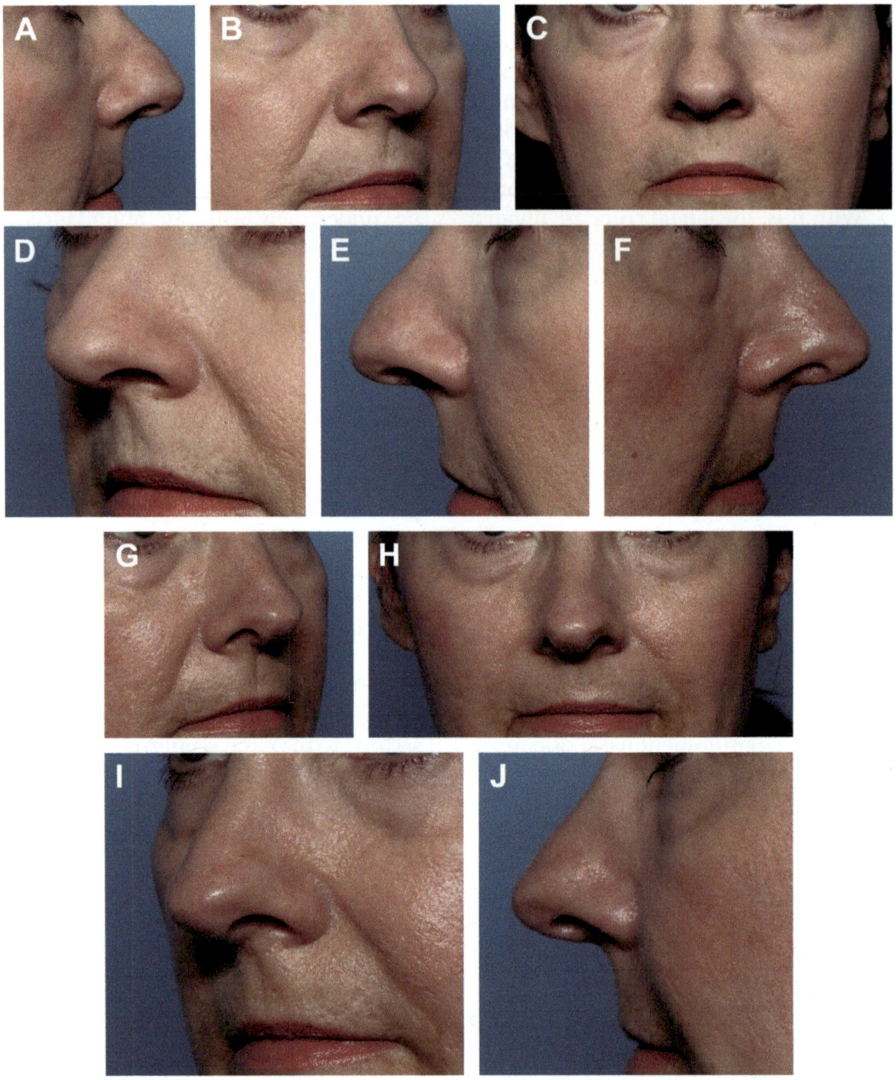

FIG. 2 Addressing the nasal tip. 56-year-old female presents with dissatisfaction with nasal tip fullness. She underwent open rhinoplasty with cephalic trim and interdomal sutures. **(A–E)** Preoperative photos. **(F–J)** At 1 year postoperatively, she demonstrates a more defined and less bulbous nasal tip.

visit. Normal saline nasal spray is prescribed for as-needed use. The patient is instructed to keep their head of bed elevated, follow strict sinus precautions, and avoid any strenuous activity that could elevate blood pressure and induce bleeding.

REHABILITATION AND RECOVERY

The patient is counseled that ecchymoses can be present for multiple weeks after surgery. The majority of edema will resolve within the first 1 to 3 months postoperatively, but complete resolution can take up to 1 year. Complete edema resolution can take even longer than 1 year if the patient is undergoing revision rhinoplasty; some rhinoplasty surgeons advocate for 1.5 years of swelling resolution. Patients may start to slowly increase their activity 1 month after surgery, but strenuous activity should be avoided for at least the first 2 months to avoid bleeding and worsening swelling.

CLINICAL RESULTS

Final results from rhinoplasty in the aging patient vary widely based on surgeon technique and patient complaints, but generally tend to be more subtle in nature. There is a paucity of clinical studies on rhinoplasty in the aging population in the literature. Cochran and colleagues [9] described their favorable rhinoplasty results in 51 patients over 65-years-old. Nearly all patients underwent open rhinoplasty. Eighteen patients required either auricular or costal grafts, a much higher proportion than the younger population. Columellar strut grafting was performed universally. Internal and external nasal valve grafts were used in 92% and 80% of the patients, respectively. A large majority of patients with edentulous maxillary arch required premaxillary augmentation. Less than a quarter of patients underwent nasal bone osteotomies due to nasal bone fragility with age.

We present 3 cases of rhinoplasty in the elderly patients (Figs. 1–3). Photo consent was obtained from all patients featured in this article. The first patient is an elderly woman who had previously undergone open rhinoplasty. We performed revision open rhinoplasty for functional and cosmetic concerns (see Fig. 1). Her postoperative results demonstrate improvements in tip and dorsal aesthetics, along with improvement in functional concerns. The second patient is a 56-year-old female who presented with chief complaint of nasal tip fullness. This was addressed with an open rhinoplasty, cephalic trim to increase tip rotation, and interdomal sutures to narrow her bulbous tip. Her 1-year results demonstrate a more youthful appearing nose with refined nasal tip and increased tip rotation (see Fig. 2). The final patient is a 49-year-old female who presented with concerns regarding her dorsal nasal hump and low radix that worsened over time. Since her nasal tip demonstrated adequate projection and rotation, a closed rhinoplasty approach was chosen to perform a conservative dorsal hump reduction and radix graft. Her postoperative results demonstrate improvements in her primary complaints and maintained tip projection and rotation (see Fig. 3).

POTENTIAL COMPLICATIONS AND LIMITATIONS

Long-standing nasal concerns become more difficult to address with increased age due to the changes to the nasal framework throughout adulthood [2]. Aging rhinoplasty produces more subtle changes that primarily address tip ptosis and obstructive symptoms.

The potential complications specific to the aging population are largely due to the loss of multiple nasal support structures as the face ages, and tip ptosis recurrence with time. Disregard for ligamentous attachments of the nasal framework can lead to further destabilization of the cartilaginous structure and loss of tip support. Excessive dorsal hump reduction can lead to open roof, inverted-V, polly beak, and rocker deformities. Nasal bone fragility can make osteotomies dangerous and unsuccessful in this patient population and should be avoided, if possible. Lateral crural cephalic trim that leaves less than 6 mm of remaining cartilaginous support can worsen existing external nasal valve collapse.

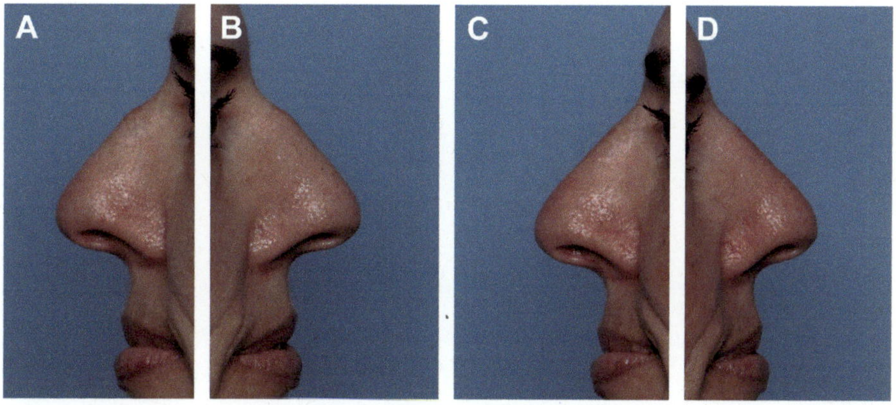

FIG. 3 Addressing the dorsal hump. 49-year-old female presents with dissatisfaction with her dorsal hump that she felt worsened over time. She underwent closed rhinoplasty with dorsal hump reduction and radix graft with morselized cartilage. (**A, B**) Preoperative photos. (**C, D**) At 4 months postoperatively, she demonstrates improved dorsal contour and higher radix.

SUMMARY

The aging rhinoplasty requires a high level of surgical skill, careful patient selection, and deep understanding of its anatomic limitations. Surgeons should take the time to discuss these limitations candidly with the patient before pursuing surgical correction. Extreme care should be taken to not over-dissect in any one plane to avoid further destabilization of the underlying nasal framework. Primarily addressing tip thickness, underprojection, and underrotation is key to improving upon age-related nasal change. The surgeon should start with surgical maneuvers to rectify tip ptosis and tip rotation to address these concerns. Results in this population tend to be more subtle in nature, but can, nonetheless, greatly impact the aesthetic appearance and function of the nose.

CLINICS CARE POINTS

- Nasal tip complex underrotation and deprojection is the hallmark of the aging nose.
- Proper patient selection and thorough preoperative discussion about surgical limitations is key to successful outcomes.
- Surgical maneuvers to address tip ptosis include columellar strut grafting, septal extension grafting, medial crura-septal fixation suture, lateral crura manipulation, alar cephalic trim, and onlay tip graft.
- Dorsal hump reduction should be conservative and performed after addressing the nasal tip complex, as this is commonly an illusion secondary to tip ptosis.
- Osteotomies should be performed under an abundance of caution, or avoided altogether.
- If external nasal valve collapse is present, lateral crural strut graft or alar batten grafting can be used.

DISCLOSURE

The authors have nothing to disclose.

REFERENCES

[1] The Aesthetic Society in collaboration with CosmetAssure. Aesthetic Plastic Surgery Stats - 2023. (2023) 25. Available at: https://cdn.theaestheticsociety.org/media/statistics/2023-TheAestheticSocietyStatistics.pdf.
[2] Rohrich RJ, Hollier LH. Rhinoplasty with advancing age. Characteristics and management. Clin Plast Surg 1996;23(2):281–96.
[3] Quatela VC, Pearson JM. Management of the aging nose. Facial Plast Surg 2009;25(4):215–21.
[4] Stupak HD, Johnson CM Jr. Rhinoplasty for the aging nose. Ear Nose Throat J 2006;85(3):154–5.
[5] Sepehr A, Chauhan N, Alexander A, et al. The effect of rhinoplasty on perceived age. Arch Facial Plast Surg 2012;14(1):68–70.
[6] Romo T 3rd, Soliemanzadeh P, Litner JA, et al. Rhinoplasty in the aging nose. Facial Plast Surg 2003;19(4):309–15.
[7] Shastri D, Tandon P, Singh A. Nasal changes in different age groups. Natl J Maxillofac Surg 2021;12(3):367–71.
[8] Boustany AN, Grover R, Alnaeem H, et al. Cosmetic rhinoplasty. Plast Reconstr Surg 2023;151(2):315e–29e.
[9] Cochran CS, Ducic Y, DeFatta RJ. Restorative rhinoplasty in the aging patient. Laryngoscope 2007;117(5):803–7.
[10] Pessa JE, Desvigne LD, Zadoo VP. The effect of skeletal remodeling on the nasal profile: considerations for rhinoplasty in the older patient. Aesthetic Plast Surg 1999;23(4):239–42.

Advances in Cosmetic Surgery 8 (2025) 177–181
ADVANCES IN COSMETIC SURGERY

Reputation Management

Best Practices to Handle Negative Reviews

Wendy Lewis, BA[a,*], Jane Yoo, MD[b,c]
[a]Wendy Lewis & Co Ltd; [b]Department of Dermatology, Icahn School of Medicine at Mount Sinai; [c]Clinical Research Center of New York

KEYWORDS
• Reputation management pearls • Monitoring your digital footprint • Strategies for elevating your reputation

KEY POINTS

- A strong online reputation and presence is an essential credential for dermatologists today.
- Every negative search result that is out there may damage your professional reputation.
- Best practices to deal with negative reviews without getting burned.

You thrived through medical school, aced your fellowships, got privileges in the prestigious teaching hospital of your choice, and are on your way to a brilliant career taking care of patients.

Then one day, when you least expect it, someone posts an anonymous review on Yelp about how badly they were treated in your practice, and you feel demoralized.

You are not alone. If you ask some of your closest colleagues, they will likely share their frustration with online reviews from anonymous sources as well as real patients. There is no need to panic, but you shoud pay attention to turn your review status around.

The advent of online review websites and social media has transformed how patients choose their doctors of all specialties. Your online presence, including before and after patient outcomes, photos, reviews, testimonials, website, and social media channels may be the first impression patients see.

Patients have more options than ever before. They are very well informed from numerous sources, including social media channels, and tend to have high expectations. They seek providers who not only demonstrate medical expertise and publish their work, but also exhibit qualities such as empathy, clear communication, and accessibility. A strong online reputation showcasing these traits can significantly influence a patient's decision to book an appointment to see you rather than a med spa across town.

DEFINING REPUTATION MANAGEMENT

Reputation management is a critical tool that can directly influence the way your brand is perceived by current patients as well as prospective ones. Having a robust presence online is an essential credential to attract the patients you want to see in your waiting room. Ideally, you can continue to take care of the patients you have currently, as well as a demographic who you want to attract.

For example, you may be seeing a lot of seniors on your schedule to treat their medical conditions and would like to transition to treat more cosmetic patients who pay for their treatments out of pocket. Being active on key social media platforms with the right tone, content, and imagery can help you to acheive that goal.

*Corresponding author. Wendy Lewis, 201 East 79th Street, 4H, New York, NY 10075. *E-mail address:* WL@Wendylewisco.com

https://doi.org/10.1016/j.yacs.2025.01.010 www.advancesincosmeticsurgery.com
2542-4327/25/

GET TO KNOW THE BASICS

Reputation management is not just about handling a one-off unflattering review. In the current climate, it is a critical success factor for all businesses to manage their online reputation.

Whenever someone searches for your name or your brand, they are likely to go directly to the first page of Google. However, if they are not impressed by what they read, they may not go any further and stop the search there if they don't like what they read. The first information they find may provide everything they need to know to want to dive a little deeper or just move on. Even a few negative comments popping up can affect your reputation and the perception of your practice.

When prospective patients read positive comments, 4–5-star reviews, photos of happy patients, and outcomes that impress them, they are more likely to want to learn more about those practices. Alternatively, if they have difficulty finding a practice that was recommended or read negative comments or complaints they may be easily turned off. Anything online that may raise doubts about your practice, results, staff, or the experience in your practice may be turning away the patients you most want to take care of.

According to Hubspot, "Reputation management is the act of managing public perceptions about a business or enterprise. This process has become more important as online conversations about businesses become the norm. When your reputation is positive, you inspire customer loyalty, a significant driver of revenue and growth. A negative reputation can be damaging to sales and customer retention, but it also helps you to learn what customers like, which can be helpful for updating business process to better meet customer needs."

Sources where consumers can find and post reviews:

(These vary based on your market)

- Better Business Bureau
- City Search
- Facebook
- Glassdoor
- Google and Google My Business
- Healthgrades
- Instagram
- RateMDs
- RealSelf
- Reddit
- Scoredoc.com
- SuperPages
- RateMDs
- TikTok
- Tripadvisor
- Trustpilot
- Twitter (X)
- Vitals
- WebMD
- WhatsApp
- Yahoo Local
- Yelp
- YouTube
- Zocdoc

PROTECTING YOUR DIGITAL FOOTPRINT

It is critically important to monitor the most important sites that matter to your brand on a routine basis and enlist someone in your practice to stay on top of it. If you are not monitoring your online presence effectively, you may not even realize that you may be losing patients to another practice in your market.

Negative reviews may originate from unhappy patients, competitors, disgruntled former employees, vendors you may have fired, former partners, and anyone whom you have had a disagreement with. If the review seems to be fake, such as a random post complaining about a treatment you do not offer, you may have some recourse, but it can be a laborious task with little yield.

Every negative search result can damage your reputation, even if ever so slightly. If you have just a few negative results in a plethora of glowing reviews, you are doing well and can take a bow. However, if several negative search results appear on the first page, it should be addressed. Focus on posting content and positive reviews so that the less impressive results get buried on the next page.

If it is positive, you may want to thank the patient for their feedback offline. If you know who the patient is, you may even send a thank you note to welcome them back. However, be mindful that in the USA and many other markets, physicians of all or most specialties are prohibited from acknowledging a doctor-patient relationship in an open forum. Failure to adhere to that restriction can have dire consequences.

Check all relevant social media platforms, including those that you may not actively use, for comments about your practice and providers. Monitor Google for negative comments about your practice name, brand, and the medical staff in your practice. Ensure that your business name, address, phone number, and other basic contact details are accurate everywhere that your business is listed or may be mentioned.

There are services that claim to make your negative reviews magically disappear, but proceed with caution as these may be a scam. Keep in mind that savvy patients may also become suspicious if you have all 5-star reviews.

STRATEGIES FOR ELEVATING YOUR REPUTATION

Original content posted on your website can be a very important reputation management tool. Your website is most likely to turn up when someone searches on Google for your name, practice, or brand name. You can acquire additional assets from media hits, articles, blogs, social channels, Google ads, and every other source where people may look for information in general.

Creating unique and relevant content throughout your website is the best practice to keep your target audience engaged and following your other channels. Make sure to link all your social media channels to your website as well, so that visitors can follow you online.

MOST VALUABLE CONTENT TO ELEVATE YOUR PRACTICE

- Organic content is king
- Short-form and long-form videos perform well
- Infographics can be good fillers
- Eye catching, unique images
- Patient photos and videos
- LinkedIn for business
- Instagram Live, Reels, Threads
- Facebook
- WhatsApp
- TikTok
- YouTube Shorts
- Pinterest

It is vitally important to actively manage your professional reputation to build trust with patients and ensure the survival and growth of your practice. In today's hyper competitive market, maintaining positive reviews enables a strong online presence that can help professionals thrive.

MONITORING YOUR REPUTATION ONLINE 24/7

If you are not being proactive to pay close attention to what patients, colleagues, vendors, and others are saying about you and your practice, you may be putting your reputation at risk unwittingly.

Regularly track mentions of your name, brand, or practice across the internet, including social media, review sites, and news articles. To be even more diligent, check potential misspellings of your name and practice name to stay on top of any potential threats that may affect your reputation.

Responding to negative reviews in an open forum may have consequences. Making the decision to respond to a negative review online is widely discouraged. As discussed previously, due to the Hippocratic Oath, physicians are prohibited from acknowledging the doctor-patient relationship. This can result in a serious violation that may cause you significant grief and a ding to your reputation. Once you post, you will own it, even if you take it down. It only takes one person to read it, and your comments may live online forever.

If you think the best way to distill an unhappy vocal patient is online, think it through before you act. It may be safer to post a very basic comment, before or instead of acknowledging a problem, but that can put you at risk. Avoid getting into a dialogue with a patient who is unhappy in an open forum. It is wise to keep all comments to a minimum and try to take it offline. Responding to negative comments can be very risky and is generally not recommended.

Reading your reviews can be extremely informative and often humbling, if you are open to making improvements. It may enlighten you to how you and your team are perceived, if you keep an open mind. These insights may be valuable to educate the whole team and position your practice as a business that is kind, caring, rational, and sensitive to the needs of patients. If a patient wants to discuss his/her circumstances with the practice, the best way to start that conversation is by getting off the internet and contacting the practice directly. The practice has not promised anything, which is wise, but it is not stonewalling, either. The outcome, favorable or unfavorable, will be determined by the private conversation that takes place between the patient and their care provider.

When in doubt about how to handle an unpleasant patient commentary online, reach out to your medical insurance carrier for assistance before taking any measures on your own. The last consideration may be enlisting an attorney with experience in defamation cases; however, this choice can come with potential risks that may escalate the situation.

BUILDING LONG-TERM TRUST WITH PATIENTS

Trust is the cornerstone of the doctor-patient relationship, and reputation plays a pivotal role in fostering that trust. A positive reputation signals a professional who is competent and trustworthy. Conversely, negative reviews or a lack of online presence can erode that trust even before a patient meets the doctor. If they have difficulty finding you or your practice online, those patients may just move on to another practice.

Proactive reputation management involves maintaining accurate information on the channels and directories that are relevant to your mission. When doctors take the time to respond to patient concerns in person, it can demonstrate commitment to superior patient care and rebuild trust and credibility.

For physicians and all health care providers, reputation management directly impacts their professional success and ability to attract new patients. In an increasingly competitive market, a robust reputation can be a differentiating factor that sets one provider apart from all the others. Positive reviews and 5-star ratings can drive more patients to your practice, and more of the patients you ideally want to treat.

Patients who feel valued and well cared for are more likely to recommend their doctor to others, both online and offline. This can generate favorable word-of-mouth advertising, amplified by a trustworthy online presence, which factors into a positive cycle of patient acquisition and retention. Happy and satisfied patients can become your number one source of referrals because they will be more trusted any paid ads, modern websites, or Google.

Reputation management does more than attract patients; it also encourages continuous improvement in health care delivery. Actively monitor feedback, as it can provide valuable insights into patient needs and areas for improvement. This kind of feedback can lead to enhanced communication, a better bedside manner, and overall improvements in patient relations and care.

Moreover, a focus on reputation underscores the importance of ethical practices and professional integrity. Physicians who prioritize their reputation are more likely to adhere to high standards of care, fostering a culture of accountability and excellence within their practices.

FIVE KEY STRATEGIES FOR REPUTATION MANAGEMENT

- Monitor your online presence: Regularly check review sites and social media platforms to stay informed about what patients are saying about your brand.
- Encourage positive reviews: Ask satisfied patients to leave reviews on reputable platforms that matter to your practice.
- Respond to feedback carefully: Address positive feedback promptly and with thanks, but be very cautious about responding to negative comments in any open forum, and take it offline.
- Engage on the social media channels your patients spend time on: Use social media platforms to share your expertise, educate patients, and promote your practice and outcomes in a positive light.
- Expand your visibility though multiple relevant channels: print, relevant social media sites, practice website, trade journals, videos, and events.

SUMMARY

Reputation management is no longer optional for doctors or most other health care providers. These may include nurse practitioners, physician assistants, registered nurses, licensed practical nurses, and advanced practice registered nurses. It is a vital component of every medical practice, just as it is for lawyers and other professionals.

A strong, positive reputation builds trust, can attract and retain patients, and drives continuous improvement in health care delivery. By proactively managing their reputations, doctors can not only ensure their success, but also contribute to a higher standard of care that will ultimately benefit their patients.

Embracing reputation management as an integral aspect of your practice will help to position you to thrive in a competitive landscape. Prioritizing patient satisfaction, ethical practices, and professional development can build lasting trust with the community you serve.

Due to social media channels and the plethora of review sites, every review that ranks less than a 4 can affect the way new patients may consider your practice. Sustaining a positive online reputation can go far to attract and retain the patients you want to have in your practice, and build trust with current and future patients.

In conclustion, if you are not monitoring how your brand comes across online to prospective patients, we can say with certainty that you are putting your practice and reputation at risk. Once your reputation has been tarnished, it may take months to many years to restore it in your community.

By taking the necessary steps to proactively managing your reputation, dermatologists and their staffs can build strong relationships with their patients and communities for their careers.

DISCLOSURE

W. Lewis: No relevant conflicts to declare. J. Yoo M.D.: No relevant conflicts to declare.

FURTHER READING

Lewis, W "Aesthetic Clinic Marketing in The Digital Age: From Meta to AI," Second Edition Date, 2024, ISBN 9780367405182, CRC Press, Taylor & Francis Available at: https://www.routledge.com/Aesthetic-Clinic-Marketing-in-the-Digital-Age-From-Meta-to-AI/Lewis/p/book/9780367405182.

Lewis W. "Textbook of Advanced Dermatology: Pearls for Academia and Skin Clinics (Part 2)" "High Yield Business tips for Dermatologists". Benthan Science 2024;274–81. Available at: https://www.benthamdirect.com/content/books/9789815238099.

Namazi, Lewis W. "Essentials for aesthetic dermatology for ethnic skin; practice and procedure" "digital marketing and social media branding". Thieme 2023;37, Part 6.

Sachdev M, Khunger N. Available at: https://www.routledge.com/Essentials-for-Aesthetic-Dermatology-in-Ethnic-Skin-Practice-and-Procedure/Sachdev-Khunger/p/book/9780367198572?source=shoppingads&locale=en-USD&gad_source=1&gclid=CjwKCAiAjp-7BhBZEiwAmh9rBY0j5ErvnxdRileRpo0vYMiPPLQEnSR6uSq1SgVdpN-4_Zi5ymiO4BoCEfYQAvD_BwE.

Lewis W. The business of dermatology: artchapter "managing your online reputation". Thieme 2020;309–17, ISBN 9783132427792.

Dover JS, Mariwalla K. Available at: https://shop.thieme.com/The-Business-of-Dermatology/9783132427792?srsltid=AfmBOopFS8j2T-wdiWQd5R2vpvCv_hozYjxwm2kxrzfd399Jzhut-QdX.

Taylor, S "Diversity, Equity, and Inclusion in Dermatology, An Issue of Dermatologic Clinics, 1st Edition" Diversity in the Dermatology Workforce and in Academic Medicine Page 8-12 ISBN 9780323939676 Date, Mar, 20, 2023 Elsevier Available at: https://www.us.elsevierhealth.com/diversity-equity-and-inclusion-in-dermatology-an-issue-of-dermatologic-clinics-9780323939676.html?qty=1.

Hanauer, DA, Zheng, K, Singer, D, et al "Public awareness, perception, and use of online physician rating sites." Date, JAMA. 2014;311:734-735PMID: 24549555. DOI: 10.1001/jama.2013.283194. Available at: https://www.jaad.org/article/S0190-9622.

Henry TA. "How to respond to bad online reviews." American Medical Association. 2016. Available at: https://www.ama-assn.org/delivering-care/patient-support-advocacy/how-respond-bad-online-reviews.

Hill, Rachel C, Grant-Kels BS, Jane M, et al. "Ethical considerations in responding to negative online reviews." Ethics Journal Club 2024. Available at: https://www.jaad.org/article/S0190-9622(24)00764-3/fulltext.

Militello, Michelle, Yang, Ronald A., Anderson, Jaclyn B., et al. Social Media and Ethical Challenges for the Dermatologist." Date, July 2021, Article_340.pdf Current Dermatology Reports (2021) 10:120–127 Available at: https://pmc.ncbi.nlm.nih.gov/articles/.

Advances in Cosmetic Surgery 8 (2025) 183–189
ADVANCES IN COSMETIC SURGERY

Social Media Dysmorphia

Roxana Shirazi, MD[a], Eric J. Beltrami, MD[b], Alexa J. Cohen, MD[b], Neelam A. Vashi, MD[c,*]
[a]Department of Dermatology, Virginia Commonwealth University School of Medicine, 9109 Stony Point Drive Box 980304, Richmond, VA 23235, USA; [b]Department of Dermatology, Boston Medical Center, 609 Albany Street, Boston, MA 02118, USA; [c]Department of Dermatology, Boston University School of Medicine, 609 Albany Street, Boston, MA 02118, USA

KEYWORDS

• Social media • Social media dysmorphia • Body dysmorphic disorder • Selfie • Filters • TikTok • Instagram • SnapChat

KEY POINTS

- Social media dysmorphia refers to body image dissatisfaction driven by idealized beauty standards on social media, amplified by filters and photo-editing tools.
- Prolonged exposure to curated images on social media fosters unhealthy self-comparisons, leading to disorted body perceptions and increased risk of body dysmorphic disorder (BDD).
- Indicators for social media dysmorphia include high social media use, presenting filtered selfies during consultations, and a history of BDD or obsessive tendencies.
- AI-powered filters, like TikTok's Bold Glamor, create hyper-realistic effects, perpetuating unattainable beauty standards and influencing patients' desires for cosmetic procedures.
- Dermatologists should educate patients on realistic outcomes, discourage realiance on filters, and recommend social media detox to improve self-image and mental health.

INTRODUCTION

Over the past decade, greater social media utilization has paralleled a heightened focus on aesthetic standards perpetuated through social media platforms. This phenomenon has resulted in the emergence of a newly recognized entity in cosmetic dermatology, social media dysphoria. Social media dysphoria describes dissatisfaction with body image relative to and as a result of beauty ideals portrayed on social media applications and their associated photo editing technology. Special consideration must be taken to recognize social media dysmorphia, adapt to what is and is not appropriate in the care of these patients, and engage in counseling regarding realistic expectations and the implications of social media on the perception of one's self. In this article, we will describe trends in social media utilization, review body dysmorphic disorder (BDD), define and characterize social media dysphoria, and discuss best practices in managing such cases clinically.

EPIDEMIOLOGY OF SOCIAL MEDIA

The earliest forms of social media, defined as interactive technologies that facilitate creating and sharing content among virtual communities and networks date back to the mid-20th century [1]. The programmed logic for automated teaching operations system, launched in 1960 at the University of Illinois, is widely considered to be the first social media platform. It revolutionized communication through online chat rooms, instant messaging, and message forums [2]. These online platforms have since evolved to allow users to share user-generated content, including digital photos and videos, and connect with other individuals and groups via

*Corresponding author. *E-mail address:* nvashi419@gmail.com

https://doi.org/10.1016/j.yacs.2025.01.008 www.advancesincosmeticsurgery.com
2542-4327/25/

ABBREVIATIONS	
AI	artificial intelligence
BDD	body dysmorphic disorder

self-created profiles. In the early 2000s, social media platforms such as Friendster and Myspace gained widespread popularity, followed by Facebook, YouTube, and Twitter. According to Statista, in 2024, over 5 billion people will be using social media worldwide. This statistical is projected to increase to over 6 billion in 2028 [3]. As of April 2024, the most popular social networking service is Facebook, with over 3 billion monthly active users. The second, third, and fourth most popular social networking services are YouTube, WhatsApp, and Instagram, respectively, all with 2 billion or more monthly active users worldwide [3].

Social media use varies widely based on demographic factors such as age, gender, race, income, and education level. In the United States, most adults use YouTube and Facebook, and about half use Instagram, whereas teens are far more likely to use Instagram, Snapchat, and TikTok. While some platforms have a nearly even gender split, others, such as TikTok and Instagram, are more likely to be used by females than their male counterparts. Hispanic adults are particularly likely to use TikTok, with 49% indicating usage. Hispanic and Asian adults also report using Instagram somewhat more frequently than Black and White adults. Adults with higher household incomes use X (formerly called *Twitter*) at somewhat higher rates, and those with higher levels of formal education are especially likely to use LinkedIn [4].

Users spend an average of 2 and half hours daily on social media and messaging apps [5]. Certain personality traits may help explain which individuals are more likely to engage in social media. A 2009 study revealed that extraversion and openness to experiences were positively related to social media use, while emotional stability was a negative predictor [6]. A 2015 study found that people with a higher social comparison orientation tend to use social media more heavily than people with a low social comparison orientation [7].

With the growing popularity of social media across a range of demographics, its impact on mental health has become increasingly significant. A 2016 systemic review concluded that social media can trigger a negative feedback loop of viewing and uploading photos, self-comparison, and disordered body perception [8]. The amount of time people spend on social media, coupled with individual personality traits, highlights how certain users may be more vulnerable to the effects of these platforms on self-image and mental health. For those inclined toward social comparison, exposure to idealized images online can heighten the risk of internalizing unrealistic standards. This comparison can foster body dissatisfaction and, in some cases, lead to more serious psychological conditions. One notable concern arising from this dynamic is BDD, a condition extensively linked in the literature to the pressures and imagery that dominate social media.

BODY DYSMORPHIC DISORDER

BDD is a psychiatric condition characterized by an excessive and persistent preoccupation with perceived flaws in physical appearance, which are often unnoticeable to others [9]. The focus of preoccupation can be any part of the body, but skin (eg, perceived acne or scarring), hair (eg, perceived thinning or excessive body or facial hair), and nose (eg, size or shape) concerns are most common. Patients with BDD engage in repetitive behaviors such as frequent checking of mirrors, comparing their appearance with that of others, excessive grooming, skin picking, reassurance seeking, taking excessive selfies, or repeatedly assessing the perceived defect [10]. To qualify for a diagnosis of BDD, the preoccupations must cause clinically significant distress or impairment in social, occupational, or other important areas of functioning [9]. Machine learning models have been shown to accurately predict the disorder, demonstrating how advancements in artificial intelligence (AI) show promise in the future of psychodermatology [11].

Currently, it is estimated that 1.7% to 2.9% of the general population is affected by BDD [12]. The prevalence rate rises to 11% to 13% among dermatology outpatients, 13% to 15% among general cosmetic surgery patients, and 20% in rhinoplasty settings [13]. There is a slightly higher prevalence among females; however, meeting the criteria for BDD is notably higher among male compared to female cosmetic surgery-seekers [13]. Age of onset most commonly occurs in early adolescence, with two-thirds of cases occurring before the age of 18 [10].

BDD is a complex psychiatric condition with multifactorial etiology, including genetic, neurobiological, and environmental factors. Research on the genetic factors underlying BDD is limited, yet heredity and genetics seem to play a role in its development. One study demonstrated that 8% of individuals with BDD have a family member also diagnosed with BDD, which is 4 to 8 times the prevalence in the general population [14]. A twin study in females who used self-report measures of dysmorphic concerns showed that genetic factors accounted for approximately 44% of the variance in dysmorphic concerns [15].

Neurobiology and imaging findings in BDD reveal structural, functional, and connectivity abnormalities in brain regions involved in visual processing, emotional regulation, and cognitive control. Positive correlations were observed between the severity of BDD symptoms and the volumes of the left inferior frontal gyrus and right amygdala [10]. These findings align with the functional hyperactivity of these regions, which are implicated in pathologic face processing. Diffusion tensor imaging studies identified fiber disorganization in white matter tracts connecting the visual and emotion/memory processing systems [16]. The affected tracts included the inferior longitudinal fasciculus, which plays a role in object and face recognition and the forceps major, which connects the right and left visual processing areas [16,17]. Poor information integration between these regions may be linked to impaired insight and contribute to difficulties in accurately perceiving visual stimuli in individuals with BDD [18]. Functional MRI studies have found that individuals with BDD show distinct brain activation patterns compared to healthy controls, including unique spatial frequency responses when viewing others' faces, heightened left hemisphere activity, and increased bilateral amygdala activation [16]. This suggests differences in visual processing that extend beyond distortions of their own appearance. Current research suggests a model for the pathophysiology of BDD that includes abnormalities in visual processing, emotional regulation, and cognitive control, correlating to dysfunction of the visual processing regions, limbic system, and frontostriatal circuits, respectively [19]. The perceptual distortions, limited insight, obsessive thoughts, and compulsive behaviors associated with BDD may stem from these aberrant neurobiological and structural findings.

Environmental factors associated with BDD include a range of adverse experiences and sociocultural influences. A meta-analysis found that various forms of adverse childhood experiences, such as abuse, neglect, and bullying, are all positively associated with BDD symptomatology [20]. In addition to childhood abuse and trauma, there is a well-documented association between social media use and BDD. Heavy usage of image-based social media platforms is significantly associated with increased BDD symptoms. A national survey found that individuals who spent 4 to 7 hours per day on Instagram and Snapchat had a higher prevalence of BDD than those who spent less than an hour per day [21]. Image-based platforms that emphasize visual content foster a culture of comparison and unrealistic beauty standards. Furthermore, frequent exposure to idealized images and edited or filtered photos can lead to negative self-appraisals and a heightened preoccupation with perceived physical flaws. The following section will explore the closely related modern phenomenon of social media dysmorphia.

SOCIAL MEDIA DYSMORPHIA, ALSO KNOWN AS *SELFIE DYSMORPHIA*

Social media does not just influence what we look like online but may more permanently rewire our brains to alter what we think we look like in real life, leading to an altered perception of body images [22]. With the accessibility of *beauty mode* on social media, filtering, contouring, and enhancing selfies is effortless. When combined with the dopamine rush from *likes* and *shares,* this can lead to withdrawal, leaving users feeling worse about themselves when they log off [23]. *Business Insider* reported that in 2018, some alleged Apple had implemented a beauty filter in selfie mode across all cameras, with no option to disable it [24]. According to the *MIT Technology Review*, TikTok was also suspected of applying an automatic facial feminizing filter during live streams [25].

With the transformative filters we have today, potential cosmetic patients can predict the outcome of an aesthetic procedure. TikTok's teenage filter removes shadow lines, boosts facial volume, and creates an even skin tone to give a youthful appearance [26]. This filter leads to an idealized artificial version of youth applying a *one size fits all* template. When comparing these photos to actual photos from one's youth, the difference between them and reality is striking. The Bold Glamor filter moves seamlessly with your face using generative adversarial networks (GAN) and smooths the skin, brightens the eyes, and sculpts facial features [27]. Notably, these filters tend to reflect current societal beauty trends, such as plump lips, larger eyes, and a slim nose. This filter has garnered significant attention due to its hyper-realistic effects, sparking concerns among experts about its potential impact on mental health and body image [28]. Adolescents are at particularly high risk for idealizing these filters and desiring them in real life given their developing self-image [29].

It is not just social media filters that are contributing to the dissonance people face when viewing themselves in real life. AI in cosmetic dermatology is growing rapidly and sometimes can assist physicians in selecting the appropriate patient for specific cosmetic procedures. While a cosmetic dermatologist or plastic surgeon may have software to display potential facial augmentation, this is now in the hands of patients who do not understand the feasibility or complexity of such alterations to their facial anatomy [30].

AI systems also play a role in social media algorithms. These algorithms personalize and curate a user's feed by learning individual preferences based on how they interact with content online. A repetitive loop is created, which exposes users to specific beauty ideals, normalizing and popularizing a certain appearance. Consequently, patients may adjust their aesthetic preferences based on these popularized standards, seeking cosmetic procedures to align with the idealized versions of beauty determined by social media algorithms [31]. Dermatologists should be able to recognize these influences and provide realistic advice to patients seeking potentially unrealistic outcomes. Although there are no formal criteria for social media dysmorphia, there are high-risk indicators that could be assessed through short questionnaires or interviews to help identify patients who may benefit from early intervention and counseling. We aim to present sample scenarios of *high-risk* behaviors to aid in establishing formal screening criteria for patients at risk of social media dysmorphia.

Screening criteria for high-risk patients for social media dysmorphia could include the following:

I. Frequency and duration of social media use
II. Bringing edited and filtered selfies to appointments and/or regular use of beauty filters or editing apps
    A. Seeking cosmetic consultations to resemble something that is not naturally occurring
III. History of BDD, eating disorders, or obsessive-compulsive tendencies
    A. Preoccupation with perceived physical flaws causes impairment in social interactions
IV. Motivation to alter appearance to *fit in* with online peers, celebrities, or influencers

CLINICAL AND PRACTICAL IMPLICATIONS OF SOCIAL MEDIA DYSMORPHIA

A patient may present to the cosmetic dermatology clinic with digital photographs for reference of their desired cosmetic outcome. In the context of social media dysmorphia, these reference photographs may be highly edited or filtered photographs of the patient or perhaps social media influencers. Seeking results equivalent to the body augmentation possible with digital image filtering can lead to patients having unrealistic expectations of what is possible with cosmetic procedures. It has been suggested that patients using SnapChat beauty filters tend to have more body dysmorphic congruent behaviors [32]. These patients may begin chasing a desired appearance that cannot be attained, or if pursued, would involve extensive interventions that may not lead to the seamless and natural appearance of these filtered images. Such *impossible* selfie consultations pose a significant challenge to the clinician managing these patients. Requests to remove nasolabial folds, enlarge the size of one's eyes, or attain a smooth face devoid of texture based on filtered or edited images of the patients or others should serve as a warning sign that a patient may have social media dysmorphia.

Once the clinician has identified a patient potentially experiencing social media dysmorphia, the consultation should consider commenting on the inability of image filtering and editing software to reliably capture realistic outcomes based on available cosmetic interventions. It is imperative to reshape the patient's goals to what is realistic based on their anatomy and which cosmetic procedures they would be appropriate candidates for. If patients express dissatisfaction with not being able to achieve results equivalent to filtering software, consider not offering cosmetic procedures to this patient as the likelihood of a satisfactory outcome for the patient is likely minimal.

Clinicians may be more likely to need to address specific requests patients may present with based on social media trends and the most commonly used filters. Enlargement of the lips with filler is a common filter enhancement, and posts regarding lip filler are highly prevalent on Instagram [33]. Cheekbone augmentation and slimming of the face are other common filter enhancements patients may desire, evidenced by the increase in patients seeking buccal fat pad treatment [34]. Flaws highlighted by the use of selfies and computer webcams, which tend to give a *fishbowl*-like appearance of the face and accentuate nose size, should also be on the cosmetic dermatologist's radar. The increased use of video conferencing during the coronavirus disease (COVID-19) pandemic may explain the greater acceptance of cosmetic procedures among patients [35].

Counseling the patient with social media dysmorphia should first consist of recognition, without judgment, that the patient's cosmetic desires have been influenced by social media posts or filters. Explaining why certain results cannot be achieved ought to be accompanied by what can be achieved, such as to give the patient confidence that they are not simply being denied care due to expressing their true expectations. Another component of counseling is education regarding preventive skin care in the long-term improvement of skin appearance and texture. The use of sunscreen and other sun protective measures, emollients and active ingredients such as retinoids for antiaging and brightening of skin, and less invasive cosmetic interventions (eg, chemical peels) are important discussion points for such patients who may not be ideal candidates for more invasive cosmetic intervention due to their social media dysmorphia [36].

Once social media dysmorphia is recognized and discussed with the patient, the clinician may recommend a *social media detox*, in which the patient is asked to forgo the use of filters, editing software, and engagement with social media personalities or influencers known to augment their photographs [37]. In doing so, the patients may begin to reframe their self-image based on reality and avoid constant exposure to an artificial, augmented version of themselves. Alternatively, the clinician may recommend the BeReal app, a social media platform designed to encourage users to share unfiltered photos of themselves. According to influencer marketing hub, BeReal is an anti-influencer social media app that may potentially address the various negative impacts associated with social media [38].

Ultimately, refusal of treatment may be necessary in patients with social media dysmorphia. It is not in the best interest of the patient nor the treating clinician to offer cosmetic procedures that cannot achieve the patients' goals as such procedures come with medical risk, financial burden, and ultimately a strained patient-physician relationship if patients were expecting results that were not attainable. Clinicians may instead offer patients to seek out a second opinion, though such patients may be susceptible to coercive marketing of cosmetic procedures by other providers. Patients should be made aware of the influence of social media on their self-perception, the realistic and unrealistic outcomes cosmetic procedures can achieve, and the safest avenues to pursue cosmetic interventions even if not offered by the clinician himself as these patients may be highly motivated to have body augmentation performed.

FUTURE DIRECTIONS

Social media users, especially those engaging with filters, editing tools, and highly edited images, should be made aware of the harmful effects these platforms can have on self-perception. Users should be educated on how the use of social media and analyzing one's digital appearance could lead to the development of unhealthy behaviors and social media dysphoria.

Dermatologists must play an active role in promoting healthy behaviors and realistic expectations by raising awareness of the negative phenomena of social media dysmorphia. While dermatologists have a significant role in combating misinformation, social media companies can enhance collaboration with physicians to promote educational content more prominently in their algorithms, thereby increasing its reach to a broader audience. Though further qualitative research is essential to establish high-risk indicators and screening criteria for social media dysmorphia to be used among dermatologists and other aesthetic health care professionals, AI-driven algorithms also hold promise for enhancing screening, diagnosis, and treatment efforts.

The dichotomy of AI, particularly in the context of social media, reveals both its potential harm and its promise. Social media, similarly to AI, offers both benefits and drawbacks by connecting and educating but can also isolate individuals and promote harmful, idealized narratives. Ultimately, how we choose to use social media and AI will shape the trajectory of our future as an entire society.

Given the dual nature of AI and social media, dermatologists must navigate their evolving influence on patient care and address emerging ethical challenges, particularly with BDD and social media dysmorphia, to provide the best possible care for patients.

CLINICS CARE POINTS

- Recognize high-risk features: Assess patients' social media use, including frequency, duration, and history of using photo-editing apps or filters. Be alert to behaviors such as bringing edited selfies to consultations.
- Screen for psychological factors: Evaluate for underlying psychiatric conditions like body dysmorphic disorder (BDD), eating disorders, or obsessive-compulsive tendencies that may contribute to unrealistic aesthetic expectations.
- Provide realistic counseling: Emphasize achievable outcomes based on anatomy and available cosmetic interventions. Avoid reinforcing unattainable ideals set by social media filters or influencers.
- Refuse unrealistic treatments: Decline cosmetic procedures where patients' expectations are not feasible to avoid dissatisfaction and harm to the patient-provider relationship.
- Cultivate ethical awareness: Be cognizant of the influence of social media algorithms and cosmetic marketing on patients' aesthetic preferences ensuring

care decisions are patient-centered rather than trend-driven.

DISCLOSURE

Dr N.A. Vashi is a consultant for L'Oreal and Janssen but these are not relevant to this project. There are no commercial or financial conflicts of interest to disclose. Additionally, there are no funding sources associated with this work.

REFERENCES

[1] Obar JA, Wildman SS. Social media definition and the governance challenge: an introduction to the special issue. Telecommun Pol 2015;39(9):745–50, Quello Center Working Paper No. 2647377. Available at: https://ssrn.com/abstract=2647377.

[2] Grainger Engineering Office of Marketing and Communications. Plato. The Grainger College of Engineering; 2020. Available at: https://grainger.illinois.edu/news/magazine/plato. Accessed November 4, 2024.

[3] Dixon SJ. Number of worldwide social network users 2028. Statista 2024. Available at: https://www.statista.com/statistics/278414/number-of-worldwide-social-network-users/. Accessed November 4, 2024.

[4] Gottfried J. Americans' social media use. Pew Research Center; 2024. Available at: https://www.pewresearch.org/internet/2024/01/31/americans-social-media-use/#fn-92491-1. Accessed November 4, 2024.

[5] Dixon SJ. Number of worldwide social network users 2028. Statista; 2024. Available at: https://www.statista.com/statistics/278414/number-of-worldwide-social-network-users/. Accessed November 4, 2024.

[6] Correa T, Hinsley AW, de Zúñiga HG. Who interacts on the web? The intersection of users' personality and social media use. Comput Hum Behav 2010;26(2):247–53.

[7] Vogel EA, Rose JP, Okdie BM, et al. Who compares and despairs? the effect of social comparison orientation on social media use and its outcomes. Pers Indiv Differ 2015;86:249–56.

[8] Holland G, Tiggemann M. A systematic review of the impact of the use of social networking sites on body image and disordered eating outcomes. Body Image 2016; 17:100–10.

[9] Substance Abuse and Mental Health Services Administration. Table 23, DSM-IV to DSM-5 body dysmorphic disorder comparison. DSM-5 changes: implications for child serious emotional disturbance [internet]. 2016. Available at: https://www.ncbi.nlm.nih.gov/books/NBK519712/table/ch3.t19/. Accessed November 4, 2024.

[10] Phillips KA, Menard W, Fay C, et al. Demographic characteristics, phenomenology, comorbidity, and family history in 200 individuals with body dysmorphic disorder. Psychosomatics 2005;46(4):317–25.

[11] Flygare O, Enander J, Andersson E, et al. Predictors of remission from body dysmorphic disorder after internet-delivered cognitive behavior therapy: a machine learning approach. BMC Psychiatr 2020;20(1):247.

[12] Hartmann AS, Buhlmann U. Prevalence and underrecognition of body dysmorphic disorder. Oxford Medicine Online; 2017.

[13] Veale D, Gledhill LJ, Christodoulou P, et al. Body dysmorphic disorder in different settings: a systematic review and estimated weighted prevalence. Body Image 2016;18:168–86.

[14] Bienvenu OJ, Samuels JF, Riddle MA, et al. The relationship of obsessive–compulsive disorder to possible spectrum disorders: results from a family study. Biol Psychiatr 2000; 48(4):287–93.

[15] Monzani B, Rijsdijk F, Anson M, et al. A twin study of body dysmorphic concerns. Psychol Med 2011;42(9): 1949–55.

[16] Feusner JD, Arienzo D, Li W, et al. White matter microstructure in body dysmorphic disorder and its clinicalcorrelates. Psychiatr Res Neuroimaging 2013;211(2):132–40.

[17] Wang Y, Metoki A, Smith DV, et al. Multimodal mapping of the face connectome. Nat Human Behav 2020;4(4): 397–411.

[18] Shin J, Rowley J, Chowdhury R, et al. Inferior longitudinal fasciculus' role in visual processing and language comprehension: a combined Meg-DTI Study. Front Neurosci 2019;13. https://doi.org/10.3389/fnins.2019.00875.

[19] Machremi E, Bakirtzis C, Karakasi M-V, et al. What scans see when patients see defects: neuroimaging findings in body dysmorphic disorder. J Integr Neurosci 2022; 21(2):045.

[20] Longobardi C, Badenes-Ribera L, Fabris MA. Adverse childhood experiences and body dysmorphic symptoms: a meta-analysis. Body Image 2022;40:267–84.

[21] Ateq K, Alhajji M, Alhusseini N. The association between use of social media and the development of body dysmorphic disorder and attitudes toward cosmetic surgeries: a national survey. Front Public Health 2024;12. https://doi.org/10.3389/fpubh.2024.1324092.

[22] Firth J, Torous J, Stubbs B, et al. The "online brain": how the Internet may be changing our cognition. World Psychiatr 2019;18(2):119–29.

[23] Truzoli R, Magistrati L, Viganò C, et al. Social media users potentially experience different withdrawal symptoms than non-social media users. Int J Ment Health Addict 2023;21:411–7.

[24] Leswing K. Some people are saying Apple's new iPhone selfie camera automatically smooths your skin in photos — and they're calling it 'beautygate'. Business Insider; 2018. Available at: https://www.businessinsider.com/beautygate-iphone-xs-camera-appears-to-apply-beauty-mode-to-selfies-2018-9. Accessed November 1, 2024.

[25] Ohlheiser A. TikTok changed the shape of some people's faces without asking. MIT Technology Review 2021.

Available at: https://www.technologyreview.com/2021/06/10/1026074/tiktok-mandatory-beauty-filter-bug/. Accessed November 1, 2024.
[26] Castellano D. The science behind TikTok's teenage look filter. Elite Facial Plastic Surgery Blog 2023. Available at: https://www.elitetampa.com/blog/teenage-look-filter-trend/. Accessed November 1, 2024.
[27] Pendergrass W. Artificial intelligence and its potential harm through the use of generative adversarial network image filters on TikTok. Issues Inf Syst 2023;24(1): 113–27.
[28] Javornik A, Marder B, Barhorst JB, et al. What lies behind the filter? Uncovering the motivations for using augmented reality (AR) face filters on social media and their effect on well-being. Comput Hum Behav 2022;128:107126.
[29] Merino M, Tornero-Aguilera JF, Rubio-Zarapuz A, et al. Body perceptions and psychological well-being: a review of the impact of social media and physical measurements on self-esteem and mental health with a focus on body image satisfaction and its relationship with cultural and gender factors. Healthcare 2024;12(14):1396.
[30] Elder A, Cappelli MO, Ring C, et al. Artificial intelligence in cosmetic dermatology: an update on current trends. Clin Dermatol 2024;42:216–20.
[31] Huang A, Fabi S. Algorithmic beauty: the new beauty standard. J Drugs Dermatol 2024;23(9):742–6.
[32] Abbas L, Dodeen H. Body dysmorphic features among Snapchat users of "beauty-retouching of selfies" and its relationship with quality of life. Media Asia 2021;49(3): 196–212.
[33] Karch J, Maymone MBC, De La Garza H, et al. Lip fillers: a cross-sectional analysis of Instagram trends. Dermatol Surg 2023;49(1):114–5.
[34] Rohrich RJ, Stuzin JM, Savetsky IL, et al. The role of the buccal fat pad in facial aesthetic surgery. Plast Reconstr Surg 2021;148(2):334–8.
[35] Khan IF, De La Garza H, Lazar M, et al. Effects of the COVID-19 pandemic on patient social media use and acceptance of cosmetic procedures. J Clin Aesthet Dermatol 2024;17(3):42–7.
[36] Ganceviciene R, Liakou AI, Theodoridis A, et al. Skin anti-aging strategies. Dermatoendocrinol 2012;4(3): 308–19.
[37] Ramadhan RN, Rampengan DD, Yumnanisha DA, et al. Impacts of digital social media detox for mental health: a systematic review and meta-analysis. Narra J 2024;4(2): e786:Epub August 7, 2024. PMID: 39280291; PMCID: PMC11392003.
[38] Mileva G. 21 BeReal statistics that will blow your mind. Influencer Marketing Hub 2024. Available at: https://influencermarketinghub.com/bereal-stats/. Accessed November 2, 2024.